L. Demling M. Classen P. Frühmorgen

Atlas of Enteroscopy

Endoscopy of the Small and Large Bowel; Retrograde Cholangio-Pancreatography

With the Collaboration of
H. Koch and H. Bauerle

Translated and Adapted by K. H. Soergel
with the Assistance of H. Pease

With 289 Illustrations, Most in Color

Springer-Verlag
Berlin Heidelberg New York 1975

Professor Dr. med. LUDWIG DEMLING, Director, University Hospital for Internal Medicine, Erlangen

Dr. med. MEINHARD CLASSEN, Associate Professor, Physician-in-Chief, Department of Medicine I, General Hospital Barmbek, Hamburg

Dr. med. PETER FRÜHMORGEN, Research Assistant, University Hospital for Internal Medicine, Erlangen

Translator and Adaptor:
KONRAD H. SOERGEL, M.D., Professor of Medicine and Chief, Department of Gastroenterology, The Medical College of Wisconsin, Milwaukee, Wisconsin

HARRY PEASE, Science Writer, Milwaukee Journal

ISBN-13: 978-3-642-61916-8 e-ISBN-13: 978-3-642-61914-4
DOI: 10.1007/978-3-642-61914-4

Library of Congress Cataloging in Publication Data. DEMLING, LUDWIG, 1921–. Atlas of enteroscopy. Translation of Atlas der Enteroskopie. Bibliography: p. Includes index. 1. Digestive organs—Exploration. 2. Intestines—Diseases—Diagnosis. 3. Endoscope and endoscopy. I. CLASSEN, MEINHARD, joint author. II. FRÜHMORGEN, PETER, 1940–, joint author. III. Title. RC 804.E6D4513.616.3'07'54.75–11 709

Typesetting, printing, and bookbinding: Stürtz AG, Würzburg

Foreword

It is my pleasure to introduce you to this new Atlas by Professor DEMLING and his colleagues on the very timely subjects colonoscopy, duodenoscopy and endoscopic cannulation of the bile and pancreatic ducts. Professor DEMLING, unlike many others who carry his teaching and administrative burdens, continues to be very personally involved in performing endoscopies. His clinic is one of the best organized and best equipped in the world. Professor DEMLING and his colleagues have been instrumental in introducing to the European continent these new techniques of duodenoscopy, colonoscopy and bile duct cannulation which were originally developed in Japan. They have added significant contributions of their own and now present to the reader a clear, concise, very well illustrated description of these methods.

Dr. CLASSEN is one of the pioneers in endoscopic cannulation. He has been kind enough to come to the United States and share his expertise with us at several Post Graduate Education programs. The students in these courses have been most enthusiastic about his presentations. Through this text he makes his extensive experience available to all endoscopists. The beginner at cannulation will find the illustrations of the various shapes the papilla may assume most helpful.

I had the pleasure this summer of teaching a course in Brazil with Dr. FRÜHMORGEN. Very few physicians have concentrated on colonoscopy to the extent that he has. Though he has been involved with the method for a relatively few years, he writes from an experience of more than 1 500 cases. He has gathered together the largest and clearest collection of colonoscopic photographs that I have ever seen. Even the experienced colonoscopist will learn from his well illustrated presentation on colonoscopic technique.

This text compliments Professor DEMLING's earlier Atlas on the Endoscopy of the Upper Gastrointestinal Tract. The English reader is indebted to Dr. KONRAD SOERGEL for his excellent translation of the text into English.

Madison, 1975 JOHN F. MORRISSEY

Preface to the German Edition

The Atlas of Enteroscopy represents a venture into new territory by describing the advances of modern gastroenterologic endoscopy in the examination of the small intestine, from duodenum to ileum, and of the entire colon. Until three years ago, large areas of the intestinal tract were not accessible to direct inspection. Today, the entire organ system, from esophagus to anus, can be visualized and biopsied, either by a combination of enteroscopy and coloscopy, or by peroral enterocoloscopy. It is now possible to inspect inflammatory and peptic lesions, tumors, diverticula, and stenotic areas and to detect their histologic features.

Another new development is the filling of the biliary and pancreatic duct systems with radiopaque contrast media by endoscopic intubation of the papilla of Vater. The pancreatic ducts have now become accessible to preoperative radiologic evaluation; this examination can be combined with selective mesenteric arteriography. Retrograde endoscopic filling of the bile ducts represents a significant advance in the differential diagnosis of obstructive jaundice: it carries a lower risk than percutaneous and laparoscopic cholangiography.

Operative endoscopy of the small and large intestine is yet another *terra nova* which has recently been entered. It includes the removal of foreign bodies, topical treatment of circumscribed lesions, coagulation of bleeding sites, and the removal of polyps with the diathermy snare.

The primary purpose of this atlas is to demonstrate the future possibilities for new clinical procedures which are based on advances in endoscopy, alone or in combination with radiologic procedures. The number of instances where the impact of these new methods can already be demonstrated is large, but a systematic description of all diseases now accessible to diagnostic and therapeutic intervention is not yet possible. The atlas represents an attempt to illustrate the giant strides taken by gastroenterologic endoscopy during the years 1970–1973. It is directed at gastroenterologists; internists, surgeons, pathologists and all those physicians who have maintained an active interest in the broadening scope of contemporary medicine.

Erlangen, Spring 1974 L. DEMLING

Contents

1. Instruments

1.1 Endoscopic Instruments

The achievement of technical perfection, as well as the development of a universal endoscope, is limited by the anatomic configuration of the organs which have to be negotiated and inspected. The commercially available duodenoscopes and coloscopes differ in specifications and design. The endoscopist has to consider their optical and mechanical qualities in choosing his instruments.

Adequate duodenoscopes and coloscopes should meet the following criteria in light of recent technical developments.

Mechanical: a tip with continuous deflection in two planes (at least 120°); durable construction; convenient arrangement and easy manipulation of external controls; automatic suction, irrigation and air insufflation; ability to obtain precisely located biopsies and material for cytologic examination even with the instrument tip deflected.

Optical: fiberoptic, high-intensity cold light source; good resolution and definition of detail; provisions for technically simple documentation by still-photography and movies, including adequate illumination.

General Design

a) Duodenoscopy: for evaluation of mucosal abnormalities in duodenal bulb and postbulbar area, forward viewing optics with good resolution even at low target distance should be used.—For retrograde pancreato- and cholangiography and for examination of certain types of scarred duodenal bulbs, the instrument should offer side-viewing optics, a directable catheter and a tip which can be deflected in two planes.

b) Coloscopy: Forward viewing optics; the instrument tip should be deflectable in 2 planes, by more than 90°.

Duodenoscopy

Bulboscopy (Table 1)

ACMI (American Cystoscope Maker, Inc., 8 Pelham Parkway, Pelham Manor, N.Y. 10803) esophago-gastro-duodenoscope, FO-7089, types J, JJ, P and F-8 (Fig. I). Forward viewing 70° (75°; F-8), fixed focus.

The instruments differ in the development of their mechanical components. All offer an extremely small tip deflection radius of 2 cm. The tip of type J can be deflected upwards by 180° and downwards by 100°. The polydirectional deflection of type P and F-8 represents a further refinement (Fig. II): the tip can be deflected by about 180° in all directions by a single lever control and describes, therefore, a hemispheric excursion. This facilitates the inversion maneuver and few blind areas remain in the stomach. Type JJ differs from type J by an additional slight bend in the distal flexible portion; it is supplied only by special order.

The optical resolution is suboptimal for photographic documentation and could be improved. The optical field of 70° (75°) with fixed focus provides a good survey view but limits the recognition of fine detail. Unfortunately, the biopsy forceps cannot be introduced when the tip is maximally deflected. Air insufflation and suction are controlled by convenient push buttons but irrigation requires attachment of a separate syringe.

Table 1. Technical data of bulboscopes

Technical data	ACMI FO-7089 A/J/JJ/P/F-8	Olympus GIF-D2	Wolf 7877	Wolf 7883	Storz Fiberscope
Working length	1050	1110	1300	1025	1120
Diameter (mm)					
Rigid tip	12.7	13.0	12.0	13.5	13.0
Flexible part	11.4 (F-8:12.0)	12.0	11.8	12.5	12.0
Length of rigid tip (mm)	44.0 (A, J, JJ); 55.0 (P) 42.0 (F-8)	22.0	23.0	20.0	40.0
Tip deflection					
Upwards	120° (A); 180° (J, JJ); 180° (P, F-8)	150°	90°	140°	130°
Downwards	120° (A); 100° (J, JJ); 180° (P, F-8)	150°	90°	140°	110°
To right	∅ (A); ∅ (J, JJ); 180° (P, F-8)	100°	90°	∅	90°
To left	∅ (A); ∅ (J, JJ); 180° (P, F-8)	100°	90°	∅	90°
Biopsy forceps deflection	∅	∅	90°	∅	∅
Focal depth (mm)	6–100	5–∞	5–50	5–∞	3–∞
Optical field	70° 75° (F-8)	75°	70°	70°	60°
Direction of view	180°	180°	100°	180°	150°
Variable focus	∅	+	∅	+	+

The F-8 Panendoscope represents the latest improvement of type FO-7089P. The optical field is 75° and the biopsy forceps can be introduced at full deflection to 180°. The focal depth is 6–100 mm.

These instruments are well suited for esophago-gastro-bulboscopy. Use of the proper technique allows inspection of the base of the duodenal bulb. An additional side-viewing instrument needs to be used only in some cases of scarred duodenal bulbs. An instrument channel is provided for obtaining bioptic and cytologic specimens and for the introduction of instruments used for operative endoscopic procedures.

Olympus Optical Corp. of America (2 Nevada Drive, New Hyde Park, N.Y. 11040): esophago-gastroscope EF-L, forward view, 60°, working length 865 mm, fixed focus (Fig. III).

Because of its shortness and the tip deflection in only one plane of 90°, this instrument is not suited for bulboscopy. It has been replaced by type EF-B2 for esophagoscopy (working length 715 mm; deflection of 50° in the lateral and 90° in the vertical plane) and by type GIF for bulboscopy.

Gastrointestinal fiberscope GIF-D2 (Fig. IV). Forward viewing, 75°; working length 1110 mm, variable focus.

This instrument fulfills most of the requirements for an esophago-gastro-bulboscope. It possesses very good optical and mechanical qualities. Air insufflation, irrigation and suction can be conveniently controlled by two trumpet valves. The variable

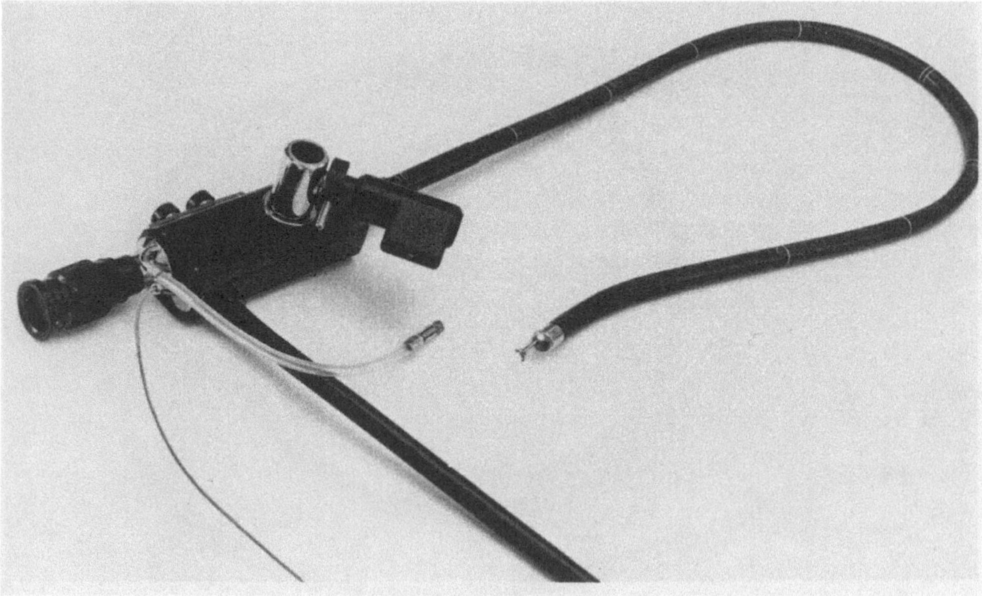

Fig. I. Panendoscope F-8 (ACMI, Inc., Pelham Manor, New York, 10803) with biopsy forceps

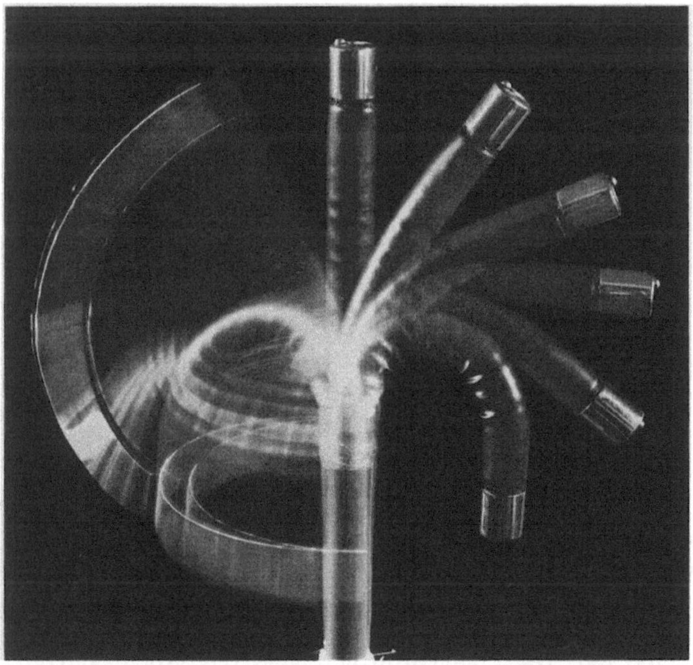

Fig. II. Polydirectional deflection of panendoscope FO-7089 P and F-8 (ACMI)

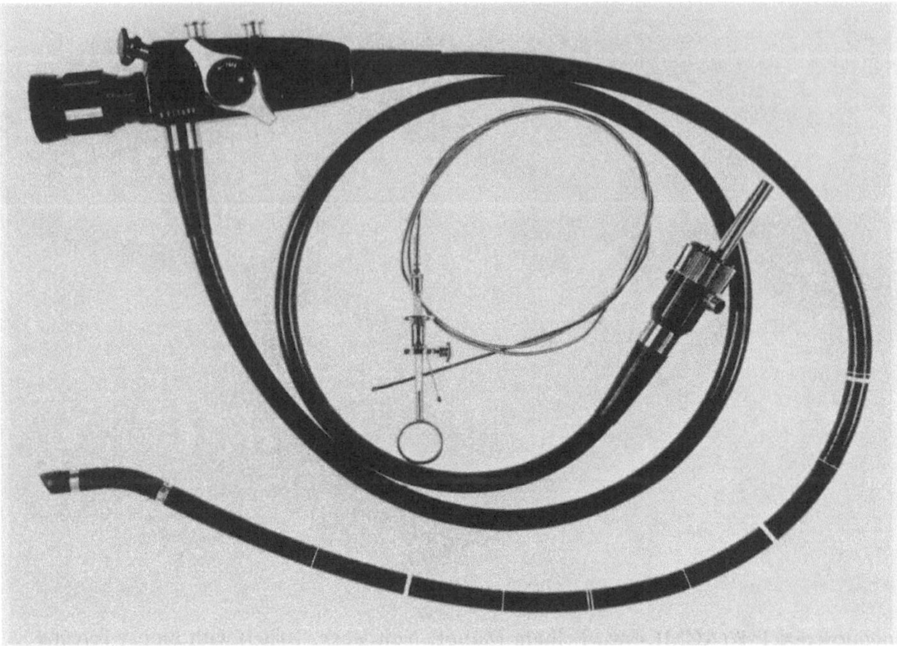

Fig. III. Esophagoscope EF-L (Olympus Optical Corp. of America, New Hyde Park, New York, 11040)

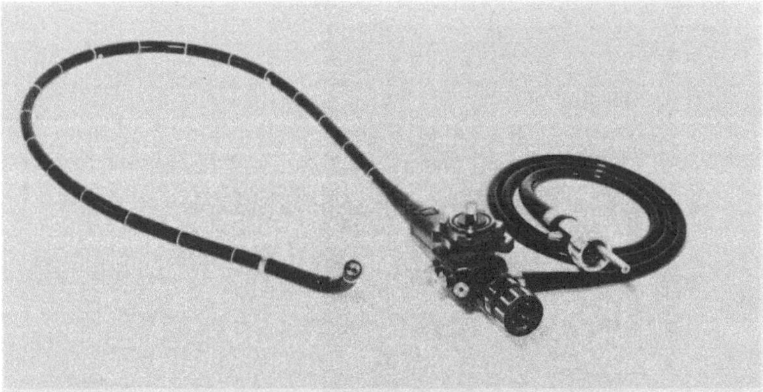

Fig. IV. Panendoscope GIF-D2 (Olympus)

focus permits excellent optical resolution and magnification when close to the target, a characteristic which is particularly valuable for inspection of the duodenal bulb. Intragastric viewing is facilitated by tip deflection in two planes, by 150° and 100°, respectively. Occasionally, however, certain parts of the stomach are viewed poorly or not at all; a side-viewing instrument should be available for such cases. The inability to direct the biopsy forceps radially is compensated by the mobility of the instrument tip in two planes. It is difficult and often impossible to introduce the biopsy instrument while the tip of the endoscope is deflected maximally.

Fa. Karl Storz (Tuttlingen, Germany): fiberscope (Fig. V). Direction of view 150°, optical field 60°, working length 1120 mm, variable focus.

Automatic air insufflation is conveniently controlled by a push-button on the instrument handle. Irrigation and suction are provided by a separate pump. A second channel serves for the introduction of flexible accessory instruments. The instrument tip can be deflected in two planes by 130° and 90°. To date, little working experience has accured with this new instrument; it is not sold in the U.S.A.

Wolf (Knittlingen, Germany): fiber duodenoscope 7877 (Fig. VI). Direction of view 100°, optical field 70°. Working length 1300 mm, fixed focus.

Air and water insufflation and aspiration are controlled by valves located on the instrument handle. A separate channel allows the introduction of flexible accessory instruments. The maximal tip deflection of 90° in two planes must be considered unsatisfactory, especially for examination of the stomach. The additional mobility of 90° of biopsy and other instruments as they emerge at the tip facilitates very precise localization of the biopsy site under direct vision.

Fiber esophago-gastro-bulboscope 7883 (Fig. VII). Forward viewing optics, 70°, working length 1025 mm, variable focus.

The instrument tip can be deflected by 140° in one plane. The biopsy forceps can be introduced at maximal tip deflection. Automatic air insufflation, irrigation and suction are controlled by conveniently arranged valves, as with type 7877. Due to limited personal experience, this instrument cannot yet be evaluated objectively. These two instruments are not sold in the U.S.A.

Deep or Postbulbar Duodenoscopy (Table 2)

Forward or side viewing endoscopes manufactured by Olympus, Machida, and ACMI are available for deep or postbulbar duodenoscopy. Forward viewing optics are recommended when the examination is

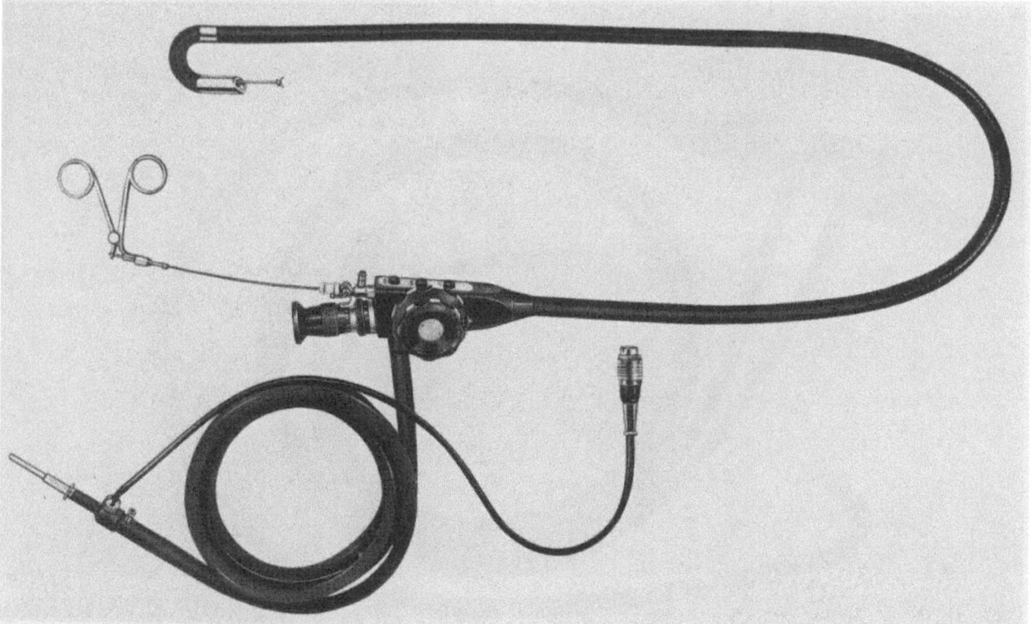

Fig. V. Fiberscope with biopsy forceps. (Storz, Tuttlingen, Germany). Not available in the United States

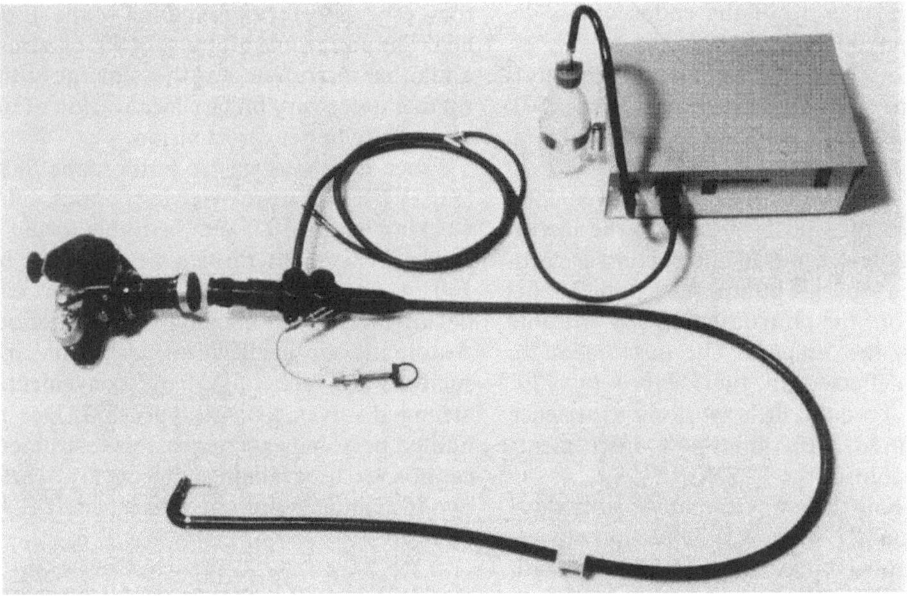

Fig. VI. Fiber duodenoscope 7877, Fa. Wolf, Knittlingen, Germany. Not available in the United States

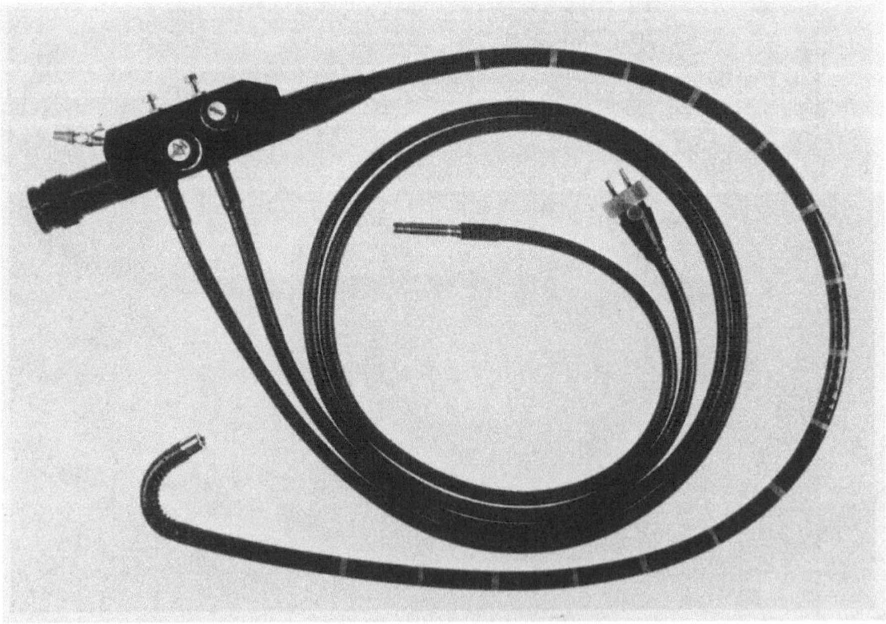

Fig. VII. Panendoscope 7883, Fa. Wolf, Knittlingen, Germany. Not available in the United States

limited to the duodenal wall, while side-viewing optics are preferred for visualization and intubation of the papilla of Vater. The direction of view of side- and forward-viewing duodenoscopes differs by 90°.

Olympus Corp. of America (New Hyde Park, N.Y. 11040): duodeno-fiberscope JF-B; the latest model is type JF-B2 (Fig. VIII). Side-viewing optics, 65°, working length 1370 mm, fixed focus. Manual control of automatic air insufflation, irrigation and suction mechanisms by two trumpet valves on the instrument handle is satisfactory. Deflection of the instrument tip in two planes (120° up and down; 90° to left and right) is directed by a convenient two-button system (Fig. IX). In addition, accessory instruments introduced through a separate channel can be deflected by up to 85°. Optical resolution and field of vision are good.

American Optical Machida Co. (P.O. Box 752; Southbridge, Massachusetts 01550): fiber duodenoscope FDS (Fig. X). Side-viewing optics, 56°, working length 1300 mm, variable focus.

Table 2. Technical data of duodenoscopes

Technical data	Machida FDS	Olympus JF-B2
Total length (mm)	1515	1520
Working length (mm)	1300	1370
Rigid tip		
Length (mm)	23.0	17.0
Diameter (mm)	11.0	10.0
Diameter of flexible part (mm)	10.5	10.0
Radius of deflection (mm)	70.0	60.0
Tip deflection		
Upwards	120°	120°
Downwards	120°	120°
To right	90°	90°
To left	90°	90°
Tip rotation to left and right	60°	∅
Optical field	56°	65°
Direction of view	90°	90°
Focal depth (mm)	3.5–∞	5–60
Biopsy forceps deflection	40°–90°	30°–85°

The instrument tip can be deflected by 120° in one plane and by 90° in the other. Despite excellent optical qualities, it is difficult to find and intubate the papilla of Vater with this instrument because the tip is quite long, resulting in a large radius of tip deflection. Introduction into the descending duodenum may be difficult. Further disadvantages are the manual air insufflation with a rubber balloon, irrigation with an attached syringe and the absence of automatic suction. Forward viewing optics with an optical field of 180° are said to be available in the near future.

An additional instrument for deep duodenoscopy is the *ACMI* F5-A gastro-duodenoscope. Working length 1200 mm, diameter of flexible part 12.7 mm. Side viewing optics, 75°, with polydirectional deflection to 100° each way. Focal depth 5–40 mm, fixed focus. Automatic air insufflation and suction through the biopsy channel. Water irrigation requires attachment of a syringe. Accessory instruments can be deflected an additional 75° beyond the instrument tip. The radius of tip deflection is fairly large which limits the usefulness of this instrument for cannulation of the ampulla of Vater and for inspection of the base of the duodenal bulb.

Enteroscopes

Only prototypes are currently manufactured by Machida and Olympus. A brief description is given in the chapter on Enteroscopy.

Coloscopy (Table 3)

Fiberoptic instruments for endoscopy of the colon are either short, for sigmoidoscopy, of long, for high coloscopy.

ACMI (8 Pelham Parkway, Pelham Manor, N.Y. 10803): coloscope F9, types S, L, and A (Fig. XI). Working length 1050, 1650, and 1600 mm. Optical field 75°. Direction of view 180°; fixed focus.

Types S and L are equipped with automatic air insufflation, facilities for suction and

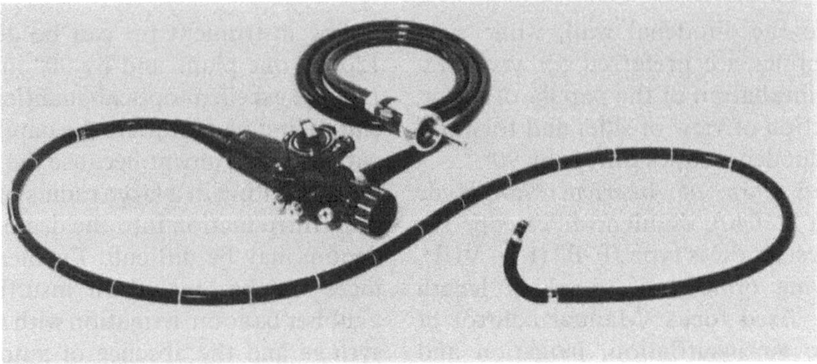

Fig. VIII. Duodenoscope JF-B2 (Olympus)

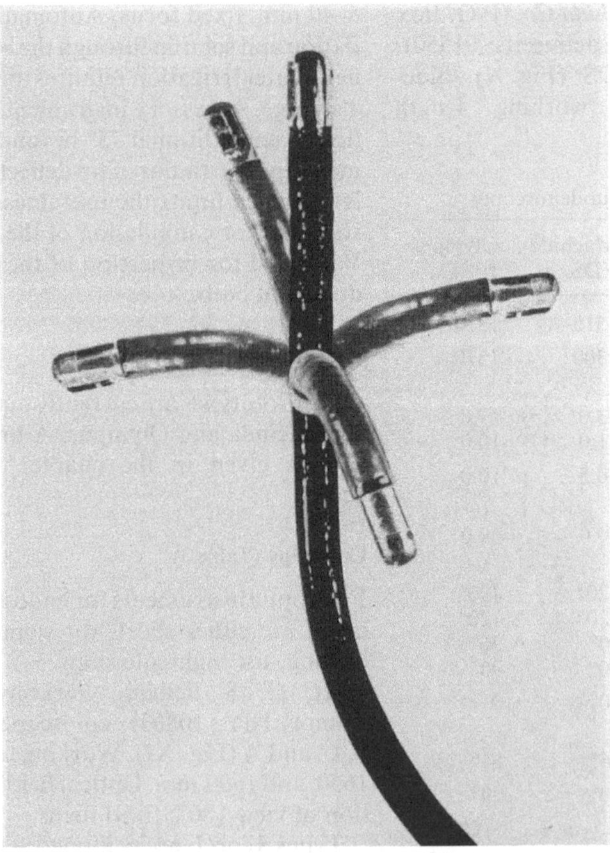

Fig. IX. Maximal tip deflection of duodenoscope JF-B (Olympus)

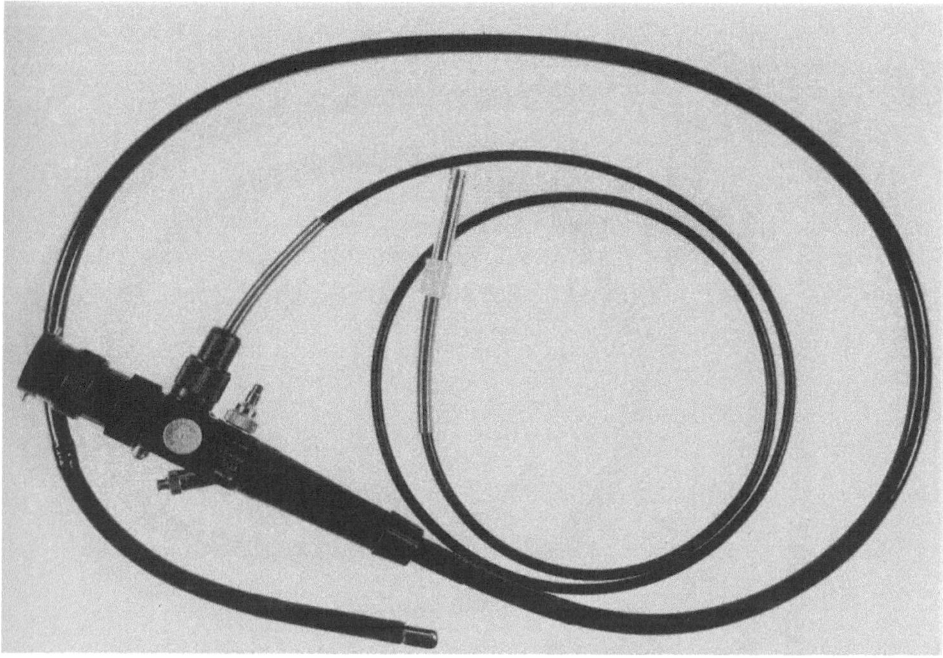

Fig. X. Duodenoscope FDS (American Optical Machida Company, Southbridge, Mass. 01550)

irrigation and an operating channel for introduction of biopsy forceps and other flexible instruments. The tip can be deflected by 180° in all planes in an extremely short radius by a single control. The F9 series represents improved versions of model FO-9000, types A, P, and PL. Type F9-A is provided with an additional large operating channel with independent suction; tip deflection is polydirectional to 160° one way.

Table 3. Technical data of coloscopes

Technical data	ACMI		Olympus CF-MB2/LB2	Machida FSS/FCS	Wolf Sigmoidoscope 7890
	F9-S/L	F9-A			
Working length (mm)	1050 (S) 1650 (L)	1600	1120 (MB2) 1870 (LB2)	800/1880	860
Diameter (mm)					
Rigid tip	15.0	18.0	14.4	14.5	15.5
Flexible part	13.0	15.8	14.0	11.6	12.5
Tip deflection					
Upwards	180°	160°	120°	120°	140°
Downwards	180°	160°	120°	120°	140°
To right	180°	160°	120°	120°	∅
To left	180°	160°	120°	120°	∅
Biopsy forceps deflection	∅	∅	18°	∅	∅
Focal depth (mm)	10–200	10–200	10–100	7–45	5–∞
Optical field	75°	75°	60°	60°	70°
Direction of view	180°	180°	180°	180°	180°
Variable focus	∅	∅	∅	∅	+

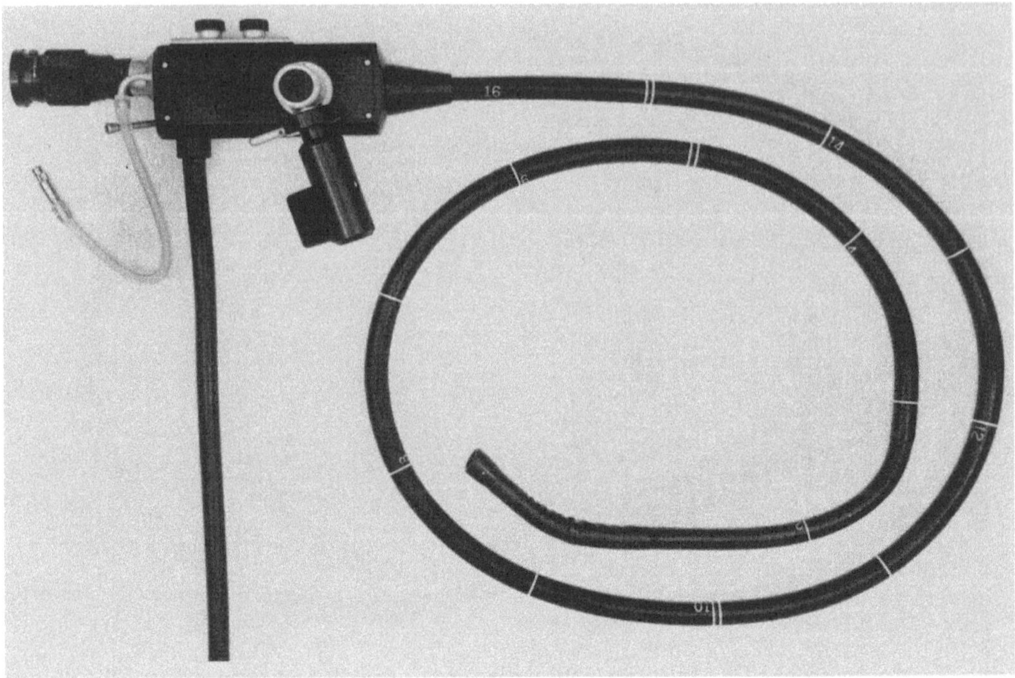

Fig. XI. Coloscope F9-L. ACMI (Pelham Manor, New York, 10803)

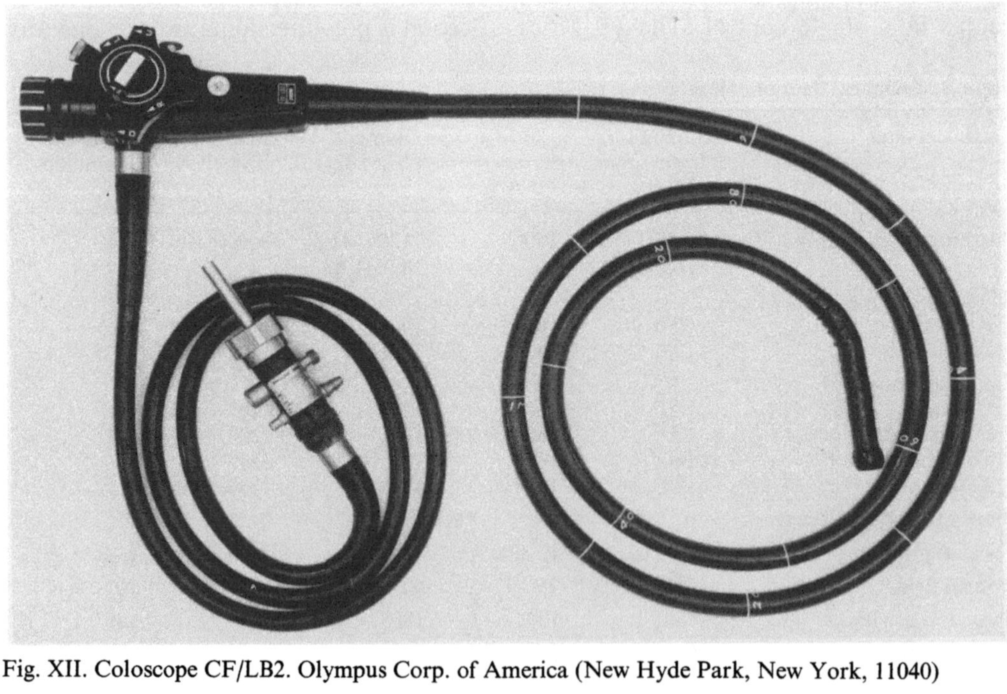

Fig. XII. Coloscope CF/LB2. Olympus Corp. of America (New Hyde Park, New York, 11040)

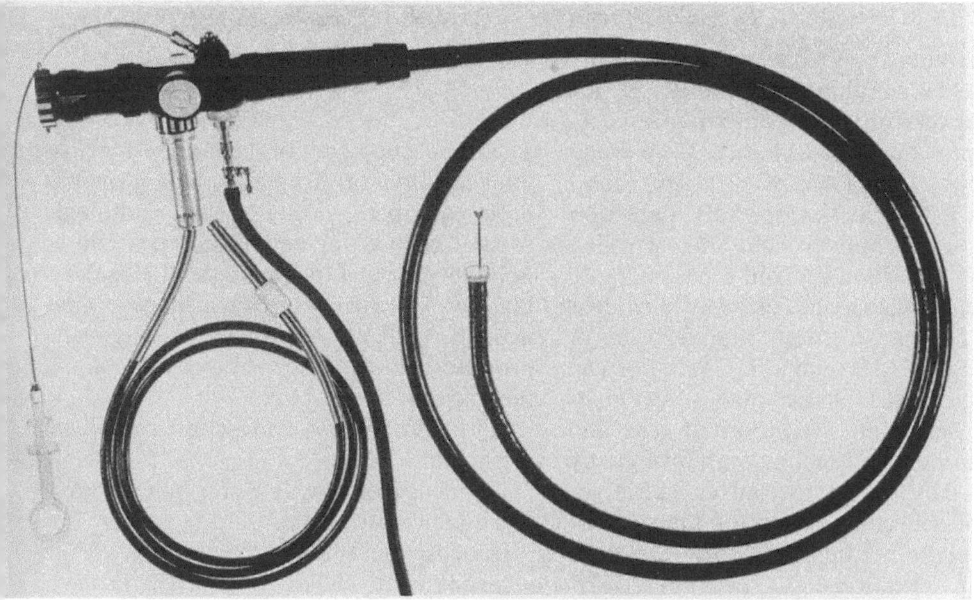

Fig. XIII. Coloscope FSS/FCS. American Optical Machida Co. (Southbridge, Mass. 01550)

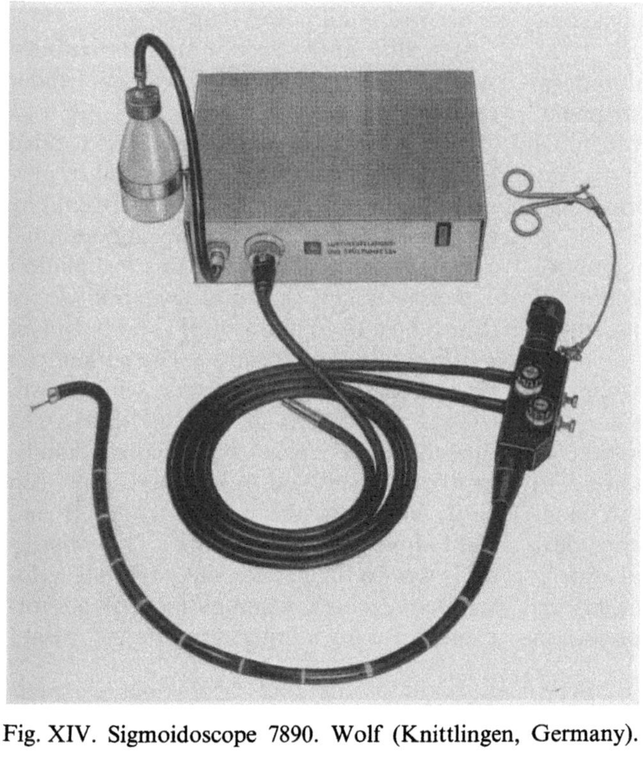

Fig. XIV. Sigmoidoscope 7890. Wolf (Knittlingen, Germany). Not available in the United States

The capability of introducing two accessory instruments simultaneously adds to the technical versatility of operative coloscopy.

Olympus Corp. of America (2 Nevada Drive, New Hyde Park, N.Y. 11040): coloscopes CF-MB2/LB2 (Fig. XII). Direction of view 180°, optical field 60°, working length 1120/1870 mm, fixed focus.

These two coloscopes differ only in their length and represent slight modifications of types CF-SB, MB, and LB. Their tips can be deflected to 120° in two planes. Automatic air insufflation, irrigation of lens and objects in view, and suction are conveniently controlled by two trumpet valves. The larger radius of deflection allows the insertion of forceps and other flexible instruments even at full tip deflection.

American Optical Machida Co. (Southbridge, Massachusetts 01150): coloscope FSS/FCS (Fig. XIII). Direction of view 180°, optical field 60°. Working length 800/1880 mm; fixed focus.

This instrument is offered in two versions, for sigmoidoscopy and high coloscopy. Tip deflection in four directions with a very short rigid tip (about half the length of the tips of ACMI and Olympus coloscopes) greatly facilitates the use of this instrument. The optical qualities are superb. Unfortunately, the coloscopes of this manufacture again are not equipped with automatic air insufflation, suction and irrigation.

Wolf (Knittlingen, Germany): sigmoidoscope type 7890 (Fig. XIV). Direction of view 180°, optical field 70°, working length 860 mm, variable focus.

The distal tip of the instrument can be deflected by 140° in two directions and can be arrested in any position. Automatic air and water insufflation and suction are conveniently controlled by two valves. A channel is available for the introduction of flexible instruments. Lacking personal experience, the optical properties of this instrument cannot be evaluated; it is not sold in the U.S.A.

1.2 Radiologic Equipment

The Endoscopy Unit of the University Hospital for Internal Medicine, Erlangen, has been equipped with a special radiologic room designed for endoscopic procedures in cooperation with the Medical Engineering Group, *Siemens AG*, Erlangen, Germany (Fig. XV). A variety of diagnostic procedures had to be considered in planning this facility:

1. Combined endoscopic-radiologic methods:
   Duodenoscopy with retrograde cholangio-pancreatography;
   laparoscopic splenoportography;
   laparoscopic cholangiography (transhepatic or via the the gallbladder).
2. Endoscopic procedures for which fluoroscopic localization of the instrument tip or a single radiograph for documentation purposes are occasionally needed:
   enteroscopy (jejuno-ileoscopy);
   coloscopy;
   peroral small bowel biopsy.

In addition, the Section of Pulmonology wished to perform bronchoscopy under fluoroscopic control.

The roentgen installation was expanded by angiographic equipment in order to provide the capability for splenoportography and for combined endoscopic-angiographic examinations. The basis of this installation is a *fluoroscopy unit with spot film device* (Sireskop and Explorator 35) and *image-intensifier television facilities*. The patient can be examined standing up or lying down. Ceiling suspension of the overhead X-ray tube facilitates access to the patient significantly. Nurses and other personnel can easily attend to the patient from left and right during the procedure. The *floating table top* is a further advantage for all endoscopic-radiologic examinations; it permits rapid centering of interesting areas for filming.

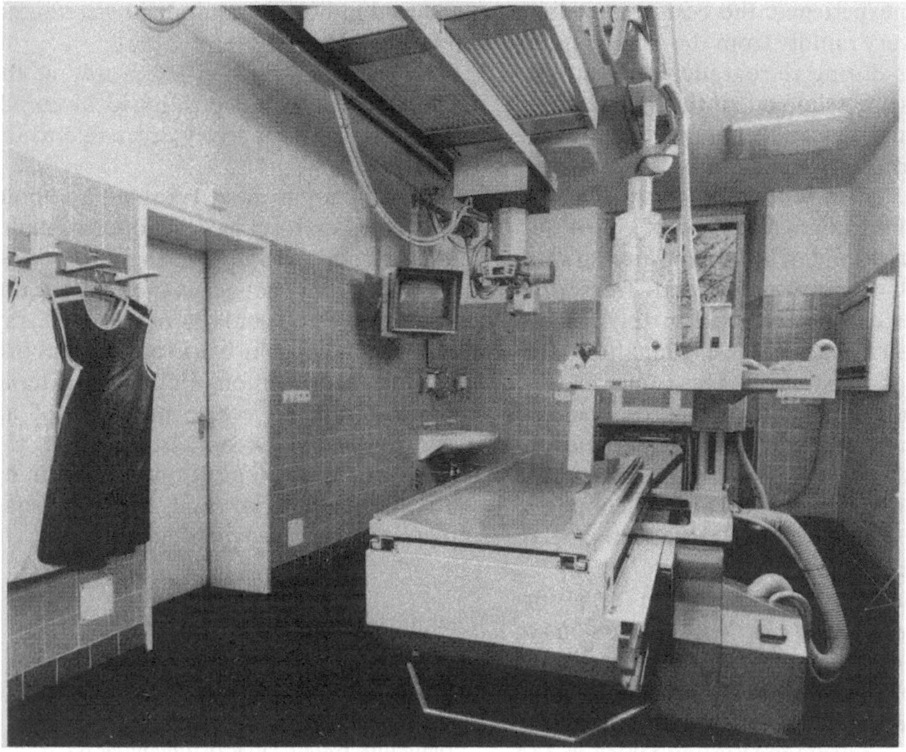

Fig. XV. Radiologic endoscopy room

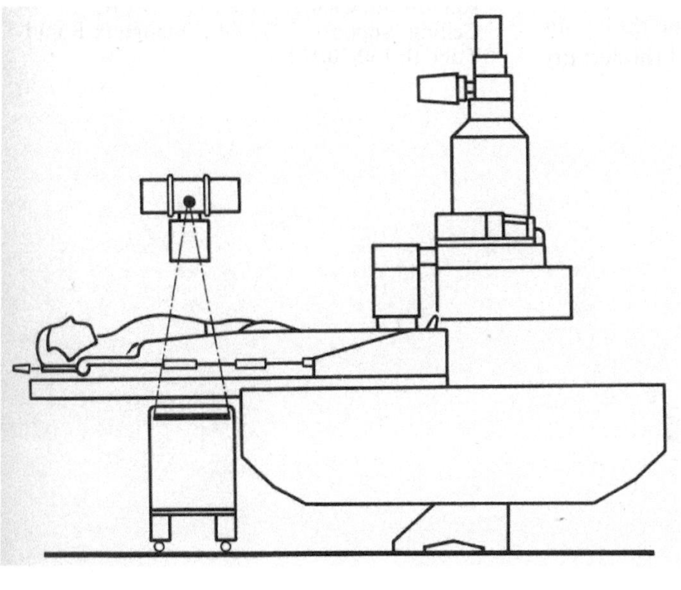

Fig. XVI. Schematic drawing of rapid film changer

In our experience, the contrast medium empties very rapidly from the small pancreatic ducts during retrograde pancreatography. This necessitated that the time required for manual cassette changing had to be shortened. To this end, an *image-intensifier roll film camera* with 70 × 70 mm film was added. This camera allows the taking of single exposures and of serial exposures at rates of 1, 2, 3, 4, and 9 per second. Interesting sequences can be recorded in this fashion during every phase of the examination without special preparation. This camera is also used to advantage during laparoscopic and transhepatic cholangiography. Serial exposures with the *ACT-rapid film changer* are still required for laparoscopic splenoportography because of the larger film size of 35 × 35 cm (Fig. XVI).

The patient is positioned in a motor-driven *rotating cradle* with excursion of more than 90° to either side for laparoscopic splenoportography and for transhepatic cholangiography. Combined with the ability to tilt the X-ray diagnostic unit Sireskop 3 to 90° head-down, this provides ideal patient mobility for laparoscopy. In order to facilitate manipulations during laparoscopy, the beam supporting the spot film device was enlarged, allowing the device to be raised by an additional 20 cm. This eliminates the necessity of moving it aside during the examination. No further alterations of the serially produced radiologic equipment were necessary.

The rotating cradle is fixed only at the foot end. The head is positioned in an adjustable shell and is freely accessible to the bronchoscopist.

The table top is moved craniad by about 100 cm for laparoscopic splenoportography and for abdominal arteriography. The ACT-rapid film changer is then placed under the table top and an overhead X-ray tube, suspended from a 3-D ceiling support, is swung into position. Following arterial catheterization or needle puncture of an organ under fluoroscopic observation, the patient can thus be positioned for filming with minimum delay and without being moved, solely by moving the table top.

Technical data

Radiologic Diagnostic Unit Sireskop 3 with Spot Film Device

Explorator 35:

Biangulix Rapid Tube Bi 150/30/50 R;
Image Intensifier Unit Sirecon 2—duplex 25/15;
Image Intensifier Roll Film Camera 70 mm, Sircam 70;
Twelve Pulse Roentgen Diagnostic Generator, Gigantos;
Motor Driven Cradle, unsupported head rest.

Angiographic Unit:

Rapid Film Changer AOT 35 × 35 cm;
Ceiling Support 3-D with Biangulix-Rapid-Tube Bi 150/30/101.

2. Duodenoscopy

2.1 Historical Development

The first attempts at inspection of the duodenum were made a few years after HIRSCHOWITZ had introduced fiberglass optics into endoscopy in 1958. HIRSCHOWITZ's initial claim that the duodenal bulb could be entered in about 50 percent of cases with the instruments available at that time could not be confirmed. In 1966, WATSON succeeded in visualizing the papilla of Vater endoscopically. Finally, in 1968 McCUNE reported the first intubation of the papilla of Vater through a duodenoscope with retrograde pancreatography. DEMLING and collaborators conducted endoscopic studies of the duodenum with various prototypes during the same year. The Japanese companies Olympus and Machida already had developed production models of duodenoscopes. Therefore, Japanese gastroenterologists including OI, KOZU and HARA were the first to perform retrograde cholangiography routinely. The initial experiences with this new method were discussed at the large international congresses of endoscopy in 1970.

2.2 Indications

Combined examination of esophagus, stomach and duodenal bulb (esophago-gastro-bulboscopy).

The fiberendoscopes with forward viewing or variable optics currently available allow inspection of esophagus, stomach and the proximal duodenum during a single procedure. This examination hardly takes longer than an ordinary gastroscopy.

We have performed this combined procedure since 1970 whenever there were abnormal radiologic findings of one of these organs, in cases of epigastric pain of uncertain etiology, and in the presence of acute upper gastrointestinal bleeding from an unknown site (emergency endoscopy). This approach has proven its value. The bleeding site was localized during emergency endoscopy in 135 of 151 patients with upper gastrointestinal bleeding. In 45 of these cases it was in the duodenum. In 11.2 percent of patients with radiologic abnormalities, additional lesions of one or two further organs were discovered during combined esophagogastroduodenoscopy [3].

The importance of enteroscopy for the diagnosis of duodenal diseases will be discussed mainly in the section on duodenal ulcer. We recommend, therefore, that all three organs be included in the endoscopic examination even when the radiologic findings give a direct indication only for, e.g., esophagoscopy or gastroscopy. This procedure is also of value as a screening method for chronic bleeding or X-ray negative dyspepsia.

Fibergastroscopes with side-viewing optics, e.g., GF-B2 (Olympus) and FGS-BL (Machida), are preferred over forward-viewing instruments for examination of cardia and fundus. Complete endoscopic instrumentation for esophagus, stomach, and proximal duodenum consists, therefore, of at least one instrument with forward- and one with side-viewing optics [8]. The newer prograde fiberendoscopes (ACMI 7089 J,

P, and F8; Olympus GIF-D2) reach to the descending duodenum, but rarely beyond.

Inspection of the Entire Duodenum requires the use of side-viewing instruments (Olympus JF-B2; Machida FDS; ACMI F5-A). We, therefore, employ this type of instrument for examination of postbulbar duodenum, proximal jejunum and the papilla of Vater. Side-viewing optics are recommended also for "retrograde" inspection of the duodenum, that is, of the afferent loop after Billroth II gastrectomy. Aspiration of secretions trough the intubated papilla of Vater is useful in the diagnosis of pancreatic and biliary tract tumors [7, 10]. Aspiration must be performed prior to the instillation of contrast medium since hypertonic materials such as Conray 60 induce cell lysis.

Radiographic Visualization of the Major Pancreatic Duct (Duct of Wirsung) is indicated for all pancreatic diseases associated with narrowing of the ductal system. This includes inflammatory and tumorous stenoses, as well as concrements in the ampulla of Vater or the major pancreatic duct. Retrograde pancreatography should always be performed after complete resolution of acute pancreatitis in order to outline the ductal anatomy.

Stenoses of the upper third of the descending duodenum represent an additional indication for retrograde pancreatography. The existence of an annular pancreas can be diagnosed conclusively in this manner. Retrograde pancreatography frequently allows delineation of the anatomic relationships between epigastric tumors, e.g., pseudocysts, and the pancreatic duct system [1, 4, 5, 9].

Retrograde cholangiography. The most important contribution of retrograde cholangiography lies in the differentiation between extra- and intrahepatic obstructive jaundice. This method is superior to oral and/or intravenous cholangiography with tomography in the demonstration of gallbladder and bile duct lesions because sufficient contrast medium can be injected for optimal visualization.

It must be emphasized again that both structures, the pancreatic as well as the common bile duct, should be examined after successful cannulation of the papilla of Vater. This is particularly true when the duct system injected first showed pathologic alterations. A possible narrowing of the common bile duct secondary to chronic pancreatitis or to pancreatic tumor can then be considered in mapping surgical strategy.

Spontaneous or operative biliary-enteric anastomoses are a further domain of duodenoscopic cholangiography [2].

Contraindications

Coagulation abnormalities, severe coronary artery disease, congestive heart failure and pulmonary insufficiency are relative contraindications. Active duodenal ulcers, contrary to previous opinion [6], do not perforate with duodenal air insufflation. At least, this complication has never been described. As mentioned above,retrograde pancreatography in patients with acute pancreatitis should be delayed until complete remission has occurred. The same precaution applies to acute bacterial cholangitis. Possible dangers of duodenoscopy and of endoscopic retrograde cholangiopancreatography (ERCP) are listed in the chapter on "complications".

References

1. Ashizawa, S., Fujino, M.: Fiberduodenoscopy. Acta, gastro. ent. jap. **2**, 137 (1972).
2. Classen, M., Frühmorgen, P., Kozu, T., Demling, L.: Endoscopic-radiologic demonstration of biliodigestive fistulas. Endoscopy **3**, 138 (1971).
3. Classen, M.: Diskussionsbemerkung. In: Grundlagen der gastrointestinalen Endoskopie (Lindner, H., Hrsg.). Gräfelfing: Demeter 1972.
4. Classen, M., Koch, H., Demling, L.: Diagnostische Bedeutung der endoskopischen Kontrastdarstellung des Pankreasgangsystems. Leber Magen Darm **2**, 79 (1972).
5. Cotton, P.: Endoscopy and cannulation of papilla of Vater; retrograde cholangio-pancreatography (ERCP). Gut **13**, 1014 (1972).

6. HENNING, N.: Diskussionsbemerkung. In: Grundlagen der gastroenterologischen Endoskopie (HEINKEL, K., Ed.). Gräfelfing: Demeter 1968.
7. KOZU, T.: Duodenoscopic collection of intraductal pancreatic juice. In: Endoscopy of the small intestine (DEMLING, L., CLASSEN, M., Eds.). Stuttgart: Thieme, 1973
8. LINDNER, H.: Instrumentarium zur Endoskopie des Ösophagus, des Magens und des Bulbus duodeni. Dtsch. med. Wschr. **36**, 1440 (1971).
9. OI, J., KOBAYASHI, S., TAKEMOTO, T.: Endoscopic pancreato-cholangiography. Endoscopy **2**, 103 (1970).
10. WITTE, S., RIEGG, H.: Cytologic findings in the bile after cannulation of the papilla of Vater. In: Endoscopy of the small intestine (DEMLING, L., CLASSEN. M., Eds.). Stuttgart: Thieme, 1973

2.3 Technique

Premedication

Bulboscopy and *postbulbar duodenoscopy* require the same patient preparation as other endoscopic examinations of the upper gastrointestinal tract. One-half to one hour prior to the procedure, the patient receives 0.5 mg atropine sulfate and 10–20 mg triflupromazine (Vesprin) intramuscularly while still on the ward. A spray of 2 ml of 1 percent tetracaine (Pontocaine HCl) or 0.5 percent dyclonine HCl (Dyclone) solution for topical anesthesia of the pharynx and meperidine (Demerol), 50–100 mg intravenously, are given immediately before the start of the examination.

When peristaltic waves obstruct the view during the procedure, propantheline Br (Pro-Banthine), 15–30 mg, may be given intramuscularly or intravenously.

Technique

Bulboscopy is performed with the patient in the left lateral decubitus position, as are all other endoscopic examination of the upper gastrointestinal tract. Special maneuvers rarely are required, since the pylorus is entered under direct vision through the forward viewing endoscope. Occasionally, however, the pylorus slides by laterally as the instrument tip is advanced and the duodenum cannot be entered right away. In these cases, the biopsy forceps can be introduced into the duodenum without difficulty to act as a guide for the endoscope.

Postbulbar Duodenoscopy, on the other hand, requires a special technique because the side viewing duodenoscopes demand that the pylorus be passed blindly (Fig. XVII).

The duodenoscope is first introduced into the gastric antrum without major technical difficulties. Air insufflation should be used sparingly at this stage in order to avoid the induction of strong peristaltic waves. The motto is "as little as possible, as much as necessary." With the pylorus in view, the instrument tip is slightly deflected craniad (upwards) and advanced as close to the pylorus as possible. Next, the tip is deflected downward, in the direction of the lesser curvature of the antrum; simultaneously, the duodenoscope is slowly pushed forward. The duodenal bulb is entered easily, usually with a perceptible jolt if one avoids that the pylorus slides by laterally during this maneuver. The optical lens lies flush against the superior part of the duodenal bulb at this stage and vision is obscured. One can, however, frequently recognize entry into the intestine by discerning the villous architecture of the duodenal wall. The lumen of the descending duodenum then comes into view after rotation of the instrument by 180°, advancing the endoscope further and insufflation of small amounts of air. Frequently one can already see a prominence on the inner part of the C-loop behind which the papilla of Vater should be sought. As the duodenoscope continues to be advanced, the plica longitudinalis, which is oriented at a right angle to the transverse folds of Kerckring, comes into view. The papilla of Vater is located near the proximal part of this fold: sometimes directly on it, sometimes adjacent to it and in some cases obscured by smaller folds in the immediate proximity.

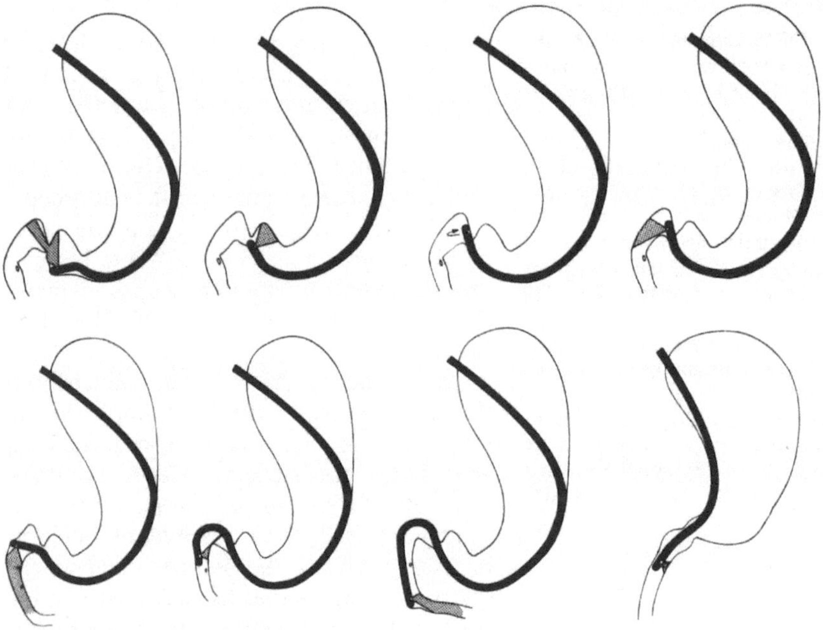

Fig. XVII. Technique of postbulbar duodenoscopy

In cases where the papilla of Vater is not spotted upon introduction of the duodenoscope into the proximal part of the descending duodenum, it is advisable to advance the instrument to the junction of the second and third portions of the duodenum. The endoscope is then withdrawn slowly with constant inspection of the medial (inner) aspect of the C-loop. This is accompanied by straightening of the instrument within the stomach, which explains the fact that it frequently has to be pulled back a considerable distance before the papilla comes into view. Its appearance is again heralded by the plica longitudinalis. The minor papilla is usually found about 2 cm above (craniad) and more towards the dorsal aspect of the duodenum. For cannulation of the major and the minor papilla—with a lower chance of success for the latter—the instrument tip has to be positioned in such a way that the protruding teflon catheter points straight at the orifice. This may require that the patient be moved into the supine or prone position.

The duodenoscope can easily be advanced to the duodeno-jejunal junction when examination of the entire duodenum is clinically indicated.

References

1. Demling, L., Classen, M.: Duodenojejunoskopie. Dtsch. med. Wschr. **95**, 1427 (1970).
2. Classen, M.: Fiberendoscopy of the Intestines, Gut **12**, 330 (1971).
3. Koch, H., Classen, M.: Endoskopie des Bulbus duodeni. Leber Magen Darm **1**, 21 (1971).
4. Koch, H., Kozu, T., Classen, M., Demling, L.: Technik der Duodenoskopie. In: Fortschritte der Endoskopie, Bd. 3, Stuttgart, New York; Schattauer 1972.
5. Kozu, T., Deyhle, P., Classen, M., Koch, H., Demling, L.: Neue Verfahren für die Intestinoskopie. Dtsch. med. Wschr. **95**, 2194 (1970).
6. Oi, O., Kobayashi, S., Kondo, T.: Endoscopic pancreatocholangiography. Endoscopy **2**, 103 (1970).

2.4 Endoscopic Orientation in the Duodenum

The four parts of the duodenum: bulb (D1), descending (D2), inferior horizontal (D3), and ascending (D4), possess some characteristic features which help the endoscopist with orientation.

The bulb is a conical structure (Fig. 1); its lumen narrows at the apex where it leads into the descending duodenum. One recognizes a convex fold emerging from a caudal and dorsal direction; shaped like a romanic arc, it resembles the gastric fold at the incisura angularis (Fig. 2).

The wall of the duodenal bulb differs from the rest of the duodenum by the absence of the folds of Kerckring. Compared to the appearance of the antral mucosa, the bulbar mucosa has a slightly darker hue. Close inspection reveals a villous surface structure characteristic of the small intestine which in the duodenal bulb may appear finger-, leaf-, or ridge-shaped. Exact localization of pathologic changes within the bulb is difficult because the flexible fiberscopes have a tendency to rotate on their long axis (torque). This problem can be overcome by instilling a few milliliters of water with the patient in the left lateral supine position; the water will collect at the lowest point, the base of the duodenal bulb.

The inferior and superior duodenal flextures serve as landmarks for orientation in the descending duodenum. Normally, the superior flexure describes an acute angle, causing the folds of Kerckring to be crowded; that is, in the longitudinal axis the distance between folds is less than at the inferior flexure. The descending duodenum assumes a cylindric shape with a circular or oval cross section upon air insufflation (Fig. 3). The experienced endoscopist finds the papilla of Vater (Fig. 4) without difficulty, usually in the second portion of the duodenum. Among 50 patients, it was located in the middle third in 54 percent, in the distal third in 30 percent, and in 16 percent in the upper third of the descending duodenum [1]. Atypical localization of the ampulla of Vater, from gastric antrum to the ligament of Treitz, is very unusual. The different shapes of the papilla are described on page 27.

In cases where a minor pancreatic (Santorini's) duct communicates with the duodenum, a small accessory papilla (papilla minor) exists 2 to 3 cm above (craniad) the papilla of Vater. The junction between the descending and the inferior horizontal parts of the duodenum is usually identified easily at the inferior flexure, but the transition from the inferior horizontal to the ascending part is rarely recognizable to the endoscopist. Arteriomesenteric narrowing of the inferior horizontal part by the superior mesenteric artery, resulting in dorsal displacement of the duodenum in thin patients, is a rare help in orientation. A crescent-shaped narrowing of the duodenal lumen is seen through the endoscope in these cases. The duodeno-jejunal flexure is easily recognized by its acute angle. According to our experience, fluoroscopy is rarely needed for endoscopic orientation in the duodenum and proximal jejunum.

References

1. Classen, M., Hellwig, H., Rösch, W.: Anatomy of the pancreatic duct. A duodenoscopicradiological study. Endoscopy **5**, 14 (1973).

2.5 Endoscopy of the Duodenum

2.5.1 Peptic Lesions and Sequelae

Duodenal Ulcer
The Significance of Endoscopic Diagnosis

Duodenal ulcer is one of the most common, if not the commonest, gastrointestinal disease. More than 96 percent are located in the duodenal bulb. Endoscopy has improved the precision of diagnosis of duodenal peptic ulcer disease. In our hospital, 30 percent of duodenal ulcers were not recognized by the radiologist [8]. When all modern radiologic techniques are employed, the rate of X-ray-negative ulcers of the duodenal bulb is lowered to 10 percent [13]. Two bulbar ulcers are present in about 20 percent of cases; about 80 percent of these lie on opposite walls ("kissing ulcers") [10] (Fig. 6).

The positive endoscopic finding ordinarily leaves no doubt about the correctness of the ulcer diagnosis. Scars hardly ever lead to confusion regarding the presence of an ulcer. The endoscopic criteria of duodenal ulcer are discussed below. The situation differs when an ulcer is identified radiologically but not found during endoscopy. Our group estimated previously that in about 10 percent of these cases the presence of an ulcer could not be excluded with certainty by the endoscopist [8]. This was due to anatomic and technical factors. Gastric outlet stenosis or heavy scarring and scarred recesses of the duodenal bulb interfere with passage of the instrument and hinder complete inspection of the bulb. In addition, the tip of the first generation forward viewing duodenoscopes was not sufficiently flexible. The use of modern instruments (e.g., ACMI F8, or Olympus GIF-D2) with tip deflection of up to 180° and the additional examination with a side viewing duodenoscope will permit the rate of endoscopic duodenal ulcer diagnosis to approach 100 percent.

The diagnosis of bleeding duodenal ulcers during emergency endoscopy is of special importance. In 22 percent of a total of 181 patients with acute upper gastrointestinal hemorrhage, a duodenal ulcer was identified as the bleeding site (Table 4). This figure emphasizes the importance of including the duodenum, especially the bulb, in the endoscopic examination when confronted with hematemesis or melena.

Beyond that, duodenoscopy for the first time permits the exact evaluation of the effect of drugs in the treatment of duodenal ulcer [1].

Table 4. Results of emergency endoscopy

Bleeding site	*n*
Esophagus	
Varices	33
Esophagitis	18
Erosions	3
Mallory-Weiss syndrome	2
Stomach	
Varices	3
Ulcer	22
Erosions	26
Carcinoma	13
Benign tumors	3
Postpolypectomy	1
Postaspiration biopsy	1
Marginal ulcer	8
Peptic jejunal ulcer	1
Duodenum	
Ulcer	40
Erosions	5
Papillotomy	1
Carcinoma	1
Total	181

Method

Forward Viewing Instruments

After passage of the pylorus and pharmacologic inhibition of muscular contractions, the instrument is advanced to the superior duodenal flexure and beyond. The proximal part of the descending duodenum and the distal (aborad) parts of the bulb are thoroughly inspected at this time. Ulcers hidden in pseudodiverticula and deep scars are brought into view with the help of the biopsy forceps: it is slowly advanced into the pouch, thereby enlarging the opening which communicates with the lumen. When indicated, one can also grasp the aborad margin of the pouch and push it aside. These manipulations should be conducted cautiously and should be omitted in the presence of clinical signs of perforation. Complete examination of the proximal duodenum is indispensible, especially when there are radiologic or clinical indications for the presence of an ulcer. The base of the bulb should be inspected thoroughly during the withdrawal of the instrument into the stomach. This region also comes into view across the pylorus for a few seconds at the time when duodenal motor function returns. The postpyloric area can be inspected in greater detail by inversion of the duodenoscope (e.g., Olympus JF-B2) within the bulb [6].

Side Viewing Instruments

Side viewing instruments, such as the JF-B2 Olympus or the FDS Machida, can usually be introduced into the duodenum at the first try, even in the presence of pyloric or bulbar narrowing. The lateral orientation of the lens system and the flexibility of these instruments whose short tip can be deflected in two planes allow inspection of scarred recesses which is frequently impossible with forward viewing duodenoscopes. In addition, this instrument type is often indispensible for the recognition of pathologic alterations at the base of the duodenal bulb. Abnormal findings in the bulb were visible only with the side viewing instrument in 12 percent of 321 patients who were examined with both types [11].

Endoscopic Appearance of Duodenal Ulcer (Figs. 5–13)

About 50 percent of duodenal ulcers are located in the anterior, 25 percent in the posterior wall, 20 percent in the superior, and 5 percent in the inferior aspect of the duodenal bulb [7, 9, 10, 14].

The duodenal ulcer looks very much like the gastric ulcer. The mucosal defect may be round, oval, or linear. Ulcers within scarred areas and in pseudodiverticula due to scarring have bizarre shapes with radial extensions like "pseudopods of an ameba" (SCHINDLER). The ulcer border is sharply demarcated and appears red, in contrast to the periphery of a scar. Longstanding ulcers have a heaped-up edge which is elevated above the ulcer base covered with necrotic debris. The macroscopic appearance of the florid ulcer is usually unmistakable. The diagnosis rests on biopsy of the ulcer border only in those rare cases where grayish-yellow necrotic material cannot be differentiated from the appearance of a scar. The mucosa adjacent to many ulcers is markedly injected, with prominence of the mucosal relief. This appearance is caused by an accompanying duodenitis which is limited to the area surrounding the ulcer [2, 3].

Endoscopic recognition of a bleeding ulcer can be very difficult, especially in the deformed, stenotic bulb. The ulcers are invariably located at or very close to the area of narrowing. Correct localization can be accomplished in the majority of instances following aspiration of the blood, irrigation, and elimination of contractions by parenteral injection of an anticholinergic drug or of glucagon.

So-called "giant ulcers" cover entire scarred areas or pseudodiverticula [15]. The radiologic differentiation from a scarred bulb and from duodenal diverticula is frequently impossible. The endoscopist does not encounter these difficulties.

Postbulbar ulcers account for only 3 percent of all duodenal ulcers [7]. Localization distal (aborad) to the papilla of Vater is extremely rare and should raise suspicion of the Zollinger-Ellison syndrome or an infiltrating tumor. Postbulbar ulcers look the same as bulbar ulcers. Ulcers on opposite walls are termed "kissing ulcers" and are detected more frequently by the endoscopist than the radiologist: Kawai found "kissing ulcers" in the duodenal bulb of 20 patients; 8 of these were detected only during endoscopy [10].

Scarring

Scars in the Duodenal Bulb (Fig. 16)

Many duodenal ulcers heal with scar formation but without changing the appearance of the bulb. We term this situation "scars in the bulb" in distinction to the more or

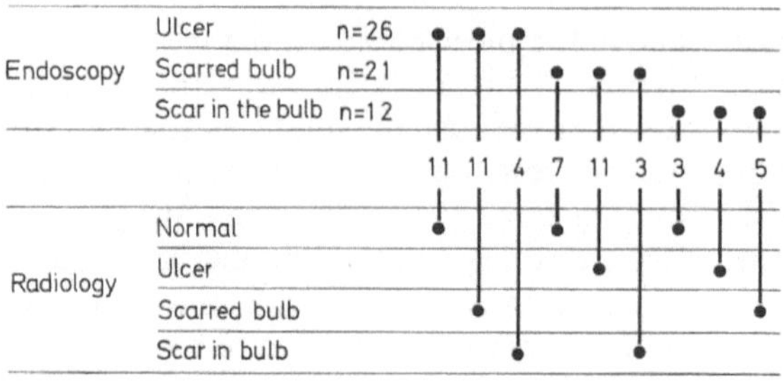

Fig. XVIII. Discordant radiologic findings with endoscopically proven bulbar ulcers and scars

less deformed "scarred bulb" (Fig. XVIII). The bulbar scar is characterized endoscopically by grayish-white tissue without inflammation of the adjoining mucosa. We assume that this type of scar, single or multiple, is the result of superficial ulcers. Radiating folds and heaped-up edges are absent.

Scarred Bulb (Fig. 17)

The spectrum of the scarred bulb reaches from the isolated deformity of one wall to the concentrically narrowed, tubular organ.

The endoscopic appearance is dominated by grayish-white scars, atypical folds and pouches. The normal recess of the bulb can, on the other hand, be shrunken or completely absent; others parts may exhibit prestenotic dilatation. Occasionally observed poststenotic dilatations are interpreted as being caused by a jet effect of the chyme which accumulates proximal to the stenosis. Duodenal motor function is diminished or absent in heavily scarred areas and is increased proximal to stenoses.

Studies conducted by our group have shown that "typical" ulcer symptoms are at least as frequent in patients with a scarred bulb as in those with an active ulcer (Fig. XIX). This observation leads to the conclusion that the scarred bulb is of greater clinical significance than previously appreciated in the vicious cycle of ulcer-scar-ulcer [5].

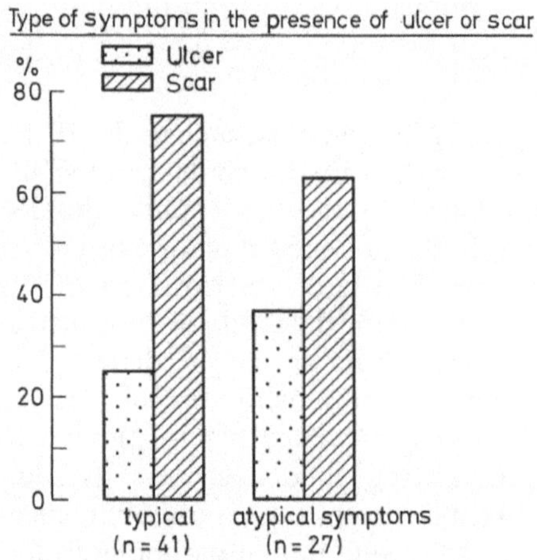

Fig. XIX. Symptoms of patients with scarred bulb and with active duodenal ulcer

Erosions (Figs. 14, 15)

Erosions are superficial defects limited to the mucosa. According to the nomenclature proposed by Kawai, gastric erosions are divided into incomplete and complete lesions according to their macroscopic appearance. Complete erosions are surrounded by a prominent halo which corresponds histologically to hyperplasia of the alveolar ridges. The elevated margin surrounds a central depression which is covered by debris due to fibrinoid necrosis. Incomplete erosions usually are small and nearly or completely level with the surrounding mucosa. In the duodenal bulb, incomplete erosions predominate by far. It is doubtful whether bulbar erosions are the site of bleeding as often as gastric erosions. So far, we have seen postbulbar erosions only in patients with the Zollinger-Ellison syndrome.

Complete erosions must be differentiated from adenomas of the Brunner's glands by obtaining target biopsies (Figs. 24, 25). The same applies to small duodenal polyps and to polypoid heterotopic mucosal tissue. Iatrogenic trauma of the duodenal mucosa caused by the endoscope may mimic the appearance of erosions.

References

1. BROWN, P., SALMON, P.R., HTUT, T., READ, A.E.: Double blind trial of carbenoxolone sodium capsules in duodenal ulcer therapy, based on endoscopic diagnosis and follow-up. Brit. med. J. **3**, 655 (1972).
2. CHELI, R.: Duodenitis. Facts and fiction. Endoscopy **3**, 2 (1971).
3. CLASSEN, M., KOCH, H., DEMLING, L.: Duodenitis. In: Inflammation in Gut. Basel: S. Karger 1970.
4. CLASSEN, M.: Evaluation of endoscopy for the diagnosis of the duodenal ulcer. Arch. Mal. Appar. dig. **61**, 21 (1972).
5. FRÜHMORGEN, P., JENNY, S., CLASSEN, M., BAUERLE, H., KOCH, H., DEMLING, L.: Anamnese bei Ulkus und Narben im Bulbus duodeni. Dtsch. med. Wschr. **6**, 188 (1972).
6. FRÜHMORGEN, P., KONISZEWSKI, G., CLASSEN, M.: Duplication of the pylorus. Endoscopy **4**, 234 (1972).
7. FUJINO, M., ASHIZAWA, S.: Fiberduodenoscopy. Acta gastro-ent. jap. **7**, 137 (1972).
8. JENNY, S., FRÜHMORGEN, P., CLASSEN, M., BAUERLE, H., FUCHS, H., DEMLING, L.: Endoskopisch-radiologische Diagnostik des Bulbus duodeni (Ulkus, Narbe). Dtsch. med. Wschr. **4**, 118 (1972).
9. KASUGAI, T., KUNO, N., AOKI, J., KIZU, M., KOBAYASHI, S.: Fiberduodenoscopy: analysis of 353 cases. Gastroint. Endoscopy **1**, 9 (1971).
10. KAWAI, K., KOHLI, J., MISAKI, F., AKASAKA, J., IDA, K.: Comparative study for duodenal ulcer by radiology and endoscopy. Endoscopy **5**, 18 (1973).
11. KISSLING, U., CLASSEN, M., DETTE, G., FRÜHMORGEN, P., DEMLING, L.: Die Ergebnisse von 1399 Untersuchungen des Bulbus duodeni. Schweiz. med. Wschr., in Druck.
12. OTTENJANN, R.: Rationelle Diagnostik des Ulkusleidens. Diagnostik **5**, 65 (1972).
13. SEIFERT, E.: Endoskopische Diagnostik der Gastritis und des Duodenalulkus. Med. Welt (Stuttg.) **23**, 1890 (1972).
14. SEIFERT, E.: Indikation und Wert der kombinierten Ösophago-Gastro-Bulboskopie. Vortr. 8. Seminar Dtsch. Ges. Gastroent. Endoskopie, in press.
15. WENDENBURG, H.H., WEHLING, H.: Über differentialdiagnostische Schwierigkeiten bei großen Divertikeln und Riesenulzera am Bulbus duodeni. Dtsch. med. Wschr. **18**, 845 (1972).

2.5.2 Duodenitis

Studies by CHELI and by our group [1–3, 5] have cast doubt on the belief that chronic duodenitis is a clinical entity. Neither does diffuse duodenitis precede or accompany duodenal ulcer disease. Inflammatory changes are seen histologically only in mucosal fragments removed from the immediate vicinity of the ulcer [1, 2].

Macro- and microscopic, diffuse duodenitis is found in the Zollinger-Ellison syndrome. The endoscopist observes the mucosa of the entire duodenum to be swollen with broadening or absence of the folds of Kerckring. The mucosa is injected and shows petechial or diffuse hemorrhages and occasionally ulcerations, scars and narrowing of the lumen as well. Any of these changes in the postbulbar duodenum should raise the suspicion of the Zollinger-Ellison syndrome.

PIEGLER described duodenal involvement by Crohn's disease in three of our eighty patients [6]. Prominent findings on endoscopy are punched out, partly superficial, ulcerations with reddish margins and fibrinoid necrosis. The duodenal wall is rigid and its structure is altered markedly by the presence of stenoses and partial or complete absence of Kerckring's folds. Duodenal motility is decreased or absent. In one of our patients with duodenal Crohn's disease, the papilla of Vater could not be identified at first. Following intravenous injection of cholecystokinin-pancreozymin, bile was seen to flow from an irregularly-shaped orifice. The diagnosis is established on clinical grounds and confirmed by histologic examination of biopsies obtained under direct vision. Mesenteric vein thrombosis is characterized by diffuse reddening and mucosal hemorrhages. Endoscopic descriptions of additional types of duodenitis accompanying parasitic infestation and other diseases [3, 4] are not yet available.

References

1. CHELI, R.: Duodenitis and duodenal ulcer. Digestion **1**, 175 (1968).
2. CHELI, R.: Duodenitis. Facts and fiction. Endoscopy **3**, 106 (1971).
3. CLASSEN, M., KOCH, H., DEMLING, L.: Duodenitis. In: Inflammation in Gut. Basel: Karger 1970.
4. DEBRAY, C., PERGOLO, F.: Les duodénites. Arch. Mal. Appar. dig. **40**, 206 (1951).
5. DEMLING, L., CLASSEN, M.: Duodenitis. In: Klinische Gastroenterologie (DEMLING, L., Ed.). Stuttgart: Thieme 1972.
6. PIEGLER, TH.: Verlauf und Prognose der Crohnschen Erkrankung. Inauguraldissertation, Erlangen 1970.

2.5.3 Duodenal Stenoses

The choice of endoscopes depends on the localization and degree of the stenosis. Stenotic areas proximal (craniad) to the papilla of Vater can be examined well with forward viewing instruments, except that narrowing at or immediately beyond the superior duodenal flexure can best be evaluated with side viewing duodenoscopes such as the Olympus JF-B2. The ascending duodenum can only be reached with the longer duodenoscopes. Severe stenoses with prestenotic dilatation can be inspected through forward viewing optics, since there is sufficient room for deflection of the instrument tip. Attempts at advancing the duodenoscope through the narrowed segment should only be made after the degree of stenosis has been assessed during pharmacologic inhibition of motor activity.

Extrinsic compression has to be differentiated from intrinsic causes of duodenal narrowing. Endoscopy can help in the diagnosis of superior mesenteric artery compression, and of stenoses caused by bands, cysts or tumors in adjacent organs. The role of endoscopy in the diagnosis of pancreatic tumors and cysts lies mainly in its combination with radiology during retrograde pancreatography. The same applies to the diagnosis of the annular pancreas. This will be discussed in detail later on. However, carcinomas of the pancreas and the extrahepatic bile ducts may infiltrate the duodenum [3]. Endoscopically, this results in extrinsic compression, stenosis and/or ulceration. The target biopsy is again the *sine qua non* for diagnosis in these circumstances. An additional cause for stenosis of the descending duodenum is chronic pancreatitis involving the head of the pancreas [2].

The endoscopic appearance of bulbar stenosis is characterized by changes which have been described in the discussion of the scarred bulb. One sees whitish scars radiating toward the luminal narrowing and scarred recesses with or without florid ulceration. Postbulbar stenosis exhibits identical alterations; additionally, the folds of Kerckring are partly or completely effaced.

Stenoses caused by operations on the duodenum or adjacent organs may assume many shapes. All degrees of duodenal stenosis may be encountered, from scars and distortion of Kerckring's folds to subtotal or total stenosis with prestenotic dilatation. Rarely, the duodenum is compressed by diverticula filled with chyme. We cannot yet state whether this can be relieved by endoscopic drainage of the diverticulum. Benign and malignant tumors frequently present with the symptoms of duodenal stenosis [4, 5]. Here, too, the diagnosis is made by target biopsy [1].

Endoscopy alone can define the degree and, combined with directed biopsy and retrograde cholangio-pancreatography, it can frequently also establish an etiologic diagnosis of duodenal stenosis.

References

1. DEMLING, L., CLASSEN, M., KOCH, H.: Endoscopy in the diagnosis of duodenal tumors. Vortr. 9. Int. Kongr. Gastroent. Asnemge, Paris, 1972.
2. DREILING, D.A., JANOWITZ, H.D., PERRIER, C.V.: Pancreatic inflammatory diseases. New York, Evanston, London: Harper & Row 1964.
3. FRANTZ, V.K.: Tumors of the pancreas. Arm. Forces Inst. Path. Washington DC., 1959.
4. MOULINIER, B., BRUHIERE, J., GRENIER-BOLCY, PH.: La fibroscopie dans les tumeurs bénignes

du duodenum. Arch. Mal. App. dig. **61**, 333 (1972).
5. VAN DAMME, J.: Tumours malignes du duodenum. Arch. Mal. App. dig. **61**, 339 (1972).

2.5.4 **Diverticula** (Figs. 21–23)

Congenital diverticula, which may contain heterotopic pancreatic tissue, are rare. Acquired diverticula predominate by far and their prevalence increases with age. They are found mainly along the concave, inner margin of the duodenum, particularly near the papilla of Vater, the inferior horizontal portion of the duodenum and at the duodeno-jejunal junction. Their diameter varies between a few millimeters and 10 cm and they occur singly or in groups. Diverticula near the papilla of Vater occasionally pull its orifice towards them so that bile and pancreatic juice empty directly into the diverticulum. In addition, the papilla itself may be located within the diverticulum. Intubation for retrograde visualization of pancreatic and bile ducts is extremely difficult or impossible in this situation.

Duodenal diverticula rarely are of clinical significance. Often they play the role of the "diagnostic scapegoat" [1] in patients with unexplained epigastric distress. Complications of duodenal diverticula, such as bleeding, ulceration, perforation and torsion are extremely rare. This also applies to the occurrence of ascending cholangitis in association with a diverticulum near the ampulla of Vater.

Endoscopically, the diverticular orifice is easily recognized by mucosal folds converging towards it. Recognition of small diverticula may require pharmacologic inhibition of duodenal motility and air insufflation. The diverticular pouch and its contents can be inspected when the communication with the duodenal lumen is sufficiently wide.

Biopsies for the diagnosis of diverticulitis and the presence of heterotopic tissue require strict indications. Although no complications have yet been reported, one should keep in mind that the wall of acquired diverticula is devoid of a muscular layer and may, therefore, be perforated with ease. It appears possible to sample diverticular contents under sterile conditions. This may lead to a better understanding of the role played by intestinal diverticula in the blind-loop syndrome.

References

1. HOEFFKEN, W.: Krankheiten des Magens und Duodenums. In: Klinische Röntgendiagnostik innerer Krankheiten (HAUBRICH, R., Hrsg.), 2. Bd.: Abdomen. Berlin-Heidelberg-New York: Springer 1966.

2.5.5 Duodenal Tumors and Heterotopias

Heterotopias

Duodenal "polyps" may harbor heterotopic gastric mucosa. BELBER observed such a solitary tumor in the duodenal bulb endoscopically [2]. We found gastric mucosa in several tiny bulbar polyps observed in one patient [1]. A possible connection between this finding and duodenal ulcer disease is being discussed since ectopic gastric mucosa is found in about one-half of duodenal ulcer patients [5]. The significance of this observation remains to be established.

Heterotopic Pancreatic Tissue may also cause polypoid projections of the duodenal mucosa. Bleeding ulcers of the overlying duodenal mucosa as well as mistaken diagnoses of duodenal carcinoma have been reported. Endoscopic experience with these lesions still is small.

Endoscopy of benign duodenal tumors is incomplete without target biopsy. Only the biopsy can conclusively establish histologic type, potential to act as bleeding site (e.g., leiomyoma) and malignant degeneration.

Benign Tumors (Figs. 24–34)

The prevalence of benign tumors of the small intestine is 0.16 percent [1, 6]: most of these occur in the ileum. Only 198 of 1399 such tumors were located in the duodenum [8]: 92 were adenomas, 35 lipomas, 32 myomas, and 12 fibromyomas. Hemangiomas, lymphangiomas, neurogenic tumors, etc. were each represented between one and ten times.

Exact information on the rate of malignant degeneration of primary benign duodenal tumors is not available. It is estimated that 7 percent of adenomatous polyps and 20 percent of leiomyomas become malignant [6]. Furthermore, it is not clear whether malignant polyps may also arise *de novo*.

According to MACHELLA [6], about 50 percent of duodenal adenomas arise from Brunner's glands. They appear as round polypoid defects radiologically. The usual endoscopic appearance is that of multiple sessile polyps [7]; biopsies show Brunner's gland structure underlying a partially rarified epithelial layer.

The Peutz-Jeghers syndrome (perioral, labial and buccal pigmentations, small intestinal polyposis, hereditary) is a rare cause of small intestinal polyposis. Malignant degeneration of these polyps has been reported. We have removed several duodenal polyps with the high frequency diathermy snare in two patients and decreased thereby the risk of intestinal obstruction by these large polyps which already had lead to several laparotomies in both patients.

The Cronkhite-Canada syndrome (ectodermal pigmentation, loss of finger and toe nails, gastrointestinal polyposis) is an even rarer condition. The histologic appearance is that of inflammatory polyposis with mucus-filled retention cysts. The potential for malignant degeneration appears extremely small.

References

1. ABU-HAYDAR, F.R.: Cit in T.E. MACHELLA [6].
2. BELBER, J.P., MUSIEK, R.: Ectopic gastric mucosa in the duodenum. Gastroenterology (abstr.) **58**, 1063 (1970).
3. CLASSEN, M.: Contribution of endoscopy to the diagnosis and management of benign peptic ulcer. In: Clinics in Gastroenterology (SIRCUS, W., Ed.). London: Saunders 1973.
4. DEMLING, L., CLASSEN, M., KOCH, H.: Endoscopy in the diagnosis of duodenal tumors. Vortr. 9. Int. Kongr. Gastr. ASNEMGE, Paris 1972.
5. JOHANNSEN, A.: Benign tumours of the duodenum composed of heterotopic gastric mucosa. Vortr. 2. Europ. Kongr. Dig. Endoskopie, Paris 1972.
6. MACHELLA, T.E.: Tumors of the small intestine. In: Gastroenterology, Bd. II (BOCKUS, H., Ed.). Philadelphia, London: Saunders 1966.
7. MOULINIER, B., BRUHIERE, J., GRENIER-BOLEY, PH.: La fibroscopie dans le tumeurs benignes du duodenum. Arch. Mal. Appar. dig. **61**, 333 (1972).
8. RIVER, L., SILVERSTEIN, J., TOPI, J. W.: Benign neoplasms of the small intestine a critical comprehensive review with reports of 20 new cases. Int. Abstr. Surg. **102**, 1 (1956).

Malignant Tumors (Figs. 35–37)

Only about 3 percent of all gastrointestinal malignancies occur in the small intestine. The prevalence of carcinoma decreases from duodenum to ileum; the reverse is true for sarcomas [2]. In a large autopsy series, the incidence of malignant duodenal tumors was 0.033 percent [1].

Carcinoma is the most frequent duodenal malignancy. The clinical manifestations are determined by its location and type (stenosing, ulcerating, or penetrating). Bile-stained vomiting occurs only with stenosing carcinomas located distal to the papilla of Vater. Bleeding is not rare. Peripapillary tumors result in intermittent obstructive jaundice, similar to choledocholithiasis.

Most carcinomas found in the duodenum arise in adjacent organs (pancreas, bile ducts, right kidney), infiltrating the duodenal wall. Endoscopy contributes to the differential diagnosis not only by inspection and biopsy but also by retrograde visualization of the pancreatic and bile ducts. Usually the endoscopist has to be content with the statement that a carcinoma is present in the duodenum. The answer to the question whether primary or secondary is found at autopsy, if ever.

The endoscopic appearance of duodenal carcinoma is characterized by atypical, convoluted folds which may narrow the lumen and ulcerate. Alternately, the tumor may exhibit a polypoid growth pattern or present as a simple ulcer [3, 4]. In two of our four patients with duodenal carcinoma, the entire duodenal bulb was covered by rigid fold formations which were superficially ulcerated.

These cases of bulbar carcinoma illustrate that one should not rely on the rule of thumb that tumors proximal to the papilla of Vater are benign. The target biopsy settles the diagnosis.

Cytologic examination of duodenal irrigation fluid or of material obtained with a brush may also be of help in tumor diagnosis [4].

Duodenal sarcomas, lymphoblastomas, and melanomas are even rarer. We have verified two duodenal lymphoblastomas by endoscopic biopsy.

The *carcinoid tumor* is usually located in the ileum but in 1.5 percent of cases it occurs in the duodenum [2].

References

1. Hoeffken, W.: Krankheiten des Magens und Duodenums. In: Klinische Röntgendiagnostik innerer Krankheiten (Haubrich, R., Ed.). 2. Bd.: Abdomen. Berlin-Heidelberg-New York: Springer 1966.
2. Kümmerle, F., J. Schier: Dünndarmtumoren. In: Klinische Gastroenterologic (Demling, L., Hrsg.). Stuttgart: Thieme 1973.
3. Oi, J., Nakayama, K.: A case of primary duodenal cancer diagnosed by duodenoscopy and scopic biopsy: Endoscopy **2**, 134 (1970).
4. Takagi, K., Ikeda, S., Nakagawa, Y., *et al.*: Retrograde pancreatography and cholangiography by fiberduodenoscope. Gastroenterology **59**, 445 (1970).

Antral Mucosa in the Afferent Loop Following Billroth II Resection (Figs. 38, 39)

The rate of recurrent ulceration following Billroth II-resection varies between 0.5 and 5 percent [1]. A frequent cause is retained antral mucosa at the proximal end of the afferent loop. This situation can be diagnosed by directed duodenoscopic biopsy, leading to properly planned surgical intervention [2].

References

1. Demling, L., Ottenjann, R., Elster, K.: Endoskopie der Speiseröhre und des Magens. Stuttgart: Schattauer 1972.
2. Pohl, W., Flachsenberg, E., Elster, K.: Endoscopic-bioptical diagnosis of antral mucosa within the duodenal stumps. Endoscopy **4**, 162 (1972).

2.6 Endoscopy of the Papilla of Vater (Major Papilla) (Figs. 40–55)

2.6.1 Anatomy

The papilla of Vater is located in the middle-third of the descending duodenum in 54 percent of cases [3]. Location in the duodenal bulb or the stomach is very rare. Aborad variants towards the inferior duodenal flexure or even to the duodeno-jejunal junction occur in 4.8 percent, according to Hess [8]. In 50 patients, we found the papilla in the distal third of the descending duodenum in 30 percent and in the proximal third in 16 percent [3].

Endoscopic Aspects

Endoscopically, the papilla of Vater may assume three different shapes [11, 13, 14]. The hemispheric type with a surface of onion skin-like layers; the papillary type which is prominent also but the surface appearance is irregular instead of showing concentric folds; the flat type hardly protrudes from the mucosal surface and is more difficult to find and intubate. The appearance of the orifice of the papilla of Vater is variable also. Slit-like and round openings of different sizes are observed. Identification of the orifice is facilitated by the presence of slender concentric folds which are paler than the surrounding mucosa. According to Kozus, an occasionally observed valvular protrusion which becomes visible during emptying of the ampulla does not represent a septum between the orifices of the common bile and the pancreatic duct. Two or more orifices may be observed on the same papilla. Independent orifices of the common bile and the major pancreatic duct are present when two adjacent papillae are found. The area surrounding the ampulla of Vater has a characteristic appearance. A bulging circular fold, the plica duodenalis major, overlies the papilla from above. Occasionally it covers the papilla completely and has to be pushed back with the biopsy forceps or a probe in order to reveal the orifice. An inconstant longitudinal fold (plica longitudinalis) approaches for 2 to 3 cm from above and continues below (aborad) the papilla where it may bifurcate. The intramural portion of the common bile duct courses toward the papilla from above and causes a protrusion of the duodenal wall into the lumen which can sometimes be easily recognized.

The experienced endoscopist recognizes the papilla of Vater without delay on the basis of the typical features just described.

Minor Papilla

The minor papilla with the orifice of the ductus Santorini (minor pancreatic duct) is located a few centimeters proximal (orad) to the papilla of Vater. Very rarely is it encountered distal (aborad) to the major papilla. The existence of a minor papilla does not necessarily mean that a ductus Santorini, indeed, exists [8].

Endoscopically, the minor papilla appears as a cone-shaped structure. The orifice is recognized—if at all—as a tiny white or reddish fleck on the tip of the cone. We succeeded in filling the entire pancreatic duct system via the minor papilla and the ductus Santorini in three cases. In patients where the two anlagen of the pancreas fail to merge during embryologic development (pancreas divisum), the duct of the dorsal anlage continues to be the major duct and ends in the papilla minor [5]. Retrograde pancreatography cannot differentiate with certainty between a separate duct system (ductus divisus) and a pancreas divisum.

The Ampulla of Vater

The common bile and the major pancreatic duct merge in a common ampulla before combined entry into the duodenum in about 75 percent of cases. The ampulla is 3–10 mm long [1] and its diameter may reach 7 mm. There are numerous variations in the manner by which these two ducts enter the duodenum [8, 10, 12]. BECKER distinguishes three major types [2]. Other classifications are those of STERLING and of COUINAUD [16, 4].

The tubular ampulla possesses a distinct system of crypts (classification according to ELIAS). In our opinion, the variable arrangement of the orifices of both duct systems and the crypt pattern of the ampulla are the main reasons for the occasional failure of retrograde cannulation, especially of the common bile duct. The ampulla is surrounded by the sphincter of Oddi which is composed of an ampullary part, the choledochal and the pancreatic duct sphincter. The main protective function of this sphincter lies in the prevention of duodeno-biliary and duodeno-pancreatic reflux.

2.6.2 The Abnormal Papilla of Vater (Figs. 56–65)

Stenosing Papillitis

HESS distinguishes a primary form of stenosing papillitis, without involvement of neighboring organs, from a secondary form [8, 9]. The latter accounts for more than 90 percent of the cases and is associated mainly with calculous disease of the biliary tract. He reported stenosing papillitis to be present in more than one-fourth of 1220 patients with cholecysto- and/or choledocholithiasis [8]. HESS' classification is somewhat controversial because it is not yet clear whether so-called secondary papillitis is cause or consequence of biliary tract calculi. Stenosing papillitis may certainly occur primarily and then initiate a sequence of events which leads to chronic pancreatitis or to ascending cholangitis and eventually, secondary biliary cirrhosis.

The spectrum of the histologic correlate reaches from edema with polymorphonuclear infiltration to fibrosis; the mucoid crypts may be cystically dilated.

Adenomyomatosis of the papilla is characterized by hyperplasia of the mucoid crypts and of the sphincter of Oddi [7]. These changes occur mainly in the elderly and are reminiscent of prostatic "hypertrophy".

Papillitis may involve the entire sphincter of Oddi resulting in a hair-thin, Y-shaped appearance of the terminal portions of the common and main pancreatic duct. Alternately, the choledochal or the pancreatic duct sphincter may be affected singly. Isolated involvement of the ampullary portion of the sphincter results in dilatation of the ampulla, the "hydroampulla" of HESS.

Acute papillitis is recognized endoscopically by edematous swelling and reddening of the papilla. The orifice may be unrecognizable unless Indocyanin Green is injected intravenously [14]. Overall, the macroscopic findings of papillitis are neither constant nor diagnostically reliable. Target biopsies reveal the changes discussed above within the mucosa. It must be kept in mind, however, that the information derived from biopsies is restricted to the ampullary part of the sphincter. Only endoscopic probing of the ampulla and retrograde instillation of contrast medium can demonstrate stenoses and dilatation of ampulla, pancreatic and/or common bile duct. The problems with this endoscopic-radiologic approach are that intubation may be impossible in the presence of ampullary stenosis and that stenosis of the choledochal or pancreatic duct sphincter may preclude filling of the respective duct. No agreement has yet been reached as to the extent to which the mucosal biopsy of the papilla surface is representative of inflammatory changes in sphincter muscle, ampullary mucosa and prepapillary portions of the pancreatic and common bile ducts. FOEDISCH denies such a correlation [7].

Concrements in the Papilla

Gallstones are much more frequently impacted in the suprapapillary portion of the choledochus than in the ampulla itself. They may grow very large and become immobilized by scar formation. In more than 40 percent of cases they also cause obstruction to flow through the main pancreatic duct [8]. A gallstone impacted within the ampullary orifice leads to the formation of a "hydroampulla". Gallstones within the papilla may also float back into the common bile duct or may cause stenosing papillitis. The resulting endoscopic appearance is that of a coarsely enlarged papilla which may display a gaping orifice. In cases where contrast medium instillation is successful, one finds delayed emptying and prestenotic dilatation in either of the two ducts, depending on size and localization of the gallstone. The presence of one or multiple small stones, however, does not necessarily impair flow through the pancreatic and common bile duct. Numerous radiographic films must be taken, especially during the emptying phase, because small stones are easily overlooked when ampulla and ducts are distended with contrast medium. Serial films with a 70 or 100 mm camera have proved useful.

Prolapse of the Papilla of Vater

We have never observed endoscopically the "prolapse" of the papilla of Vater described by the radiologist in the presence of stenosing papillitis and carcinoma of the papilla. Perhaps this finding simply represents enlargement of the papilla caused by these diseases.

A similar appearance may result from the prolapse of a polyp through the papillary orifice with resulting obstruction to the flow of bile and pancreatic juice.

Carcinoma of the Papilla of Vater

The prognosis of this tumor is relatively favorable due to its slow growth and its tendency to metastasize late. According to HESS, it accounts for about 5 percent of all tumors of the gastrointestinal tract. The radio of carcinoma of the pancreas to that of the ampulla is 3:2 [8]; 80 percent are adenocarcinomas and 20 percent are scirrhous carcinomas. Clinical manifestations include dyspeptic complaints, weight loss, occult or manifest gastrointestinal bleeding, the symptoms of cholangitis, cholecystitis or pancreatitis and, in the initial phases, intermittent jaundice.

The endoscopist sees polypoid tumor formations replacing the papilla which may be ulcerated. Even within extensive tumor formations, an orifice may be visible which can be intubated for retrograde instillation of contrast medium. This observation is consistent with the clinical experience that obstructive jaundice occurs after the appearance of pain, weight loss and fever in three-fourths of the patients. The diagnosis is established by histologic examination of biopsies obtained under direct vision. In cases where the tumor involves the head of the pancreas, the primary site cannot be determined with certainty, despite all diagnostic maneuvers. Other malignant tumors of the papilla of Vater, e.g., sarcomas, are extremely rare and have not yet been observed endoscopically.

References

1. ANACKER, H.: Erkrankungen der Leber und des Gallenwegssystems. In: Klinische Röntgendiagnostik innerer Krankheiten (HAUBRICH, R., Ed.). 2. Bd. Berlin-Heidelberg-New York: Springer 1966.
2. BECKER, V.: Pankreas (Inselapparat ausgenommen). Spezielle pathologische Anatomie, 6. Bd. Berlin-Heidelberg-New York: Springer 1973.
3. CLASSEN, M., HELLWIG, H., RÖSCH, W.: Anatomy of the pancreatic duct. A duodenoscopic-radiological study. Endoscopy **5**, 14 (1973.)
4. COUINAUD, CL.: Anatomie de l'abdomen. Paris: G. Doin & Cie. 1963.
Fiberduodenoscopic observation on the dy-
5. DOERR, W.: Spezielle pathol. Anatomie II. Heidelberger Taschenbücher, 70. Bd., Teil A. Berlin-Heidelberg-New York: Springer 1970.
6. ELIAS, H.: Die Gallenwege. Ed. C.H. Boehringer Sohn. Ingelheim 1967.
7. FÖDISCH, H.: Feingewebliche Studien zur Orthologie und Pathologie der Papilla Vateri. Stuttgart: Thieme 1972.
8. HESS, W.: Die Erkrankungen der Gallenwege und des Pankreas. Stuttgart: Thieme 1961.
9. HESS, W.: Die chronische Pankreatitis. Bern. Stuttgart: Huber 1969.
10. HOLLE, G.: Die Bauprinzipien der Vaterschen Papille und ihre funktionelle Bedeutung unter normalen und krankhaften Bedingungen. Dtsch. med. Wschr. **85**, 644 (1960).
11. KOZU, T., OI, I., SUZUKI, S., TAKEMOTO, T.: Fiberduodenoscopic observation on the dynamics of the duodenal papilla. Endoscopy **2**, 99 (1970).
12. MILLBOURN, E.: On the excretory ducts of the pancreas in man, with special reference to their relations to each other, to the common duct and to the duodenum. Acta anat. (Basel) **9**, 1 (1950).
13. OGOSHI, K., TAKITA, Y., HARA, Y.: Endoscopic observation of the duodenum and pancreatocholedochography using duodenal fiberscope under direct vision. Gastroent. Endoscopy (Tokyo) **12**, 83 (1970.
14. OI, I., TAKEMOTO, T., KONDO, T.: Fiberduodenose: Direct observation of the papilla of Vater. Endoscopy **2**, 101 (1969).
15. SAFRANY, L., BARNA, L., TÖRÖK, I.: Differential diagnosis of cholostatic jaundice by fiberduodenoscopic retrograde cholangiography, Vortr. 2. Europ. Kongr. Dig. Endoskopie. Paris 1972.
16. STERLING, J.A.: The common channel for bile and pancreatic ducts. Surg. Gynec. Obstet. **98**, 420 (1954).

2.7 Retrograde Cholangiography

Normal Cholangiogram (Fig. 66)

Retrograde cholangiography has a success rate of 60–75 percent [5–7, 15]. Reasons for the relatively high failure rate include the variability of the papillary architecture and of the course of the terminal portions of both duct systems, as well as pathologic alterations of the papilla itself.

The normal roentgenographic pattern of the intra- and extrahepatic bile ducts is well described in the literature on intravenous and transhepatic cholangiography [1, 2, 19, 20].

While we use Conray 60 as contrast medium for retrograde cholangiography, our British colleagues recommend less concentrated media in order not to obscure small gallstones [3, 6].

2.7.1 Bile Duct Stones

Gallstone disease is very common. In Central Europe, 10–15 percent of all adults are so afflicted [8, 11], causing death in about 15 percent of these [11]. According to HESS, 26 percent of patients with cholecystolithiasis will develop choledocholithiasis [11].

The endoscopic-radiologic procedure is indicated mainly in those situations where the diagnosis cannot be established by standard radiologic examinations. This occurs most often in the presence of hepatic excretory insufficiency and of gallstones located in the common hepatic or bile duct. The procedure frequently can provide the surgeon with the important information whether gallstone disease is limited to the gallbladder or whether it involves the common bile duct. In addition, retrograde cholangiography is able to detect concrements in the intrahepatic bile ducts which occur in 27 percent of patients with choledocholithiasis [13]. Primary intrahepatic concrements, usually found at the bifurcation of the common hepatic duct, can also be demonstrated with this duodenoscopic-radiologic procedure.

Retrograde cholangiography is perferred over percutaneous transhepatic and laparoscopic cholangiography after gallbladder puncture because it is less traumatic [14]. The exact localization of pathologic alterations occasionally requires the use of two procedures [5]. Retrograde visualization should, however, always precede the two other methods [3, 5, 6].

The indications for retrograde cholangiography should be broadened because more than one-third of common duct stones cause no typical symptoms and a further one-sixth do not reveal themselves by abnormal biochemical or radiologic tests. HESS is correct in stating that a common duct stone is the more dangerous the fewer symptoms it causes and the longer it remains undiagnosed and untreated [11].

During retrograde cholangiography, stones in the bile ducts are frequently seen only after partial emptying of the contrast medium into the duodenum. The differential diagnosis includes air bubbles trapped in the contrast medium, bile duct tumors, and external compression (carcinoma of the head of the pancreas).

Occasionally it is possible to displace an ampullary concrement toward the liver by forceful injection of contrast medium, resulting in preoperative alleviation of jaundice [5].

2.7.2 Inflammation of the Biliary Tract (Figs. 74, 75)

Cholecystitis

In patients with acute cholecystitis the gallbladder does not fill during retrograde cholangiography, presumably due to swelling of the cystic duct. The common bile duct may be moderately dilated in the absence of demonstrable stenoses or concrements.

The extrahepatic bile ducts visualize well in patients with chronic cholecystitis. The wall of the shrunken gallbladder occasionally is impregnated with calcium (porcelain gallbladder). Retrograde cholangiography for cholecystitis is indicated only in those cases where routine radiologic methods fail due to the simultaneous presence of hepatocellular disease or extrahepatic obstruction.

Cholangitis

Cholangitis is accompanied by gallstone disease in 70 percent of cases; in 10 percent it is caused by stenosing papillitis [2]. Radiologic findings include concrements, narrowing of the lumen and deviations or acute angulations of the choledochus due to involvement of adjacent organs by the inflammatory process. One should, however, remember that deep inspiration may produce transient angulation of the common bile duct. The most reliable clues to the existence of established cholangitis are diffuse alterations in duct caliber which are especially pronounced with primary sclerosing cholangitis. Mucoviscidosis creates a similar appearance. Retrograde cholangiography demonstrates these changes more clearly than intravenous cholangiography.

2.7.3 Tumors of Gallbladder and Bile Ducts (Figs. 77–79)

Papillomas and Adenomas of the Gallbladder rarely cause symptoms and usually represent incidental radiologic findings.

Carcinoma of the Gallbladder is one of the rarer tumors.

In ILLINGWORTH's autopsy series, it was present in 0.42 percent of cases, accounting for 2.8 percent of all malignancies [12]. Gallstones and chronic cholecystitis exist in 80 percent of cases [9].

The tumor metastasizes by the hematogenous route, along the common bile duct into the liver by lymphangitic spread, and by direct extension into neighboring organs, occasionally with fistula formation.

The mechanism of obstructive jaundice which may be due to duct compression by tumor or by lymph node metastases is clarified by the combined endoscopic-radiologic approach. The differential diagnosis includes primary carcinoma of the bile ducts and of the head of the pancreas. Only 73 cases of benign tumors of the extrahepatic bile ducts were described until 1962 [11]. They include papillomas, adenomas, fibromas and postoperative neuromas. The clinical symptomatology consists of cholangitis and obstructive jaundice.

Our Japanese colleagues diagnosed a papilloma of the choledochus prolapsing through the papilla of Vater by duodenoscopic biopsy [10].

Carcinoma of the Bile Ducts occurs mainly in males, in contrast to carcinoma of the gallbladder. Both tumors are either squamous, scirrhous, or adenocarcinoma, with the latter form predominating.

Tumor location and growth pattern determine the clinical picture. Involvement of one of the hepatic ducts interferes with drainage of the corresponding hepatic lobe, while tumors at the hepatic duct junction and distal to that point may cause complete biliary obstruction. Clinical key findings are jaundice (typically intermittent) and hydrops or empyema of the gallbladder. A schematic presentation by EDMONDSON illustrates the location of malignant tumors of the bile duct system as detected in 50,000 autopsies [9].

It is sometimes impossible to instill contrast medium beyond the tumor stenosis during retrograde cholangiography. Spot films reveal only an irregular narrowing. In these cases, the endoscopic approach is complemented by percutaneous transhepatic cholangiography or instillation of contrast medium into the gallbladder during laparoscopy. When retrograde instillation is successful, the contrast medium outlines the exophytic tumor growth in the presence of prestenotic dilatation. Cytology might become a further aid in the diagnosis of these tumors.

The differential diagnosis should include benign tumors of the bile ducts, concrements and, in the presence of narrowing of the intrapancreatic portion of the common bile duct, infiltrating carcinoma of the pancreas. The exact preoperative diagnosis usually is only of academic interest since the clinical presentation of obstructive jaundice mandates surgical intervention in any case. Unnecessary operations in high-risk patients are avoided by the demonstration of hepatic metastases by liver scan, ultrasound, or during laparoscopy. SHERLOCK discussed the difficulties in differentiating between primary biliary cirrhosis and carcinoma of the hepatic duct junction, especially in cases where the tumor has a smooth surface and causes only partial obstruction

[17]. We found such changes of the hepatic ducts in a patient carrying a diagnosis of primary biliary cirrhosis for two years. The correct diagnosis of hepatic duct carcinoma was established only at laparoscopy.

While retrograde cholangiography does not yield a precise diagnosis in all cases of obstructive jaundice, it does contribute to assessment of the indications for surgical intervention. Preoperative localization of the level of obstruction is of additional help in the planning of the operation.

2.7.4 Sequelae of Operations on the Biliary Tract (Figs. 80–86)

Postcholecystectomy Syndrome

Among the organic causes of symptoms following cholecystectomy are residual gallstones, biliary tract strictures, incomplete removal of gallbladder and cystic duct and chronic pancreatitis. In most cases, the term "postcholecystectomy syndrome" is used to designate so-called biliary dyskinesias as well as persisting symptoms unrelated to the biliary tract for which surgery had been performed unnecessarily.

Organic causes of the postcholecystectomy syndrome are convincingly demonstrated during retrograde visualization of the biliary tract. Cystic duct remnants, with or without calculi and/or infection, residual gallstones and strictures are recognized without difficulty. We pay particular attention to the papilla of Vater, especially after transduodenal probing of the common bile duct during the original surgical procedure. This may result in papillary stenosis and retention of the contrast medium in the bile ducts for more than 60 minutes.

Biliary-Enteric Anastomoses

Perforation by gallstones may lead to spontaneous fistulization between the biliary tract and the small intestine. Most fistulas are created deliberately in order to bypass an obstruction to bile flow which defies surgical correction.

These anastomoses consist mainly of side-to-side or, occasionally, end-to-side connections of the choledochus with the duodenal bulb, the descending duodenum or the jejunum. Cholecystoenteric anastomoses are avoided because of the increased risk of postoperative cholangitis.

Duodenal anastomoses with the biliary tract are easily identified and probed during endoscopy. Instillation of contrast medium for visualization of the bile ducts succeeds without difficulty. Our group was able to demonstrate the advantages of this method over the usual radiographic procedures [4]. It allowed the demonstration of residual stones and of stricture of the anastomotic opening as the cause of postoperative distress in many patients.

Food rests accumulated in the retroduodenal pouch formed by the terminal choledochus in one of our patients with a wide side-to-side choledochoduodenostomy. This pouch could be inspected through the anastomosis and was visualized radiologically after installation of contrast medium.

In another patient it was possible to remove the retained arm of a T-tube from the distal common bile duct by a combination of irrigation and forceps extraction. The piece was withdrawn into the stomach from where it was allowed to pass down the intestinal tract [5].

The value of the endoscopic-radiologic approach to biliary-enteric anastomoses rests on the fact that the area is examined by two different methods which complement each other. The cause of symptoms and objective abnormalities can thus be established and the indications for relaparatomy are made more precise.

2.7.5 Diseases of the Liver (Fig. 76)

Retrograde cholangiography is able to contribute to the evaluation of those hepatic diseases which are accompanied by changes in the bile ducts. Acute infectious hepatitis does not represent an indication for duodenoscopy since OI was unable to demonstrate any abnormalities by this method. Although transmission of infectious hepatitis by the duodenoscope has not yet been reported, this possibility has to be considered seriously. As a precautionary measure, we do not perform duodenoscopy in patients with HAA-(Australia antigen) positive hepatitis.

Hepatic Abscess

To our knowledge, retrograde cholangiography has not yet been performed in the presence of a hepatic abscess. We would avoid retrograde cholangiography when an abscess is suspected for the same reasons that contraindicate this procedure in the presence of all febrile infections of the biliary tree (see chapter on complications).

Hepatic Cysts

Nonparasitic hepatic cysts are caused by abnormal development of the intrahepatic ducts. Other probable causes of intrahepatic cysts are localized occlusion of intrahepatic bile ducts, congenital ectasia of hepatic lymphatics and of mucoid glands of the bile ducts, and trauma.

Only those cysts which communicate with the bile ducts or the digestive tract can be demonstrated by retrograde cholangiography. No actual experience has yet been gained with this method.

Hepatic Tumors

Carcinomas of the Liver are divided into malignant hepatomas and malignant cholangiomas (bile duct carcinomas) according to their tissue of origin. Experience with these tumors, as well as with benign hepatic tumors and hepatic metastases, during retrograde cholangiography is still meager. Figures 87–89 demonstrate a malignant cholangioma presenting as a large cystic tumor in the left hepatic lobe which was resected. The tumor cavity had previously been anastomosed with the duodenum. This anastomosis enabled us to perform duodenoscopic biopsy of the lesion and to define it by instillation of contrast material.

References

1. ADOLPH, K.: Gallengangs- und Pankreasdiagnostik. Stuttgart: Enke 1968.
2. ANACKER, H.: Erkrankungen der Leber und der Gallenwege. In: Klinische Röntgendiagnostik Innerer Krankheiten (HAUBRICH, R., Ed.). New York: Springer 1966.
3. BLUMBART, L.H., COTTON, P.B., BURWOOD, R., LAWRIE, B., SALMON, P., DAVIES, G.T., BEATES, J.S.M., SKIRVING, A.: Endoscopy and retrograde choledochopancreatography in the diagnosis of the jaundiced patient. Lancet **2**, 7790 (1972).
4. CLASSEN, M., FRÜHMORGEN, P., KOZU, T., DEMLING, L.: Endoscopic-radiologic demonstration of biliodigestive fistulas. Endoscopy **3**, 138–142 (1971).
5. CLASSEN, M., DEMLING, L.: Retrograde Cholangiographie beim Verschlußikterus. Radiologe **13**, 35 (1973).
6. COTTON, P.B.: Endoscopy and cannulation of the papilla of Vater and retrograde cholangiopancreatography (ERCP). Gut **13**, 1014 (1972).
7. DEYHLE, P., FUMAGALLI, J., PAEZ, C., JENNY, S., PRETER, B., JENNY, M., AMMANN, R.: Klinischer Wert der endoskopisch-retrograden Pankreato-Cholangiographie. Dtsch. med. Wschr. **97**, 1139 (1972).
8. DOERR, W.: Spezielle pathologische Anatomie II. Heidelberger Taschenbücher, 70. Bd., Teil A. Berlin-Heidelberg-New York: Springer 1970.
9. EDMONDSON, H.A.: Tumors of the gallbladder and extrahepatic bile ducts. Armed. Forces Inst. Path. Washington, D.C. 1967.
10. HARA, Y.: Personal communication.
11. HESS, W.: Die Erkrankungen der Gallenwege und des Pankreas. Stuttgart: Thieme 1961.
12. ILLINGWORTH, C.F.: Carcinoma of the gallbladder. Brit. J. Surg. **23**, 4 (1935).
13. NORMAN, O.: Studies on the hepatic ducts in cholangiography. Acta radiol. scand. (Suppl.) 84, (1951).
14. OGOSHI, K., NURA, M., HARA, Y., NEBEL, O.T.: Endoscopic pancreatocholangiography in the evaluation of pancreatic and biliary disease. Gastroenterology **64**, 210 (1973).
15. OI, I.: Duodenoscopy during pancreatic diseases. Arch. Mal. Appar. dig. **61**, 349 (1972).
16. SALMON, P.: Endoscopy in the diagnosis of obstructive jaundice. In: Endoscopy of the small Intestine (DEMLING, L., CLASSEN, M., Eds.). Stuttgart: Thieme 1973.
17. SHERLOCK, S.: Diseases of the liver and the

biliary system, 4. ed. Oxford: Blackwell 1968.
18. VENNES, J.A., SILAVIS, S.E.: Endoscopic visualization of bile and pancreatic ducts. Gastroint. Endosc. **18**, 149 (1972).
19. WANNAGAT, L.: Laparoskopische Cholezysto- und trans-hepatische Cholangiographie. In: Klinische Gastroenterologie (DEMLING, L., ed.). Stuttgart: Thieme 1972.
20. WENZ, W., KOLIG, G.: Fehler und Gefahren der perkutanen transhepatischen Cholangiographie. Röntgenfortschritte **103**, 713 (1963).

2.8 Retrograde Pancreatography

2.8.1 Anatomy and Topography of the Pancreas (Figs. 90–92)

The pancreas is situated retroperitoneally and courses diagonally from the descending duodenum cephalad and to the left towards the splenic hilus. The body of the pancreas measures 1.5–4.5 cm, average 3.3 cm in the craniad-caudad direction; the ventrodorsal diameter is 2–3 cm [2, 3, 36]. The choledochus is either located dorsal to the head of the pancreas or traverses it.

The body of the pancreas lies dorsal to the stomach; its caudal limit borders on the duodeno-jejunal junction. The tail of the pancreas courses ventrally past the upper pole of the left kidney toward the hilus of the spleen; it is in close proximity to the splenic flexure of the colon and to the diaphragm.

The main pancreatic duct (Wirsung) is oriented in the longitudinal axis of the organ. It shows a steep, craniad ascent within the head of the pancreas. The angle of ascend decreases gradually at about the midline as the duct continues toward the tail of the pancreas. This cranio-convex curve may be missing, in which case Wirsung's duct ascends continuously from the papilla of Vater to the spleen. A second variant is the "inverted U" course of the main pancreatic duct: it ascends normally within the head of the pancreas, then follows a horizontal course for a short distance, only to descend back to the level of the papilla.

The diameter of the main pancreatic duct measures 3.4–4.8 mm in the head, 2.9–3.4 mm in the body and 2.0–2.3 mm in the tail of the pancreas. The smaller values were obtained in Japan [20] while the higher diameters were obtained by us [9]. According to our measurements the length of Wirsung's duct, which gives an estimate of the length of the entire pancreas, is normally about 20 cm. This value may well represent an underestimate to the extent that parts of the pancreas are not aligned at a right angle to the X-ray beam. The minor pancreatic duct (Santorini) drains the dorsal pancreas anlage. It is joined by the Ramus capitis inferior within the head of the pancreas which drains the caudally situated uncinate process. COTTON found an accessory papilla (papilla minor) in 24 percent of his patients [10]. This papilla may exist in the absence of a minor pancreatic duct.

Fifteen to thirty first order ducts branch off from the major pancreatic duct; each of these is supplied by several second order ducts which, in turn, branch into third order canaliculi.

Contradictory information exists about the anatomic location and number of the orifices of the common bile, major and minor pancreatic ducts (see chapter on papilla of Vater). According to ANACKER, the common bile and major pancreatic ducts enter the duodenum jointly with formation of a single ampulla in 80 to 90 percent of cases. Their orifices are separate in less than 5 percent of cases; even rarer is the existence of separate openings of each of the three ducts [2].

Emptying of Contrast Media from the Pancreatic Ducts

Abnormalities of the pancreatic duct system appear to be reflected not only by variations in caliber but also by the time interval needed for emptying of retrogradely instilled contrast medium. In collaboration with WORMUTH, we found that the normal emptying time is less than ten minutes. This interval was invariably exceeded in the presence of chronic pancreatitis and of pseudocysts [44].

2.8.2 Congenital Abnormalities of the Pancreas (Figs. 54, 55, 93–95)

The *Annular Pancreas* results from failure of the ventral pancreas anlage to rotate during embryologic development. As a result, the pancreas surrounds the duodenum completely or incompletely and may cause jaundice and duodenal obstruction at any age. An increased incidence of pancreatitis with this condition has not been documented [24].

The Pancreas Divisum, resulting from partial or total failure of both pancreas anlagen to fuse, has already been discussed on page 28.

Pancreatic Cysts probably represent small ducts without communication with the rest of the duct system. DOERR and BECKER consider the cause to be abnormal composition of pancreatic secretions with formation of intraductal plugs leading to retention behind obstructed ducts [4, 12]. In any event, these cysts represent developmental abnormalities; they may be single or multiple and their size varies greatly. They are lined by epithelium and are, therefore, true cysts in contrast to the pseudocysts. We have no experience with the appearance of these cysts on the retrograde pancreatogram.

The alterations caused by *Pancreatic Pseudocysts* are discussed on page 37. We cannot yet define the clinical significance of multiple, pea-sized pancreatic cysts found in several of our older patients without symptoms of pancreatic disease. It remains to be seen whether these cysts represent the same lesion as is frequently found at postmortem pancreatography in older persons without manifest pancreatic disease [1, 41].

We observed the pancreatic duct changes of *Cystic Fibrosis* (mucoviscidosis) in a ten year-old patient. They consisted of variations in caliber without obvious cystic dilatations. The contrast medium was retained abnormally long within the pancreas. The intrahepatic duct system, by contrast, did show cystic changes.

2.8.3 Pancreatitis (Figs. 96–117)

During a symposium in Marseille, France, in 1963 an attempt was made to arrive at a uniform nomenclature of pancreatic inflammatory diseases. A clinical classification was decided upon without regard to etiology:

1. Acute pancreatitis;
2. Acute recurrent pancreatitis;
3. Chronic recurrent pancreatitis;
4. Chronic-progressive pancreatitis.

A number of other classification systems exist but will not be mentioned further [4, 5, 9, 12, 28, 33, 40].

Indications and Findings

Retrograde pancreatography should be attempted during the symptomfree interval of *Acute Recurrent Pancreatitis* in order to identify changes of the papilla of Vater or of the pancreatic ducts (stenoses, concrements) [15, 38]. LEGER and LATASTE, as well as DOUBILET, MULHOLLAND and POPPEL reported that inflamed areas of the parenchyma can be recognized by the patchy escape of contrast medium from the ducts during operative pancreatography [13, 22, 23]. This claim does not appear to be sufficiently supported.

It should be remembered that operative pancreatography is usually carried out without fluoroscopic observation. The amount of contrast medium needed for complete filling of the duct system can, therefore, not be determined precisely. When this amount is exceeded, focal—not diffuse—staining of the parenchyma by contrast medium occurs in one or another part of the pancreas. This phenomenon is observed in patients with and without a history of pancreatitis. However, we cannot disprove this claim directly since we consider acute pancreatitis to be a contraindication for ERCP.

Pseudocysts in communication with the

duct system are demonstrated directly by retrograde pancreatography, as mentioned previously. Pseudocysts without patent communication and inflammatory masses may compress the pancreatic ducts and lead to discontinuity in the column of contrast material. Pseudocysts which begin to fill during retrograde instillation of contrast medium should definitely not be filled completely. Proof of existence and exact localization are sufficient. The danger of producing bacterial infection of the pseudocyst should not be underestimated (see chapter on complications).

Duodenoscopy in the presence of *Chronic Pancreatitis* at present serves mainly for the radiologic demonstration of the duct system. In the near future, however, it will be possible to combine this procedure with manometric measurements of the papilla and the pancreatic ducts. It is conceivable that knowledge of the regulation of ampullary contraction and of pancreatic secretory pressures will yield a better understanding of pancreatic pathophysiology. Further diagnostic advances may come from the cytologic study of pancreatic secretion aspirated through the papilla [21, 43], from transduodenal pancreatic needle biopsy [6] and from laparoscopic observation of the pancreas [26, 32]. We will restrict this discussion to retrograde pancreatography which should be considered a routine diagnostic method. The diagnostic yield is higher than that of operative pancreatography mainly because more advanced radiologic equipment (TV-monitoring with spotfilm of abnormal areas; roentgen cinematography; serial films with a high-speed camera) can be employed. Operative pancreatography is, therefore, essential only in cases where descending visualization of the duct system is required as accomplished by needle puncture of the distal duct or after resection of the pancreatic tail. Further, it is indicated in cases where duodenoscopic intubation was unsuccessful.

The statement by Hess that operative pancreatography yields reliable information about changes affecting the main pancreatic duct [18] and that it is valuable in designing the appropriate operative approach can be applied as well to the endoscopic-radiologic method under discussion. It is questionable, however, whether the duct abnormalities so identified allow conclusions to be drawn about their pathogenesis.

Pathologic alterations of the pancreatic duct system were demonstrated in all our 64 patients with chronic pancreatitis. Marked variations in caliber or multiple strictures with prestenotic dilatation were seen in 73 percent, an appearance properly termed a "chain of lakes" or "string of pearls" [3, 18]. Dilatation of the duct system involves mainly the primary and secondary branches; the main pancreatic duct appears to become involved later in the course of the disease. Both, papillary stenosis and calcifications, were present in 19 patients; in seven cases there was an abrupt stop of the column of contrast medium. A patient with a Billroth II gastric resection showed a very small but otherwise normal appearing duct system. This may have represented a pancreas divisum with additional inflammatory or degenerative changes causing excretory insufficiency.

We do not attempt to fill the pancreatic acini, even when pancreatic carcinoma is suspected. Preliminary experience indicate that retrograde pancreatography does not contribute to the diagnosis of pancreatic malignancies beyond the demonstration of changes affecting the excretory ducts.

Stenoses and kinks of the retro- or intrapancreatic portion of the common bile duct occurring with chronic pancreatitis are a domain of retrograde cholangiography [7, 8]. The long tubular stenosis associated with chronic pancreatitis begins at the point where the choledochus reaches the dorsal aspect of the pancreas and ends at the papilla. One may also find short strictures at the craniad (superior) border of the pancreas with normal diameter of the terminal choledochus, as well as a ring-like stenosis of the intrapancreatic part of the choledochus which may be an early stage of tubular stenosis according to HESS [18].

Retrograde cholangiography yielded abnormal findings in 28 of 64 (48 percent) of our patients with chronic pancreatitis. Papillary stenosis was present in ten cases, stenosis of the intrapancreatic or retroduodenal parts of the choledochus in thirteen, and gallstones in five. Abnormalities of the biliary tree were identified in twelve additional patients by intravenous cholangiography or at operation; these included three patients with gallstones and nine with common bile duct stenosis. Twenty-four of our patients with chronic pancreatitis have not yet been operated upon. It is conceivable that further biliary tract pathology will be found at the time of surgery. In summary, we can state that at least 40 of our 64 patients (62 percent) with chronic pancreatitis had proven abnormalities of the biliary tract. This fact supports our claim that retrograde cholangiography should be performed on all patients with pancreatitis.

Based on our present experience, chronic pancreatitis may be accompanied by the following changes of the pancreatic ducts:

1. Papillary stenosis with dilatation of the entire pancreatic and, occasionally, biliary duct system.

2. Stenoses of the main pancreatic duct with abrupt stop of the column of contrast medium.

3a. Caliber variations resembling a baroque column, caused by a serpentine course of the pancreatic duct.

3b. Multiple strictures with marked prestenotic dilatation of the pancreatic duct.

4. Calcifications (intraductal with alcoholic pancreatitis [27]).

5. Pseudocysts.

Numerous other workers have either accepted this system of classification or assess these criteria similarly [10, 11, 20, 25, 30, 34, 35, 37, 39, 42].

A few criteria previously considered typical of chronic pancreatitis [18] had to be revised during the evaluation of retrograde pancreatograms:

1. Filling of first, second and third order ducts with contrast medium is normal, provided their course and caliber is regular.

2. The same applies to "reflux into the parenchyma" which can be induced during every pancreatography.

The incidence of a normal duct system in the presence of chronic pancreatitis is not known.

2.8.4 Tumors of the Pancreas
(Figs. 118–126)

Benign Tumors (adenomas, cystadenomas, fibromas, myxomas, etc.) are rare. The changes observed during retrograde pancreatography consist of duct displacement and obstruction of the pancreatic and/or common bile duct. Hamartomas of the pancreas cause similar abnormalities according to STADELMANN [37].

The early diagnosis of *Carcinoma of the Pancreas* is one of the most important indications for endoscopic-radiologic pancreatography. Routine roentgenologic methods usually detect only advanced stages of this tumor [38].

We have performed duodenoscopy in 21 patients with histologically verified carcinoma of the pancreas. The carcinoma originated from the head of the pancreas in 19 patients, and from the body and tail in one each. With tumors in the head of the pancreas, the following abnormalities of the choledochus were detected: complete stenosis in four, tubular stenosis in three, and circumscribed stenosis or external compression in three. One of these patients already had undergone a choledochoduodenostomy. Retrograde cholangiography was technically unsuccessful in eight patients with carcinoma of the head of the pancreas. Retrograde pancreatography was not accomplished in nine, which was due to technical reasons in three (T-tube in the papilla; duodenal stenosis; etc). Among the remaining twelve patients, four had normal appearing pancreatic duct systems and only one exhibited diffuse dilatation of the main duct in the body and tail of the pancreas. The single carcinoma of the tail of the pancreas was palpable through the abdominal wall. Retrograde pancreatography, performed four months prior to autopsy, showed changes limited to an irregular outline of the pancreatic duct in the tail region. At autopsy, the pancreatic duct was grossly infiltrated by tumor, sparing only the portion within the head of the pancreas.

The radiologic findings of the pancreatic and common bile duct in the presence of carcinoma of the pancreas can be summarized as follows:

1. Irregular contours;
2. External compression;
3. Stenoses with prestenotic dilatation;
4. Abrupt stoppage of the column of contrast medium;
5. Displacement;
6. Alterations of the parenchymal structure observed during pancreatography.

The frayed outline of the pancreatic duct represents an important diagnostic clue. Stenoses with prestenotic dilatation and interruptions of the contrast column cannot be differentiated with certainty from alterations caused by chronic pancreatitis, cysts, and inflammatory masses. More reliable criteria for differential diagnosis will have to be derived from examination of a large number of patients. The difficulties in differential diagnosis are further compounded by the presence of histologically verified pancreatitis which coexists with pancreatic carcinoma in at least 10 percent of cases [14]. In view of the small number of patients examined to date it appears too early to establish a classification of pancreatic duct changes due to carcinoma of that organ [17, 28].

When in doubt, the entire diagnostic repertoire (arteriography, splenoportography, ultrasound study, isotope scanning, etc.) needs to be employed for tumor diagnosis. The diagnostic usefulness of ancillary procedures during duodenoscopy, such as cytologic examination of secretions aspirated from the ampulla or the pancreatic duct and transduodenal needle biopsy of the pancreas, cannot be evaluated as yet. Initial reports suggest that laparoscopic inspection and palpation of the pancreas may be of value in the diagnosis of cancer [26, 32]. The diagnosis of cancer of the pancreas continues to be established only after the tumor has become inoperable; this was true in 20 of our 21 patients. The challenge lies in detecting this tumor before it causes obvious clinical symptoms.

Oi described irregular contours, dilatations, compression and necrotic cavities of pancreatic ducts and parenchyma in patients with sarcomas of the pancreas [31].

Islet Cell Tumors cause external compression or occlusion only when of sufficient size and when located near a pancreatic duct. One of our patients with the Zollinger-Ellison syndrome had a normal retrograde pancreatogram. Safrany was able to localize the tumor by retrograde pancreatography in a patient with this syndrome [34].

References

1. Adlung, J., Gürich, H., Ritter, U.: Über Veränderungen am Pankreasgangsystem. Med. Welt. (Stuttg.) **20**, 387 (1969).
2. Anacker, H.: Krankheiten des Pankreas. In: Klinische Röntgendiagnostik Innerer Krankheiten (Haubrich, H., Ed.), Bd. II. Berlin-Heidelberg-New York: Springer 1966.
3. Anacker, H.: Die pathologischen Veränderungen des Pankreasgangsystems im Röntgenbild. Röntgenfortschr. **96** (1962).
4. Becker, V.: Pankreas (Inselapparat ausgenommen). Spezielle pathologische Anatomie, 6. Bd. Berlin-Heidelberg-New York: Springer 1972.
5. Becker, V.: Pathogenese und pathologische Anatomie der chronischen Pankreatitis. Schweiz. med. Wschr. **100**, 1194 (1970).
6. Classen, M., Koch, H., Frühmorgen, P., Grabner, W., Demling, L.: Results of retrograde pancreaticography. Acta gastroent. jap. **7**, 131 (1972).
7. Classen, M., Demling, L.: Duodenoskopie und retrograde Cholangio-Pankreatikographie in der klinischen Routine. Vortr. Bad Mergentheimer Stoffw. Tagg. 1972 (Boecker, W., Ed.). Stuttgart: Thieme 1973.
8. Classen, M., Demling, L.: Retrograde Cholangiographie beim Verschlußikterus. Radiologe, **13**, 35 (1973).

9. CLASSEN, M., HELLWIG, H., RÖSCH, W.: Anatomy of the pancreatic duct. A endoscopic-radiologic study. Endoscopy, **5**, 14 (1973).
10. COTTON, P.B.: Endoscopy and cannulation of the papilla of Vater; retrograde cholangiopancreatography (ERCP). Gut **13**, 1014 (1972).
11. DEYHLE, P., FUMAGALLI, J., PAEZ, C., JENNY, S., PRETER, B., JENNY, M., AMMANN, R.: Klinischer Wert der endoskopisch-retrograden Pankreato-Cholangiographie. Dtsch. med. Wschr. **97**, 1139 (1972).
12. DOERR, W.: Spezielle pathologische Anatomie. II. Heidelberger Taschenbücher, 70. Bd., Teil A. Berlin-Heidelberg-New York: Springer, 1970.
13. DOUBILET, H., POPPEL, M., MULHOLLAND, J.: Pancreatography. Radiology **64**, 325 (1955).
14. GAMBILL, E.E.: Pancreatitis associated with pancreatic carcinoma: A study of 26 cases. Proc. Mayo Clin. **46**, 174 (1971).
15. GULBIS, A., CREMER, M., ENGELHOLM, L., PEETERS, J.P., DUMONT, N.: La Cholangio-Wirsungography retrograde. Vortr. 2. Europ. Kongr. Dig. Endoskopie, Paris 1972.
16. GÜLZOW, M.: Zur Einteilung der Pankreatitiden. Dtsch. Z. Verdau.- u. Stoffwechselkr. **26**, 3 (1966).
17. HARA, Y.: Personal communication.
18. HESS, W.: Die chronische Pankreatitis. Bern, Stuttgart: Huber 1969.
19. HEULLY, F., GAUCHER, P., LAURENT, J., JEANPIERRE, R., VICARI, F., BAS, M., PONSARD, D., WATRIN, B.: Valeur de la Wirsungographie per — duodenoscopique dans le diagnostic des neoformations pancreatiques. Vortr. 2. Europ. Kongr. Dig. Endoskopie, Paris 1972.
20. KASUGAI, T., KUNO, N., KIZU, M., KOBAYASHI, S., HATTORI, K.: Endoscopic pancreatocholangiography I and II. The endoscopic pancreatocholangiogram. Gastroenterology **63**, 227 (1972).
21. KOZU, T., OI, I., TAKEMOTO, T.: The cytology of the intrapancreatic juice taken by duodenoscopic cannulation into the duodenal papilla. 2. Europ. Kongr. Dig. Endoskopie, Paris 1972.
22. LATASTE, J., NEVEUX, R.: L'intervention chirurgicale précoce dans les pancréatitis aigues. Presse méd. **74**, 1875 (1966).
23. LEGER, H., LEGER, L., CACHIN, M., FUMERY, J., HECTOR, A.: L'exploration radio-chirurgical des faux kistes du pancréas. Presse méd. **94**, 2136 (1957).
24. LEHMANN, E.D.: Annular pancreas as a clinical problem. Ann. Surg. **115**, 572 (1942).
25. LIGUORY, C.: Personal Communication
26. MEYER-BURG, J.: The inspection, palpation and biopsy of the pancreas by peritoncoscopy. Endoscopy **4**, 99 (1972).
27. NAKAMURA, K., SARLES, H., PAYAN, H.: Three dimensional reconstruction of the pancreatic ducts in chronic pancreatitis. Gastroenterology **62**, 942 (1972).
28. OGOSHI, K., TAKITA, Y., HARA, Y.: Endoscopic observation of the duodenum and pancreatocholangiogram using duodenofiberscope under direct vision. Gastroent. Endoscopy **12**, 83 (1970).
29. OGOSHI, K., HARA, Y.: Retrograde pancreatocholangiography. Japan. J. clin. Radiol. **17**, 455 (1972).
30. OI, I.: Fiberduodenoscopy and endoscopic pancreatocholangiography. Gastroent. Endoscopy **17**, 59 (1970).
31. OI, I.: Duodenoscopy during pancreatic diseases. Arch. Mal. Appar. dig. **61**, 349 (1972).
32. OTTENJANN, R.: Personal Communication.
33. RITTER, U.: Erkrankungen des exkretotischen Pankreas. Stuttgart: Thieme 1971.
34. SAFRANY, L.: Endoscopy and retrograde Cholangio-Pancreatography after Billroth II operation. Endoscopy **4**, 198 (1972).
35. SALMON, P.: Personal Communication.
36. SCHOLZE, H.: Die Pankreatitis. Stuttgart: Enke, 1972.
37. STADELMANN, O., DEYHLE, P., HÜGEL, H., LÖFFLER, A., MIEDERER, S.E., FUMAGALLI, J.: Endoscopic pancreaticography in the diagnosis of tumours. In: Endoscopy of the small intestine (DEMLING, L., CLASSEN, M., Eds.) Stuttgart: Thieme 1973.
38. VASILENKO, V. CH., VASILJEV, J.V.: Duodenoscopy in diagnosis of tumors of the duodenopancreatic area. Vortr. 2. Europ. Kongr. Dig. Endoskopie, Paris 1972.
39. VENNES, J.A., SILVIS, S.E.: Endoscopic visualization of bile and pancreatic ducts. Gastroint. Endoscopy **18**, 149 (1972).
40. WANKE, M.: Experimentelle Pankreatitis, proteolytische und biliäre Form. Stuttgart: Thieme 1968.
41. WATER, J., WEILL, J., BUCHSER, M., WEILL-BUSSONI, M.: Postmortale Angiographie. Arch. Mal. Appar. dig. **54**, 1219 (1965).
42. WIESNER, W., WEISS, H.D., ANACKER, H.: Erste Erfahrungen mit der duodenoskopischen retrograden Pankreatikographie in der Diagnostik der chronischen Pankreatitis. Dtsch. Med. Wschr. **97**, 991 (1972).
43. WITTE, S., RIEGG, H.: Cytologic findings in the bile after endoscopic cannulation of the papilla of Vater. In: Endoscopy of the small intestine (DEMLING, L., CLASSEN, M., Eds.). Stuttgart: Thieme 1973.
44. WORMUTH, J., CLASSEN, M.: Unpublished observations.

2.9 **Complications** (Figs. 127–130)

Complications During Insertion of the Instrument

The danger of endoscopic perforation exists in the presence of duodenal stenosis. The actual perforation risk of duodenoscopy is, however, very small indeed. None has occurred during 2,500 esophago-gastro-bulboscopies and 700 duodenoscopies performed during the past three years. Only a total of two endoscopic perforations of the duodenum have been reported so far.

PALME *et al.*, described small intestinal volvolus, which they attributed to air insufflation, after duodenoscopy in a patient who had undergone prior intestinal surgery [9].

Cholangiopancreatography (ERCP)

Submucosal deposition of contrast material occurs occasionally next to the papilla when the catheter has not completely passed through the papillary orifice. These deposits disappear completely within an hour and are harmless according to our experience and that of OI.

The older catheters used for contrast medium instillation had a metal tip which occasionally was left behind within the papilla, fortunately never within the ducts themselves. These detached tips were passed spontaneously. Currently manufactured catheters no longer have metal tips.

Rupture of the pancreatic duct by a far advanced catheter led to formation of a transient pseudocyst in one case [5] and to extravasation of contrast medium into the omentum in another [11].

The clinical significance of the frequently observed rise in serum amylase after retrograde pancreatography has not yet been completely evaluated [7]. It is certain that this phenomenon is related to the degree of filling and possibly to the presence of preexisting pancreatic disease. We have documented that filling of the acini (parenchymography) is followed by a significantly higher complication rate (acute pancreatitis) then filling limited to the duct system [10] (Table 5). Earlier observations that pancreatitis occured even in about 8% of those patients without parenchymography were possibly related to the use of an inadequate X-ray machine. There is general agreement that clinically relevant pancreatitis occurs after about 2 percent of retrograde pancreatographies (ERP). Pseudocysts of the pancreas represent a real danger: ERP may be followed by bacteremia and sepsis. DEYHLE observed a patient with a pseudocyst who developed fatal pancreatic necrosis after ERP [4]. We lost a patient due to the same complication.

Table 5. Complications of ERP

	Uncomplicated	Hyperamylasemia only	Clinical Symptoms	Total
Acini filled	30	34	23	87
Acini not filled	156	32	26	214
Total	186	66	49	301

The incidence of fever, cholangitis and sepsis following ERCP is 1–2 percent in different centers. Cholangitis after retrograde cholangiography occurs mainly in patients with impaired bile flow due to strictures, stones or tumors, This complication may develop as late as 36 hours after the procedure; the patients should, therefore, be observed carefully for this period of time. For this reason, we believe that ERCP should not be done on out-patients. It is not yet completely clear whether the catheter inoculates bacteriae into the bile ducts or whether existing biliary tract infection is activated and spread by the instillation of contrast material. Prophylactic administration of broad-spectrum antibiotics has been recommended in order to prevent this complication [3, 6]. We believe that the risks of this measure outweigh its advantages. Antibiotic therapy limited to patients in whom retrograde cholangiography revealed biliary tract obstruction appears to be more reasonable. We recommend immediate surgical correction of the obstructing lesion in addition to antibiotic therapy in cases where retrograde cholangiography is followed by fever. This also applies to pancreatic pseudocysts. We have not lost a patient since institution of this policy.

Transmission of viral hepatitis by fiberscopes has not yet been reported. This possibility must, however, be considered especially since effective instrument sterilization is not yet possible. We support, therefore, COTTON's recommendation not to perform fiberendoscopy in icteric patients with a positive Australia antigen (HAA) test [1, 2].

Macroscopic damage to the papilla by the instillation catheter is slight. Minor bleeding is seen occasionally. OI considers severe bleeding from the papilla as a clue to the presence of a carcinoma of the bile ducts or of the pancreas [8]. As long as long-term follow-up observations are not available, we recommend against the widespread use of papillary biopsy, especially from the orifice of the papilla. In addition, there are no studies on the effect of different contrast media and of the injection pressure. Careful roentgenologic studies and serial tests of pancreatic function are required in patients who have undergone retrograde pancreatography in order to demonstrate the safety of this procedure conclusively.

References

1. COTTON, P.B., SALMON, P.R., BLUMGART, L.H., BURWOOD, R.J., DAVIES, G.T., LAWRIE, B.W., PIERCE, J.W., READ, A.E.: Cannulation of papilla of Vater via fiber-duodenoscope. Lancet **1972I**, 53.
2. COTTON, P.B.: Endoscopy and cannulation of the papilla of Vater; retrograde cholangiopancreatography. Gut **13**, 1014 (1972).
3. CREMER, M.: Personal communication.
4. DEYHLE, P., FUMAGALLI, J., PAEZ, C., JENNY, S., PRETER, B., JENNY, M., AMMANN, R.: Klinischer Wert der endoskopischen retrograden Pankreato-Cholangiographie. Dtsch. med. Wschr. **97**, 1139 (1972).
5. GAUCHER, P., *et al.*: Analyse critique des aspects radiologiques fournis par la Wirsungographie et la cholangiographie per — duodenoscopique chez les malades atteints de pancreatitic chronique. Vortr. 2. Europ. Kongr. Dig. Endoskopie, Paris 1972.
6. GULBIS, A., CREMER, M., ENGELHOLM, L., PEETERS, J.P., DUMONT, N.: La Cholangio-Wirsungographie retrograde. Vortr. 2. Europ. Kongr. Dig. Endoskopie, Paris 1972.
7. OGOSHI, K., HARA, Y.: Retrograde pancreatocholangiography. Japan. J. clin. Radiol. **17**, 455 (1972).
8. OI, I.: Duodenoscopy during pancreatic diseases. Arch. Mal. Appar. dig. **61**, 349 (1972).
9. PALME, G., MEYER-BURG, J., DRESSLER, S.: Volvuluskomplikation im Gefolge einer Duodenoskopie. Endoscopy **4**, 49 (1972).
10. RUPPIN, H., CLASSEN, M.: Unpublished observations.
11. STADELMANN, O., *et al.*: The efficiency of duodenoscopy in the clinical diagnostic procedure. Vortr. 2. Europ. Kongr. Dig. Endoskopie, Paris 1972.

3. Jejuno-Ileoscopy

The term "enteron" refers to the entire alimentary canal. The designation "enteroscopy" as suggested by CLASSEN should, however, be restricted to endoscopy of jejunum and ileum and exclude duodeno- and coloscopy. This definition appears useful and has found wide acceptance. OI and TAKEMOTO, the pioneers of duodenoscopy, were the first to attempt peroral jejunoscopy with long instruments. Shortly thereafter, our group reached the terminal ileum and the anus with an enteroscope. The optical properties of the instruments at our disposal were excellent from the very beginning. This enabled us to inspect the entire alimentary tract with exception of the flexure regions [3]. OGOSHI and HARA [9] and YANAGATA's group [14] also began to develop peroral enteroscopy at about the same time.

3.1 Indications

Enteroscopy is indicated when inflammation or tumor of jejunum and ileum are suspected.

3.2 Technique and Results

Forward viewing instruments are usually employed. Depending on the indication and the clinical situation, the enteroscope is introduced into the small intestine via the rectum or perorally. A high degree of instrument flexibility is a prerequisite for safe passage of the small intestine. This property, on the other hand, interferes with the introduction of the instrument by either route [9]. This has led to the use of stiffening wires in an attempt to reduce the length of the endoscope coiled in stomach or sigmoid colon. This expedient has, indeed, allowed the introduction of the enteroscope to one meter beyond the ligament of Treitz and a 30 percent success rate in intubation of the terminal ileum via the rectum [6]. Distal jejunum and proximal ileum cannot yet be reached in this fashion.

Another possibility is the method of transintestinal intubation developed by BLANKENHORN [2] which TORSOLI *et al.* [11, 13], OI and HIRATSUKA [7, 8, 10] and we [3–5] have employed for various endoscopic procedures. Two to five days prior to the examination, the patient swallows a teflon tube with a leading rubber ballon filled with mercury or lead shot. After the tube has passed the anus, it is used for introduction of the instrument. The end-to-end connection between endoscope and transintestinal tube is not without dangers since the tube has to be tied to the outer rim of the endoscope tip. This results in imperfect alignment of the endoscope when pulled aborad by the transintestinal tube. We have discontinued this procedure after witnessing an intestinal perforation. Following a suggestion by PAOLUZZI [11] and by HIRATSUKA [7], we now employ the "monorail" or "ropeway" method. The transintestinal tube is used as a guide by pulling it through the instrument channel of the enteroscope. This procedure has proved to be of value

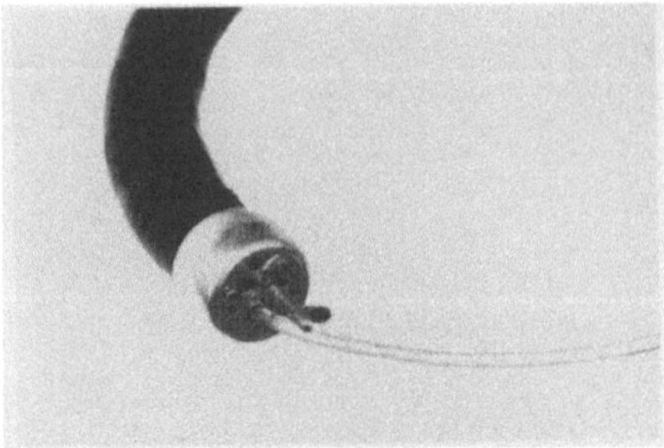

Fig. XX. Tip of the two-channel enteroscope; Olympus (prototype)

in terms of level of intubation and diagnostic yield. The method was refined further by the addition of a second instrumentation channel to the existing Olympus enteroscope (Fig. XX) which allows biopsies to be taken with the transintestinal tube in place. We are now able to advance this instrument to the terminal ileum in 5–15 minutes, provided no organic stenoses are present. Peroral coloscopy during the same sitting has little practical vaulue because the instrument length of two meters would cause too much foreshortening (accordion-pleating) of the entire intestinal tract. Our current procedure for complete enteroscopy, for instance in cases of occult bleeding, is as follows: the enteroscope is guided to the terminal ileum over the transintestinal tube; the entire small intestine is then inspected carefully during withdrawal of the fiberscope; finally, the transintestinal tube is used as a guide for complete coloscopy. The latter step has the advantage that the coloscope quickly reaches the cecum and that it is nearly always possible to enter the terminal ileum. Inspection of the terminal ileum should always be carried out with the coloscope because the ileocecal valve cannot be identified with certainty by the peroral approach.

Level of Intubation

Figure XXI illustrates the level of small intestinal intubation according to the different methods. The ileum is usually reached after

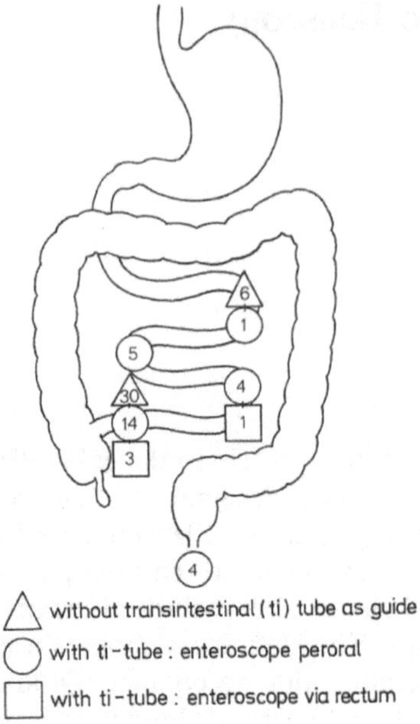

Fig. XXI. Level of intubation with the enteroscope in the small intestine

passage of a transintestinal tube. We consider peroral inspection of the ileum to be complete only when the cecum or ascending colon were seen, indicating progression across the ileocecal valve. This criterion and the high incidence of Crohn's disease in our patient material are the reasons why the small intestine was not considered to have been "seen" completely during every examination.

3.3 Diagnostic Yield (Figs. 137–139)

Crohn's Disease

Additional skip lesions were identified or suspected lesions excluded in six of nine patients with Crohn's disease of the duodenum or colon. Diffuse jejuno-ileitis was detected in a patient with diarrhea and protein-losing enteropathy; biopsies revealed Crohn's disease. Two patients with ileocecal resection and with hemicolectomy, respectively, were shown to have X-ray-negative recurrences of Crohn's disease.

Tumors

Intestinal polyps were found in two patients with the Peutz-Jeghers syndrome. Duodenal polyps were ablated endoscopically with the diathermy snare and then retrieved in both patients. One of these already has undergone five laparotomies for obstructive ileus. These examples illustrate that enteroscopy can be of therapeutic value.

Bleeding Sites

A bleeding site could be identified in only three of twelve patients with occult gastrointestinal blood loss. Two of these were sigmoid polyps; one patient had hemangiomata in duodenum and jejunum. Admittedly, all three lesions were within reach of the duodenoscope or coloscope. These rather disappointing results may have been due to excessive delay between the last bleeding episode and enteroscopy. The two to three days required for passage of the transintestinal tube are a distinct disadvantage in this context.

3.4 Complications

At another clinic, transintestinal intubation caused paralytic ileus in a patient who eventually died despite surgical intervention. One of our patients developed incomplete ileus due to knotting of the transintestinal tube within the intestine; the tube was extracted without difficulties. We have caused a perforation of the terminal ileum during introduction of the enteroscope by the transintestinal tube. We believe that this complication was caused by a technical factor. The enteroscope was connected end-to-end with the transintestinal tube which was fixed to the external rim of the instrument tip. This may have caused the tip to deviate from the direction of traction. The problem can be avoided by threading the transintestinal tube through the instrument channel.

3.5 Summary

1. Enteroscopy is especially valuable for detection of localized intestinal inflammatory disease.
2. The value of enteroscopic inspection, biopsy and, possibly, removal of small intestinal tumors cannot be questioned. Of these, 62 percent of benign tumors, 51 percent of carcinomas, and 70 percent of sarcomas are located in the proximal and distal parts of the small intestine [1, 12].
3. The results to date have been obtained with prototype instruments which require a transintestinal tube for passage of the entire small bowel. This technique is not only uncomfortable for the patient but may interfere with the rapid diagnosis of bleeding sites.

References

1. Abu-Haydar, F.R.: Cit. in T.E. Machella: Tumors of the small intestine. In: Gastroenterology (Bockus, H., Ed.). Philadelphia, London: Saunders 1966.
2. Blankenhorn, D.H., Hirsch, J., Ahrens, E.H., Jr.: Transintestinal intubation: technic for measurement of gut length and physiologic sampling at known loci. Proc. Soc. exp. Biol. (N.Y.) **88**, 356 (1955).
3. Classen, M., Frühmorgen, P., Koch, H., Demling, L.: Enteroskopie: Fiberendoskopie von Jejunum und Ileum. Dtsch. med. Wschr. **97**, 409–411 (1972).
4. Classen, M., Frühmorgen, P., Koch, H., Demling, L.: Peroral enteroscopy. Paper pres. 14th Japan. Congr. Gastroint. Endoscopy, Tokyo 1972.
5. Classen, M., Frühmorgen, P., Koch, H., Demling, L.: Peroral and peranal endoscopy of the small bowel. In: Endoscopy of the small Intestine (Demling, L., Classen, M., Eds.). Stuttgart: Thieme 1973.
6. Deyhle, P., Jenny, S., Ammann, R., Siegenthaler, W.: Illeoskopie. Dtsch. med. Wschr. **97**, 1679 (1972).
7. Hiratsuka, H.: Fibercolonoscopy in the diagnostic intestinal string derivation. Method and clinical report on ileocoecal observation. 2nd World Congress of Gastroint. Endoscopy, Rome-Copenhagen 1970.
8. Hiratsuka, H.: Personal communication.
9. Ogoshi, K., Hara, Y.: A new fiberscope for

the small intestine. Paper pres. 14th Japan. Congr. Gastroint. Endoscopy, Tokyo 1972.
10. Oi, L., Hiratsuka, H., Takemoto, T.: Fiberjejunoscopy. Symposion Fiberjejunoscopy. New Fields of Gastroint. Endoscopy, Carlsbad 1971.
11. Paoluzzi, P.: Total colonoscopy by a "monorail" method. World Congress of Gastroint. Endoscopy. Rome-Copenhagen 1970.
12. River, L., Silverstein, J., Tobe, J. W.: Benign neoplasms of the small intestine, a critical comprohensive review of 20 new cases. Int. Abstr. Surg. **102**, 1 (1956).
13. Torsoli, A., Arullani, P., Casali, C.: An application of transintestinal intubation to the study of the colon. Gut **8**, 192 (1967).
14. Yamagata, S.: Personal communication.

4. Coloscopy

4.1 Historical Development

Until a few years ago, preoperative endoscopic inspection of the colon ended in the distal sigmoid. The anatomy of this organ limited further progress of the rigid sigmoidoscope. Clinical history and radiologic studies provided the only additional help in arriving at therapeutic decisions when surgical intervention was deemed unwarranted. The need for nonoperative inspection of the proximal colon could only be fulfilled with the arrival of suitable flexible fiberendoscopes on the market. The first fibercoloscope was developed in 1964 in Japan and initial experiences were reported at the First Congress of the International Society for Endoscopy in Tokyo in 1966. An instrumentation channel permits the removal of tissue particles for cytologic and histologic examination. This is an important addition to direct visual inspection and photography.

The first successful attempts at introduction of measuring devices, biopsy instruments and flexible endoscopes into the colon with the help of a transintestinal tube described by BLANKENHORN [2] were carried out in 1966 by MATSUNAGA [12], COLAGRANDE [3] and PROVENZALE [16]. The method was refined in 1967 by FOX [8], and TORSOLI *et al.* [1, 17] who reported their initial, successful coloscopies in Prague in 1968. Further improvements came from DEYHLE [7] and OTTENJANN [15] in 1969 and from NAGASAKO and collaborators in 1970 [13].

The mechanical characteristics of the fully flexible coloscopes presently available permit inspection of the entire colon and the terminal ileum [14] in a high percentage of cases without prior transintestinal intubation [4–6, 9–13, 18]. The indications for coloscopy have been extended beyond exclusively diagnostic considerations to include the removal of polyps for diagnostic, prophylactic or therapeutic reasons, foreign body removal, topical injections, and electrocoagulation of circumscribed bleeding sites.

References

1. ARULLANI, P., PAOLUZI, P., CAPURSO, L.: Endoscopy of the colon. Proc. 1st. Europ. Congr. Digestive Endoscopy. Praque 1968: Basel-New York: Karger 1969.
2. BLANKENHORN, D.H., HIRSCH, J., AHRENS, E.H. JR.: Transintestinal intubation: technic for measurement of gut length and physiologie sampling at known loci. Proc. Soc. exp. Biol. (N.Y.) **88**, 356 (1955).
3. COLAGRANDE, C., ARULLANI, P., CASALE, C.: A suction biopsy procedure for obtaining specimens of mucosa from the right and left colon. Amer. J. dig. Dis. **2**, 389 (1966).
4. DEMLING, L., FRÜHMORGEN, P.: Coloscopy-technique and clinical results. Vortrag V. Congreso Latino Americano de Proctologia, Mexico, Mai 1972.
5. DEYHLE, P.: Duodenoskopie-Koloskopie. Vortrag. EECO Symposion, München 1970.
6. DEYHLE, P., PAUL, F.: Die Endoskopie des proximalen Dickdarms. Therapiewoche **20**, 1803 (1970).
7. DEYHLE, P., OTTENJANN, R.: Zur transintestinalen Intubation. Vortr. 3. Kongreß der Deutschen Gesellschaft für Endoskopie, Erlangen 1969. In: Fortschritte der Endoskopie (OTTENJANN, R., Hrsg.), Bd. 1. Stuttgart-New York: Schattauer 1970.
8. FOX, J.A., KREEL, L.: Technique of retrograde colonic intubation and its initial application to high colonique biopsy. Gut **8**, 77 (1967).
9. FRÜHMORGEN, P., CLASSEN, M.: Enteroscopy (small intestine—large intestine). Acta Hepato-gastroenterologica. **1**, 1 (1974).

10. FRÜHMORGEN, P., ZEUS, J., CLASSEN, M.: Klinische Wertigkeit der Koloskopie. In: Fortschritte der gastroenterologischen Endoskopie, Bd. 4 (LINDNER, H., Ed.). Baden-Baden-Brüssel: Witzstrock 1973.
11. FRÜHMORGEN, P.: Vorbereitung und Technik der Koloskopie. Fortschr. Med., **5**, 190 (1974).
12. MATSUNAGA, F., TAJIMA, T.: Diagnosis of colon polyps and polyposis with Fibercolonscope. Vortr. Weltkongress Gastroenterologie, Kopenhagen 1970.
13. NAGASAKO, K., ENDO, M., TAKEMOTO, T., KONDO, T., KIMURA, K.: The insertion of fibercolonoscope into the cecum and direct observation of the ileocecal valve. Endoscopy **2**, 123 (1970).
14. NAGASAKO, K., YAZAWA, C., TAKEMOTO, T.: Observation of the terminal ileum. Endoscopy **1**, 45 (1971).
15. OTTENJANN, R., DEYHLE, P., PAUL, F., STADELMANN, O.: Die Sondierung des proximalen Colon. Endoscopy **1**, 70 (1969).
16. PROVENZALE, L., CAMERADA, P., REVIGNAS, A.: La coloscopia total transanale mediante una metodica originale. Rass. med. sarda **69**, 149 (1966).
17. TORSOLI, A., ARULLANI, P., PAOLUZI, P.: Transintestinal intubation as guidance method for colonic biopsy, endoscopy and intraluminal studies. In: Fortschritte der Endoskopie (OTTENJANN, R., Ed.), Bd. 1. Stuttgart-New York: Schattauer 1969.
18. WATANABE, H.: Fibercolonoscopy. Gastroenterologia Japonica **2**, 141 (1972).

4.2 Anatomy and Physiology

Successful high coloscopy and ileoscopy by the rectal route without assistance by a transintestinal tube requires knowledge of the topographic anatomy and technique of insertion and a high degree of mechanical perfection of the instrument.

Familiarity with the anatomy is a prerequisite for the procedure to be efficient and without complications. Wide variations in the course of the colon, especially the sigmoid (length of 15 to 110 cm), require different techniques of instrument insertion. Many types of transitions exist between the two extremes of the very short colon with high-lying cecum and a nearly straight sigmoid and the very long colon (dolichocolon) with low-lying cecum and tightly looped transverse colon and sigmoid. Accordingly, the total length of the colon differs greatly from patient to patient. BLANKENHORN [2] estimated its length to by 91–125 cm during transintestinal intubation. According to our experience, the limits are between 90 and 180 cm without straightening of the organ.

The intraperitoneal location of cecum, transverse colon and sigmoid with variable length of the mesocolon causes the wide variability of the colon's course but favors introduction of the instrument by making it possible to straighten out loop formations (Figs. 157, 159). Rectum and descending and ascending colon are, with rare exceptions, located retroperitoneally and therefore, immobile. Occasionally, the cecum may be retroperitoneal also (cecum fixum). Tenia, haustra (Fig.s 161, 236) and variations in luminal diameter (cecum: about 8.5 cm; sigmoid: about 2.5 cm according to BOCKUS [1]) help with orientation during progress of the coloscope through tight loops and flexures.

The orifice of the ileocecal valve (Bauhin's valve) is found at the medial aspect of the mid-cecum, about 8 cm craniad to the lower limit of the cecum; its appearance is variable (Figs. 158, 180, 181). Viewed from the cecum, the ileocecal junction resembles a mouth with semilunar lips (Fig. 180a). The proximal (craniad) extends about 1.5 cm over the distal (caudad) lip, frequently allowing only a trangiential view of the former. The ileocecal valve may appear flat (Fig. 180c) or may protrude far into the cecum, simulating a polypoid tumor (Fig. 180b). A prominent tentorial fold exists medially between cecum and ascending colon (Fig. 158) and can frequently be seen endoscopically; the ileocecal valve is situated under it. The appendiceal orifice can be inspected and intubated about 4–6 cm distal to the ileocecal valve, provided the colon is well prepared (Figs. 158, 185, 186).

The main functions of the normal colon are absorption of water and electrolytes, secretion of mucus and transport of undigested food residues. Propulsion of luminal contents occurs by local accordion-like, as well as by peristaltic contractions [3].

References

1. Bockus, H.L.: Gastroenterology, Vol. II. Philadelphia. London: Saunders 1964.
2. Blankenhorn, D.H., Hirsch, J., Ahrens, E.H. Jr.: Transintestinal intubation: technic for measurement of gut length and physiologic sampling at known loci. Proc. Soc. exp. Biol. & Med. (N.Y.) **88**, 356 (1955).
3. Tuelove, S.C.: Movements of the large intestine. Physiol. Rev. **46**, 455 (1964).

4.3 Indications

Coloscopy is technically demanding and requires considerable personnel time. It should, therefore, be employed only after the possibilities of simpler diagnostic measures have been exhausted; the indications need to be stated clearly (Table 6).

Absolute indications include questionable and nondiagnostic radiologic findings; abdominal symptoms (diarrhea, passage of blood, pus or mucus, tenesmus) not explained by other investigations; follow-up of conditions known to be premalignant and of patients operated for malignant colon tumors.

Patients with recurrent hemorrhages of the gastrointestinal tract should only be coloscoped after less demanding diagnostic methods have been employed, including endoscopy of the proximal portions of the alimentary canal.

Follow-up observations and evaluation of therapy results may be indicated with intrinsic colonic diseases and in connection with "operative" coloscopy (polypectomy, electrocoagulation).

Further indications for periodic coloscopic examinations are patients with known premalignant conditions in whom colectomy is not, or not yet, planned. This group includes familial polyposis, villous adenomas, the Gardner syndrome and, in our opinion, the Peutz-Jeghers syndrome. All patients with ulcerative colitis for more than ten years and with polyps greater than 10 mm in diameter should also be followed coloscopically, the latter after coloscopic polyp removal.

Table 6

Indications for coloscopy:
1. Questionable or unclear radiologic findings;
2. appropriate clinical signs or symptoms with negative barium enema;
3. preoperative histologic verification of the diagnosis;
4. prophylaxis (premalignant conditions; postoperative colon);
5. recurrent bleeding from the lower intestinal tract;
6. evaluation of course and results of therapy;
7. "operative" coloscopy.

4.4 Contraindications

There are absolute and relative contraindications (Table 7).

Table 7. Contraindications

I. Absolute contraindications:
1. Uncooperative patient
2. Florid colonic inflammation (fulminating ulcerative colitis, Crohn's colitis and diverticulitis)
3. Peritonitis

II. Relative contraindications:
1. Bleeding disorders (biopsies and polypectomy contraindicated)
2. Cardiac or pulmonary decompensation
3. Severe coronary artery disease

Coloscopy requires more patient cooperation and understanding of the procedure than any other endoscopic examination. Patients unwilling or unable to cooperate should, therefore, not be coloscoped. It is obvious that the presence of very active inflammatory disease of the colon or adjacent structures contraindicates coloscopy.

Bleeding disorders, cardiac and pulmonary decompensation and severe coronary artery disease are considered relative contraindications.

4.5 Baseline Studies

A thorough clinical history is especially important for directing attention to the eventual diagnosis and for the recognition of possible contraindications. The patient should be asked about bleeding episodes, abdominal pain, bowel habits and medication intake (laxatives, anticoagulants). Preceding anoscopy and proctoscopy are desirable because the distal rectum and anal canal frequently cannot be examined adequately with the fiberscope. In addition, this technically simple method will reveal abnormalities in rectum and distal sigmoid which may obviate the need for coloscopy. Double contrast barium enema preceding the coloscopy serves to identify those patients in whom the procedure is specifically indicated. Blood group and coagulation status (prothombin time, partial thromboplastin time, platelet count) should be determined routinely because the need for biopsy and polypectomy is not always apparent prior to coloscopy (Table 8).

Table 8. Studies preceding coloscopy

Clinical history
Rectoscopy, anoscopy
Barium enema (double contrast)
Blood group and coagulation status (for biopsies, polypectomies)

4.6 Patient Preparation

Coloscopy of a less than optimally cleansed colon is worthless since retained feces will obscure focal lesions and heavy staining cannot be washed off the lens. This is especially important when the purpose of the coloscopy is to rule out the presence of abnormalities. We also consider it necessary that the patient be fully informed about purpose and procedures of the examination since ignorance frightens and the direction of approach is potentially embarrassing.

The preparation of the colon differs for sigmoidoscopy and for high coloscopy. For the former, we give sweet tea during the preceding day and a cleansing enema of lukewarm water without added glycerol (smearing of the lens!) on the night before. Laxatives are not necessary.

We previously prepared patients for high coloscopy by a three to five day period of clear liquid diet and daily high cleansing enemas. The same good results are now achieved by a 24-hour preparation: on the day preceding the coloscopy, we give clear liquids, 125 ml of 25 percent magnesium sulfate in the morning and afternoon, and two high cleansing enemas of lukewarm water.

The frequently recommended zero-residue "elemental" diet (Vivonex) meets with poor acceptance, coats the colonic mucosa with dark, sticky material and is, furthermore, quite expensive.

Premedication is not required; rarely is an analgetic needed during the examination. Those few patients—about 10 percent—who experience unbearable discomfort receive meperidine (Demerol), 50–100 mg, intravenously.

4.7 Technique of Examination

4.7.1 Coloscopy

The procedure is best conducted with the patient in the supine position. Although coloscopy can be performed by a single examiner, the presence of an assistant has proved to be valuable. Assistance is required in any event for obtaining biopsies and for polypectomy.

While fluoroscopic control is rarely needed for fiberoptic sigmoidoscopy, it should be available for high coloscopy to monitor the straightening of loops by the coloscope and for occasional localization of the instrument tip. Straightening of the sigmoid should be attempted in all cases in order to improve the mobility of the instrument beyond the sigmoid. Without good mobility, "blind" areas will be encountered, especially within tight loops and flexures. The course of the sigmoid colon is determined by the fixation of the mesosigmoid and can be divided into two categories: the common eta- and the rare sigma-shape. Straightening maneuvers of the sigmoid are greatly facilitated by firm knowledge of these two shapes and their variations (Fig. 159).

The instrument tip is coated with olive oil and is introduced without speculum with the patient lying on his left side. Use of a speculum causes unnecessary discomfort at the start of the procedure, inducing a defensive attitude in the patient which makes the following coloscopy more difficult. The next steps depend entirely on the topographic and anatomic situation which varies widely from patient to patient. A uniform technique can neither be described nor recommended. Whenever possible, the coloscope should be advanced with the lumen in direct view (Fig. 161). Unfolding of the colonic lumen is achieved by air insufflation and turning of the patient. The volume of air insufflated should be kept as low as possible (danger of perforation with diseases affecting the colonic wall; abdominal distress) and the amount of air present in the colon should be minimized by alternating air insufflation with suction. The patient is turned from the left lateral to the supine position when the lumen can no longer be kept in view during further advancement of the instrument. Correct timing of this change in position depends on the course of the colon and is important for a successful examination. In patients with tightly looped sigmoids, the above maneuvers may still not bring the lumen into view. In these cases, the instrument may be advanced very carefully as long as the mucosa sliding by the lens maintains its reddish color and the normal vascular architecture remains visible (Fig. 162). The coloscope must, however, be withdrawn immediately by a few centimeters as soon as the mucosa turns pale red or whitish-yellow or when the patient complains of increasing pain. Another attempt at insertion is then made after the patient is rotated on the table and, if possible, the position of the tip has been verified by fluoroscopy.

The tightly looped sigmoid (Figs. 167–169), a serpentine transverse colon (Fig. 172a) or one descending towards the pelvis (Fig. 171) and acute flexures (Fig. 170c) in that order cause the greatest difficulties. A spiral- (Fig. 167a) or eta-shape (Fig. 166a) may require that the sigmoid be straightened before the instrument tip reaches the descending colon or the splenic flexure. Without straightening, one of the sigmoid loops may be pushed as far as the lower costal margin because the pressure exerted on the instrument handle is dissipated in the curves taken by the fiberscope and is not transmitted to the tip. Rotation of the coloscope by 180° to the right will change the eta-shape of the sigmoid into the alpha-shape (Fig. 170) which allows easier progress of the instrument. We have had good success with early straightening of the sigmoid when the tip is only in the distal part of the descending colon. In the absence of adhesions, the sigmoid is straightened without any rotation maneuvers, simply by withdrawing the coloscope a few centimeters (Fig. 166).

In most cases, however, the splenic flexure can be reached by continuous advancement of the instrument. The tip of the coloscope is then "hooked" in the transverse colon which is the optimal position for straightening of the sigmoid (Fig. 164b). The sigmoid should always be straightened at this stage for the following reasons: to spare the patient pain caused by traction on the mesosigmoid and to gain the instrument length needed for further advancement. Straightening of the sigmoid after fixation of the instrument tip at a flexure or in the distal descending colon is accomplished by simultaneous careful withdrawal and rotation (Fig. 164) under fluoroscopic control. The direction of rotation is chosen so that the sigmoid loop straightens rather than forming a tighter loop (Fig. 159).

We then insert a self-made teflon-coated stiffening probe with a flexible tip through the instrumentation channel until the proximal descending colon is reached. This serves to maintain the straightening of the sigmoid and to improve transmission of force from instrument handle to the tip (Fig. 160). This stiffening probe is withdrawn during further advancement of the coloscope in order to keep the tip of the probe from reaching the splenic flexure. Another possibility for achieving partial stiffening consists of the introduction of a plastic tube, about 40 cm long, over the straightened coloscope [2]. Passage of the sigmoid is the most difficult part of coloscopy. Loops of the transverse colon (Figs. 171–175) can be passed by the technique already mentioned and are straightened after "hooking" of the coloscope tip in the hepatic flexure. The cecum can then be reached. We have performed 1523 coloscopies by this technique and currently are reaching the cecum in 98 percent of cases (Table 9).

Inspection and intubation of the ileocecal junction requires medial deflection of the instrument tip while the main part of the coloscope is in a convex position (Figs. 177, 181). Turning of the patient to the right or left may help to bring the orifice in an optimum viewing angle. Again, no firm rules apply due to the large variations in topographic arrangement. We succeed in intubating the terminal ileum during 30 percent of *all* high coloscopies. The actual success rate is higher (about 80 percent) since intubation was not always attempted. The greatest length of ileal intubation achieved was 50 cm (Fig. 178).

Table 9. Abnormal findings during coloscopy

Coloscopies	1.523	
Polyp(s)		367 patients
Carcinoma		71 patients
Ulcerative colitis		93 patients
Crohn's colitis		76 patients
Miscellaneous		277 patients
		884 patients

In cases where the orifice of the ileocecal valve cannot be visualized well by the method just described, an attempt can be made at medial inversion of the instrument tip at the lowest part of the cecum (Fig. 176a). The instrument is then withdrawn and the tip slightly straightened at the level of the valve for intubation of the ileum (Fig. 177). Waiting for spontaneous opening of the valve orifice facilitates intubation greatly.

NAGASAKO divides the gross appearance of the ileocecal valve into a papillary, a labial, and an intermediate type [1] (Fig. 180). Experience has taught us, however, that the appearance of the valve frequently changes during the examination and that this classification only characterizes a functional state (Fig. 181).

It is occasionally possible to find the orifice of the appendix, to probe it and to instill water-soluble contrast medium into it, provided the colon is well cleansed (Figs. 185–187). Selective visualization is, however, rarely indicated (see also page 68).

Inspection of prestenotic areas, the interior anal ring and the ileocecal (Bauhin's) valve may require inversion of the coloscope. To this end, the tip is maximally deflected while the coloscope is being advanced: the colonic wall acts as the fulcrum, allowing further passive deflection of the tip to 180° (Figs. 176, 190).

The experienced examiner reaches the cecum within 4 to 45 minutes with an average of about 20 minutes. The duration of the entire procedure depends on the number of biopsies and photographs obtained; it varies between 15 and 60 minutes. Thorough inspection and biopsies are carried out during withdrawal in cases where the colon was viewed only for orientation purposes during the intubation. This is all the more effective because all loops have been straightened and no "blind" areas remain. The stiffening probe should be removed at this stage. Retained fecal matter can be flushed away by irrigation from areas of interest. Simethicone preparations (Mylicon) are useful for eliminating troublesome bubble formation.

Number and location of biopsies depend on the clinical indication and the gross findings during coloscopy (Figs. 140, 151). Several biopsies should be obtained of circumscribed lesions and at least six when carcinoma is suspected. In the presence of diffuse alterations, the colon should be biopsied at several levels in order to assess severity and extent of the disease. Material for cytologic and bacteriologic examination can be obtained by brushes introduced through the instrumentation channel (Figs. 141, 152).

References

1. Nagasako, K., Endo, M., Takemoto, T., Kondo, T., Kimura, K.: The insertion of fibercolonoscope into the cecum and direct observation of the ileocecal valve. Endoscopy **2**, 123 (1970).
2. Nagy, G.S.: Fibrecolonoscopy. Med. J. Aust. **1**, 378 (1973).

4.7.2 "Operative" Coloscopy

An operation is defined as a medical procedure involving the bloody or non-bloody severing of tissue. Purely diagnostic endoscopic procedures with biopsies fall, therefore, under this definition. It follows that restriction of the term "operative endoscopy" to therapeutic endoscopic procedures is, actually, incorrect [12].

Coloscopic Polypectomy

The interpretation given by the pathologist is limited by the sites from which tissue particles were obtained. The problem is that the biopsies may not be representative of the whole lesion. It follows that polypoid lesions of the gastrointestinal tract should be removed *in toto*. This concept could not be realized at first due to technical limitations.

Numerous attempts at mechanical removal of larger polyps by forceps or snare had to be abandoned because of considerable bleeding which proved difficult to control (Fig. 191). Mechanical removal of polyps by biopsy forceps should, therefore, be restricted to lesions of up to 5 mm in diameter.

Simple electrocoagulation of polypoid lesions (Fig. 192) [23] cannot be recommended because no tissue is obtained for histologic examination.

The risk of bleeding was decreased considerably with the use of the high-frequency diathermy snare for sigmoid polypectomy in 1949 [22] and, with modified instrumentation, for coloscopic polypectomy in 1971 [4, 5, 8–10, 20].

The symmetrical (Fig. 144) and asymmetrical closed snares presently available allow only the ablation of small and medium-sized polyps. Endoscopic resection of large pedunculated and lobulated polyps with these snares is technically very difficult or impossible.

We have developed an open high-frequency diathermy snare which can be rotated by about 120°. This instrument permits the endoscopic electro-resection of large pedunculated and lobulated polyps of the gastrointestinal tract (Figs. 145, 198).

While proctoscopic polypectomy is an established, low-risk procedure, additional problems arise when polyps are removed from areas where the colonic wall is thinner, especially in the intraperitoneal parts of the colon. The danger of thermal injury to the bowel wall with consequent perforation exists, particularly during ablation of sessile polyps.

Polypectomy with the high-frequency diathermy snare currently has to be considered the method of choice. Two different types of electrical current are used: sinusoidal and spark gap. The former is a continuous, undamped high-frequency current (Fig. 193 a). It serves mainly for cutting and causes very little coagulation. The latter is a pulsed high-frequency current with damped oscillations and high peak voltage (Fig. 193 b). It generates heat and coagulates the cut surfaces. During polypectomy, both types of current are mixed for optimum results (Fig. 193 c). The cut surface is coagulated, bleeding is prevented, and the polyp becomes available for histologic study. Examination of the entire lesion is desirable because biopsies obtained by forceps may miss focal carcinomas or components of polyps of mixed histologic type.

We use closed (Fig. 144) and open (Fig. 145) high-frequency diathermy snares for coloscopic polypectomy. Ablation is carried out after CO_2 insufflation in order to avoid explosion of the methane-oxygen mixture present within the colon (Fig. 150).

We begin by "lassoing" the polyp with the snare; it is placed around the stalk and tightened until the polyp shows a livid discoloration. The snare is then tightened further with simultaneous coagulation (frequency 0.5–1.2 megaHz; output up to 80 W). The polyp is gradually pulled towards the lumen during the cutting maneuver (Fig. 194) without touching the opposite wall.

The open snare is introduced straight through the instrumentation channel and is allowed to curve near the base of the polyp. The stalk can be surrounded regardless of the maximum diameter of the polyp (Fig. 198) and is cut at the base.

Energy sources are the Erbotum R 3 (Fa. Erbe, Tübingen, West Germany) (Fig. 150) and the model SSE 2 (Valleylab, Boulder, Colorado). Ablated polyps are retrieved with the biopsy forceps during simultaneous suction or with a grasping instrument developed by SEIFERT (Fig. 146).

We have removed 282 polypoid lesions (227 pedunculated 55 broad-based) from all areas of the colon (Fig. XXII). All lesions were recovered and examined histologically [10]. Nine polyps were removed in one sitting from one patient, and three from another. One perforation was observed. The largest lesion measured 5 cm, the largest base, 3 cm in diameter (Figs. 199–201).

Follow-up coloscopy of the iatrogenic ulcer was performed in 16 polypectomized patients. The iatrogenic ulcer healed within one to three weeks, average two weeks; a scar was present in 11 and no residual changes were found in 4 patients. In one case healing was delayed until six weeks after ablation of a broadbased polyp (stalk diameter: 1 cm) (Figs. 197, 204, 205).

The diagnostic yield was high (Tables 10, 11). Two patients were found to have polypoid adenocarcinoma; segmental resection was carried out. In 15 cases, polypoid adenomas with focal carcinoma were re-

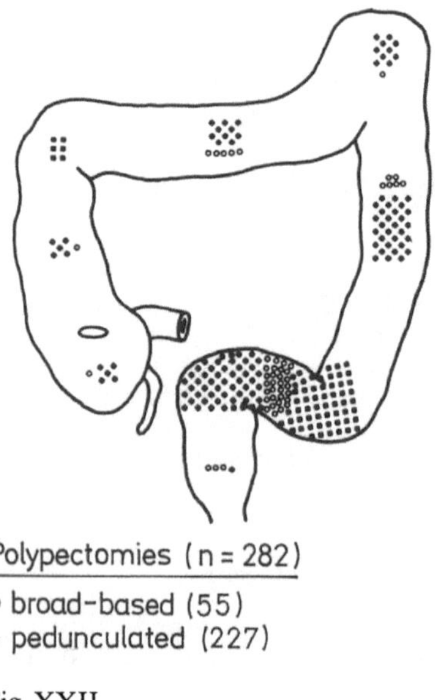

Fig. XXII

Table 10. Histologic diagnosis of 282 polypoid lesions removed via the coloscope

I.	Adenomas	
	a) polypoid	165
	b) polypoid with focal carcinoma	15
	c) papillary	8
	d) villous	9
II.	Peutz-Jeghers polyps	18
III.	Carcinomas	2
IV.	Hyperplastic polyps	57
V.	Pseudopolyps	4
VI.	Carcinoid	1
VII.	Lipoma	1
VIII.	Cronkhite-Canada-polyp	1
IX.	Angiofibroma	1

Table 11. Size and histologic diagnosis of 282 polypoid lesions removed via the coloscope

Size (cm)	Benign	Focal Cancer	Cancer	Total
<1	103	2	0	105
1–2	127	8	1	136
>2	35	5	1	41
Total	265	15	2	282

moved (Figs. 187, 202) and did not require further therapy.

The endoscopic removal of polypoid lesions from the entire colon is a low-risk procedure without major technical difficulties provided the operator is experienced, the proper technique is followed and contraindications (bleeding diathesis; base of the polyp greater than 3 cm in diameter) are observed. It represents a significant advance in preoperative tissue diagnosis and, in some cases, in therapy and prophylaxis. Compared to surgical polypectomy, the endoscopic procedure requires much shorter hospitalization and is less costly. More important, however, is the lower complication rate. While we have encountered one complication (1 perforation), only one bleeding episode occurred after 390 endoscopic polypectomies carried out at different centers [17]. By contrast, the operative mortality of exploratory laparotomy with colotomy is reported as 0.5 percent [23] and that of hemicolectomy as 1.4 percent [13].

Foreign Body Removal

Retrieval of foreign bodies from the colon must be a rare event since they usually leave the colon spontaneously. In those cases, however, where mechanical properties or pathologic changes cause retention of a foreign body, the endoscopist can avoid surgical intervention.

Deyle successfully extracted a tube which had entered the transverse colon via a colostomy. We have removed an incarcerated transintestinal tube with attached rubber balloon from the upper sigmoid with the coloscope (Fig. 206).

Injections

Injections through an endoscope have, so far, only been used in the local therapy of gastric ulcers and of early carcinomas. We have attempted to sclerose five solitary hemangiomas in the cecum and transverse colon. A metal needle at the tip of a flexible teflon tube was inserted through the instrumentation channel and a solution of phenol in peanut oil was injected (Figs. 149, 207). This attempt succeeded in only two instances and we decided to proceed with electrocoagulation.

Electrocoagulation

Electrocoagulation of circumscribed colonic bleeding sites with a flexible coagulation probe (Fig. 147) has not yet reached the stage of general clinical use. The method should not be used routinely until sufficient animal experiments and clinical experience have accumulated (Figs. 14, 18, 21). Improved results may come with the use of a laser beam; our first trials have been encouraging.

One patient with recurrent intestinal bleeding had unsuccessful attempts at injection of three hemangiomas in the cecum. These were obliterated coloscopically (Fig. 156) with a flexible coagulation probe while one of the lesions was bleeding (Fig. 208). The patient has been asymptomatic during a 1-year follow-up.

In our opinion, however, light coagulation

using an argon laser beam, as we have recently carried out at our department for the first time ever, is more successful and safer.

Angiography

Congenital and acquired vascular anomalies of the colon can rarely be diagnosed clinically or radiologically. These malformations frequently cause recurrent—often severe—bleeding episodes. Early surgical therapy is possible only when a preoperative diagnosis is established. Mesenteric angiography is the method of choice in these cases.

Varices of the colon, usually caused by portal hypertension, are rarely recognized antemortem. Only 11 cases have been reported to date, each manifested by intestinal bleeding [1, 2, 6, 7, 15, 16]. We were able to diagnose varices of the distal descending colon in one other patient by coloscopy and to demonstrate them further by endoscopic angiography (Fig. 209). The patient was 43 years old with a ten-year history of recurrent bleeding per rectum. The bleeding site could not be identified by repeated proctoscopic and radiologic examinations. We entered one of the varices with a thin needle during coloscopy and injected contrast material in order to determine their extent and to identify a possible site of venous obstruction. The angiographic and clinical findings, combined with subsequent splenoportography, did not reveal a localized obstruction of the inferior mesenteric vein. A primary vascular anomaly was the most likely diagnosis [11].

References

1. Brill, D.R., Bolasny, B., Vix, V.A.: Colonic varices. Amer. J. Digest. Dis. New series. Vol. **14**, No. 11, 801 (1969).
2. Case records of the Massachusetts General Hospital (Case No. 40102). New Eng. J. Med. **250**, 434 (1954).
3. Classen, M., Frühmorgen, P.: Operative endoscopy in the gastrointestinal tract. Acta Hepatogastroenterologica **19**, 124 (1972).
4. Deyhle, P., Seuberth, K., Jenny, S., Demling, L.: Endoscopic polypectomy in the proximal colon. Endoscopy **2**, 103 (1971).
5. Demling, L., Ottenjann, R., Elster, K.: Endoskopie und Biopsie der Speiseröhre und des Magens. Stuttgart: Schattauer 1972.
6. Feldman, M., Smith, V.M., Warner, C.G.: Varices of colon: Report of three cases. J. Amer. med. Ass. **179**, 729 (1962).
7. Fleming, R.J., Seaman, W.B.: Roentgenographic demonstration of unusual extra-esophageal varices. Amer. J. Roentgenol. **103**, 281 (1968).
8. Frühmorgen, P., Zeus, J., Demling, L.: Endoskopisch-operative Behandlung polypoider Läsionen des Dickdarms. Leber-Magen-Darm **4**, 166 (1973).
9. Frühmorgen, P.: Operative Endoskopie im Kolon. Fortschr. Med. **16**, 685 (1973).
10. Frühmorgen, P., Demling, L.: Koloskopische Polypektomie. Dtsch. med. Wschr. **98**, 1455 (1973).
11. Frühmorgen, P., Fritsch, E.v.: Coloscopic-angiographic demonstration of colonic varices. Endoscopy, in preparation.
12. Frühmorgen, P., Classen, M.: Endoskopie und Biopsie in der Gastroenterologie. Berlin, Heidelberg, New York: Springer 1974.
13. Judd, E.S.: The risk of surgery of the colon: current trends in hospital mortality rates. Proc. Mayo Clin. **36**, 492 (1961).
14. Koch, H., Pesch, H.-J., Bauerle, H., Frühmorgen, P., Rösch, W., Classen, M.: Erste experimentelle Untersuchungen und klinische Erfahrungen zur Elektrokoagulation blutender Läsionen im oberen Gastrointestinaltrakt. In: Fortschritte der Endoskopie (Ottenjann, R., Ed.). Stuttgart-New York: Schattauer 1973.
15. Levy, J.S., Hardin, J.H., Shipp, H., Keeling, J.H.: Varices of cecum as unusual cause of gastrointestinal bleeding. Gastroenterology **33**, 637 (1957).
16. Lopata, H.I., Berlin, L.: Colon varices: rare causes of lower gastrointestinal bleeding. Radiology **87**, 1048 (1966).
17. Ottenjann, R.: Colonic polyps and coloscopic polypectomy. Endoscopy **4**, 212 (1972).
18. Paul, F., Seifert, W., Krause: Therapie blutender Magenwandläsionen mittels endoskopischer Elektrokoagulation. Vortr. V. Kongreß Deutsche Gesellschaft für Endoskopie. Erlangen 1972.
19. Seifert, E.: A new flexible forceps for the removal of polyps from the gatrointestinal tract after successful endoscopic polypectomy. Endoscopy **4**, 226 (1972).
20. Seifert, E.: Endoscopic polypectomy. Gastroenterologia Japonica 5.
21. Stadelmann, O., Raschke, Müller, Löffler Miederer: Endoskopische Elektrokoagulation: Voruntersuchungen und erste klinische

Erfahrungen. Vortr. V. Kongreß Deutsche Gesellschaft für Endoskopie, Erlangen 1972.
22. TURELL, R.: Sigmoidorectal electrosurgical snare. N.Y. med. J. **49**, 2311 (1949).
23. TURELL, R., HALLER, J.D.: Adenomas of the colon and rectum. In: Diseases of the colon and anorectum (TURELL, R., Ed.). Philadelphia, London. Toronto: Saunders 1969.

4.8 Findings

4.8.1 Developmental Abnormalities

Atresias and other anomalies of anus, rectum, or sigmoid, caused by maldevelopment during the sixth to seventh week of gestation, are infrequent and are even rarer in the proximal colon. The anomalies consist mainly of partial or complete stenosis, rectal prolapse, presence of a cloaca, duplications and fistulas to other pelvic organs. Their location and type can usually be determined by radiologic methods. Classifications of these developmental abnormalities have been published by LADD and GROSS [1] and by PARTRIDGE and GOUGH [2]. Anomalous positions of the colon are the result of malrotation and fixation; they, too, are rare.

References

1. LADD, W.E., GROSS, R.E.: Congenital malformation of the anus and rectum. Amer. J. Surg. **23**, 167 (1934).
2. PARTRIDGE, J.P., GOUGH, M.: Congenital abnormalitis of the anus and rectum. Brit. J. Surg. **49**, 37 (1961).

4.8.2 Tumors of the Colon

Gross appearance, number and location of colonic tumors give little information about their histologic type and, hence, their clinical significance. Even multiple biopsies may not be representative of the whole lesion.

The published prevalence of benign colon tumors at autopsy varies between 7 and 52 percent [2]. More precise figures are available for malignant tumors. About 14 percent of all malignant tumors are situated in the colon [2, 14]. The fact that about 80 percent of these tumors are within reach of the procto-sigmoidoscope is of special importance for early diagnosis [6, 12]. Unfortunately, too many classification systems of malignant colon tumors exist, causing confusion and making comparison of different series impossible [5].

The benign and malignant polyps diagnosed coloscopically in our patients are listed in Table 12 according to size. Table 12 shows our entire polyp material, regardless of whether the lesion was removed endoscopically or only diagnosed by endoscopic biopsy.

Table 12. Size and histologic type of colonic polyps diagnosed by coloscopy ($n=414$)

Size (cm)	Benign	Focal Cancer	Cancer	Total
<1	230	3	0	233
1–2	124	8	1	133
>2	40	2	6	48
Total	394	13	7	414

Benign Tumors

Adenomatous polyps are by far the most common benign colonic tumors. The polyps are multiple in about 20 percent and single in about 80 percent of cases.

The frequently used term "polyp" simply describes a sessile or pedunculated tumor protruding from the surface of the mucosa. In order not to prejudge a certain growth pattern, the descriptive expression "polypoid lesion" should be used until a histologic diagnosis is available.

Optimal radiologic technique applied to a well-prepared colon is able to detect colonic tumors a few millimeters in size. Up to 50 percent of small polypoid lesions, however, are missed by routine diagnostic radiology or cannot clearly be differentiated from fecal matter, necessitating repeat examinations. Further difficulties of radiologic polyp detection exist in patients with diverticulosis (Fig. 210). The coloscopist is capable of finding even the smallest polyps and of differentiating them from fecal matter with little or no radiation exposure to the patient.

Benign Epithelial Tumors

All benign epithelial colonic tumors are polypoid and 95 percent are adenomas. An increased incidence of coexistent carcinoma has been reported (sentinel polyps) [2, 13] (Fig. 225).

The adenomatous polyp is the most frequent type of colonic tumor; villous papilloma and papillary adenoma represent structural variations of this lesion.

The adenomatous polyp is neoplastic and has the potential for malignant degeneration. Dedifferentiation or atypia of the epithelium, however, is a normal finding in these polyps. Carcinoma should only be diagnosed when the process invades the lamina propria after penetration of the muscularis mucosae [9]. This decision can only be made when the entire polyp is available for examination; tissue fragments obtained by biopsy are insufficient.

Step sections of the entire adenomatous polyp not infrequently reveal foci of malignant cells. Simple removal of the lesion is sufficient provided the stalk is free of malignant invasion [14].

The question as to whether and how often adenomatous polyps develop malignant degeneration remains unanswered to this day [9, 12, 14]. On the other hand, there is no doubt about the increasing incidence of carcinomatous polyps with increasing polyp size [10, 12]. We believe that removal, especially of larger adenomas, is of prophylactic value in addition to providing optimal diagnosis. Polyps greater than 10 mm in diameter should, therefore, always be ablated. Small polypoid lesions are removed or, at least, biopsied. Adenomatous colon polyps either are asymptomatic or occasionally may cause rectal bleeding. They rarely manifest themselves by obstruction or intussusception. There are no characteristic symptoms.

Villous papillomas represent a special category; 70 to 95 percent are encountered in rectum and sigmoid. Their usual endoscopic appearance is that of a broad-based, papillary, spongy and vascular tumor. They may, however, also give the same gross appearance as adenomatous polyps; the differentiation cannot be made without histologic study [11]. At least six biopsies should be obtained. Mucoid diarrhea with secondary hypokalemia and rectal bleeding may occasionally give a clue to their presence. The radiologic interpretation of these tumors is usually that of carcinoma, necessitating further endoscopic-bioptic investigation. As a rule simple endoscopic polypectomy is insufficient because of a tendency for local recurrences and the coexistence of invasive carcinoma in 8 to 16 percent of cases [8]. Local surgical resection is the recommended therapy.

Benign Nonepithelial Tumors

Endometriosis, hemangiomas [1], lipomas, neurofibromas and myomas are rarely found and will not be discussed further in this context.

Carcinoid

Carcinoid of the colon occurs mainly in appendix, cecum and rectosigmoid. The endoscopic picture of a broad-based lesion elevating the mucosal surface is rarely encountered (Fig. 216).

Polyposis

This group includes diseases characterized by multiple polyps [3], such as familial polyposis (adenomatosis), the Gardner and the Cronkhite-Canada syndrome [16].

Juvenile, Peutz-Jeghers, benign lymphoid, metaplastic and hyperplastic polyps are not true neoplastic tumors (see page 60).

Familial polyposis (adenomatosis) of the colon (Fig. 217) is inherited as a dominant trait and must be considered a premalignant condition. The polyps appear during puberty and their number varies between a few and several hundred covering the entire colon. The dominant clinical symptom is mucoid, bloody diarrhea. Therapy consists of total colectomy or of proctocolectomy depending on the extent of the disease. Intestinal polyposis coexisting with mesenchymal tumors of other organs, especially the skin, is a variant of familial polyposis (Gardner syndrome); these polyps also have an unquestioned potential of malignant degeneration (Fig. 218).

Malignant Tumors

Malignant tumors cause few or no symptoms at a stage when they still are curable. The technical and temporal demands of coloscopy are still too high to incorporate this procedure into mass screening programs of entire population segments. The contributions which coloscopy does offer to early cancer detection consist of the endoscopic examination of suspicious radiologic and clinical findings and of serial examinations of patients with premalignant conditions and after cancer surgery. The distribution pattern of malignant colon tumors (70 percent occur in rectum and sigmoid) facilitates prophylactic screening (digital examination; proctosigmoidoscopy) [6, 7].

Malignant Epithelial Tumors

The large majority of malignant colon tumors are adenocarcinomas which rarely exhibit a mucoid or scirrhous pattern. The exophytic, cauliflower-like or polypoid type which obstructs the lumen late (Figs. 219, 220) should be distinguished from the circular type which cause obstructive symptoms early in its course (Figs. 222, 223). The typical endoscopic signs are rigidity of the wall, discoloration of the mucosa, and a tendency to fragmentation during palpation and forceps biopsy. Ulcerations and mucosal friability may be encountered depending on the growth pattern. Passage of an area heavily involved or stenosed by cancer with the coloscope may be difficult or impossible. Blind advancement and excessive force should be avoided because of the dangers of perforation and bleeding.

Clinical manifestations usually occur at a stage when the carcinoma cannot be missed radiologically or endoscopically. Stenosis of the colon as identified by radiologic methods may, however, be caused by several different processes which can usually be defined by endoscopic biopsy. The main problem in differential diagnosis is the separation of carcinomatous (Figs. 227, 228) from inflammatory (Figs. 229, 231) stenoses.

Small carcinomas, up to 15 mm in diameter, cannot always be differentiated from benign tumors during barium enema examination [15]. In these cases, the endoscopic-bioptic clarification of the diagnosis is of particular importance (Table 13). In some cases where the coloscopist diagnoses carcinoma, the biopsies do not show malignant changes. This is caused by difficulties in reaching the tumor with the biopsy forceps. Surgical exploration should be carried out in such cases. The difficulties in distinguishing radiologically between malignancy and stenosis due to diverticulitis and other localized inflammatory processes has already been alluded to. Intramural lesions and diseases of neighboring organs affecting the colon (Fig. 230) are beyond the reach of the biopsy forceps and require exploratory laparotomy.

High coloscopy is very helpful in establishing the diagnosis of polypoid lesions of the ileocecal area which are reported as "rule out carcinoma" by the radiologist. In several cases such lesions were identified as an ileocecal valve which was enlarged due to Crohn's disease of the ileum or colon

Table 13. Radiologic and coloscopic diagnosis of 59 carcinomas of the colon with method of histologic verification

Diagnosis	Radiology	Coloscopy	Biopsy	Surgical Specimen
Malignancy/ suspicious of malignancy	52	59	45	59
Not malignant	6	—	12	—
Normal	1	—	2	—

(Fig. 251). Other patients with polypoid tumors of the cecum were spared exploratory laparotomy when endoscopic biopsy showed the lesions to represent large inverted appendiceal stumps (Fig. 189).

Malignant Nonepithelial Tumors

This group consists of the malignant variations of the benign nonepithelial tumors listed above; these and primary sarcomas of the colon are extremely rare [14].

Atypias of the Epithelium

The histologic diagnosis of "early carcinoma" applies when the epithelial atypia and dedifferentiation characteristically found in adenomatous polyps is demonstrated within the *flat* mucosa of the colon [5]. Identical alterations may be present in patients with longstanding idiopathic ulcerative colitis; the risk of malignant degeneration after five years of this disease is 17 percent and after fifteen years it is 25 percent. Other authors have reported the prevalence of carcinoma to be about 45 percent in patients with ulcerative colitis for more than nine years who underwent colectomy [4].

Pseudotumors

Benign lymphoid polyps (nodular lymphoid hyperplasia) are found almost exclusively in ileum and rectum and usually are asymptomatic. The pathologist requires an intact polyp for establishing an exact diagnosis. These hypertrophic lymph follicles frequently are multiple and are considered benign. Endoscopically, they appear as small submucosal tumors covered by normal mucosa (Fig. 232).

Hyperplastic (metaplastic) polyps (Figs. 233, 234) may occur in large numbers and cannot always be differentiated from familial polyposis by their radiologic and gross appearance. The polyps are sessile, rarely larger than 10 mm and have a characteristic histologic appearance. The presence of multiple hyperplastic polyps does not, however, exclude the coexistence of adenomatous polyps.

Juvenile polyposis is found in children five to nine years of age. These are completely benign lesions (hamartomas) which regress spontaneously. Removal is only indicated in those rare instances where massive bleeding, obstruction or rectal prolapse occur.

Involvement of the colon by the Peutz-Jeghers syndrome is characterized by the presence of papillomatous tumors (Fig. 203a and b) with a typical feathery arrangement of the muscularis mucosae (Fig. 203c). Peutz-Jeghers polyps are mainly located in the upper gastrointestinal tract. The colon is involved in only 50 percent of cases, in contrast to the pattern of familial polyposis.

Multiple so-called inflammatory or pseudopolyps (Figs. 235, 246) should not be considered true tumors. They represent hyperplastic mucosal rests which arise during the course of inflammatory colon disease and may persist during remission.

None of these lesions nor heterotopic rests has ever been observed to undergo malignant degeneration. An increased incidence of primary adenocarcinoma of the colon in patients with the Peutz-Jeghers syndrome has, however, been reported [17].

References

1. Bartelheimer, W., Ottenjann, R., Remmele, W.: Coloscopic recognition of hemangioma in the colon ascendens. Endoscopy **4**, 109 (1972).
2. Bockus, H.L.: Gastroenterology. Vol. II. Philadelphia, London: Saunders 1964.
3. Bussey, H.J.R.: Gastrointestinal polyposis. Gut **11**, 970 (1970).
4. Counsell, P.B., Dukes, C.E.: The association of chronic ulcerative colitis and carcinoma of the rectum and colon. Brit. J. Surg. **39**, 485 (1952).
5. Elster, K.: Histopathologie der tumorösen Kolonerkrankungen, Leber, Magen, Darm **3**, 111 (1973).
6. Frühmorgen, P.: Krebsfrüherkennung im Kolon. Fortschr. Med. **31**, 1130 (1972).
7. Frühmorgen, P., Classen, M., Demling, L.: Krebsdiagnostik im Gastrointestinaltrakt. Fortschr. Med. **26**, 1011 (1973).
8. Kaye, J.J., Bragg, D.G.: Unusual roentgenologic and clinicopathologic features of villous

adenomas of the colon. Radiology **91**, 799 (1968).
9. MORSON, B.C., BUSSEY, H.J.R.: Predisposing causes of intestinal cancer. Current Problems in Surgery, Febr. 1970. Chicago: Year Book Medical Publ. 1970.
10. OTTENJANN, R.: Colonic polyps and coloscopic polypectomy. Endoscopy **4**, 212 (1972).
11. PARTURIER-ALBOT, M.: Endoscopic aspects of rectal villous tumors. Endoscopy of the digestive system. Proc. Ist Europ. Congr. Digestive Endoscopy, Prague 1968. Basel: Karger 1969.
12. POTET, F., SOULLARD, J.: Polyps of the rectum and colon. Gut **12**, 468 (1971).
13. RAVDIN, I.S.: Polyps of the colon significance and managements. J. nat. med. Ass. (N.Y.) **52**, 387 (1960).
14. TURELL, R., HALLER, J.D.: Adenomas of the colon and rectum. In: Diseases of the colon and anorectum (TURELL, R., Ed.). Vol. I, Philadelphia, London, Toronto: Saunders 1969.
15. WELIN, S., ANDRÉN, L.: Dickdarm und Enddarm. In: Lehrbuch der Röntgendiagnostik (SCHINZ, R.H., *et al.*, Eds.), Bd. V: Abdomen. Stuttgart: Thieme 1965.
16. WITZEL, L., CLASSEN, M., ROESCH, W., DEMLING, L.: Cronkhite-Canada-Syndrom. Fallbericht und Übersicht, Dtsch. med. Wschr. **96**, 989 (1971).
17. DODDS, J.J., SCHULTE, W.J., HENSLEY, G.T., HOGAN, W.J.: Peutz-Jeghers syndrome and gastrointestinal malignancy. Amer. J. Roentgenol. **115**, 374 (1972).

4.8.3 Inflammatory Diseases

Idiopathic Ulcerative Colitis

The etiology of this disease with its intermittent or chronic course remains essentially unknown [5, 6]. Autoimmune mechanisms and additional pathogenetic factors, such as psychogenic events, are currently favored. The prevalence is unquestionably increased in highly developed countries [2, 6].

The rectum and entire colon are involved in about 90 percent of cases. Disease initially limited to the rectum may spread retrogradely over varying distances. Ulcerative colitis without rectal involvement occurs but rarely. The differentiation from Crohn's colitis (granulomatous colitis) is particularly difficult in these cases. A few centimeters of terminal ileum may be involved; this is termed "backwash-ileitis."

The diagnosis has to be established on the basis of clinical and proctoscopic findings during the acute phase. Coloscopy is contraindicated at this florid stage because of pain and the danger of perforation. During remission, however, barium enema as well as coloscopy should be performed in order to assess localization, severity and extent of involvement, to obtain tissue for histologic confirmation of the diagnosis, and to detect complications (strictures, carcinoma, abscesses and fistulas). The importance of coloscopy is emphasized by two observations: 1. the frequent lack of correlation between severity and extent of disease and clinical symptoms; 2. radiologic methods cannot determine the extent of mucosal involvement with the necessary certainty. Carefully performed procto-sigmoidoscopy is the method of choice for confirmation of the diagnosis during the acute phase of the disease.

The increased risk of carcinoma in this disease is unquestioned. Although the reported figures vary, it is certain that the incidence rises with increased duration of the disease. COUNSELL and DUKES, for example, found carcinoma in 45.5 percent of colons resected from patients with ulcerative colitis of longer than nine years' duration [3]. Carcinoma develops mainly during remission and it is not yet clear whether it arises in atrophic mucosa, in pseudopolyps, or in true adenomatous polyps.

The endoscopic appearance of acute ulcerative colitis is protean. The early stages are characterized by the absence of a vascular pattern, by fine granularity, hyperemia and increased friability (Figs. 238, 239). Florid ulcerative colitis shows irregular ulcerations, edematous and dark-red mucosa, hyperemia, superficial necrosis, pronounced friability and deposition of mucus, pus and fibrin (Figs. 240–243).

Toxic megacolon (paralytic ileus) is a serious complication with poor prognosis due to the danger of spontaneous perforation.

During the chronic stage the mucosa appears pale-red to pink (Figs. 244–247) and is finely granular and atrophic. Pseudopolyps (regenerating mucosa or remaining islands of normal mucosa) develop in 74 percent of cases [1] (Fig. 246) and may cover large areas of the colon. They represent fibrous polypoid lesions. Radiologic differentiation from familial polyposis may occasionally be impossible; endoscopic biopsy can resolve this issue. Narrowing of the lumen, loss of haustra and distensibility, shortening, and, rarely, localized stenoses [4] are typical of the later stages and can adequately be delineated by the radiologist.

Complications: massive bleeding, perforation and toxic megacolon during the acute stages. Strictures, ileus, carcinoma and, rarely, abscesses and fistulas during the chronic phase.

Diagnosis: clinical findings and carefully performed procto-sigmoidoscopy without air insufflation during the florid stage. Barium enema and, perhaps, coloscopy with biopsy during remission. Biopsies frequently reveal chronic inflammatory changes during asymptomatic intervals when the mucosa appears normal to inspection.

Differential diagnosis: Crohn's disease of the colon, diverticulitis, polyposis, carcinoma, amebic colitis and, rarely, intestinal tuberculosis and radiation colitis.

References

1. Bockus, H.L.: Gastroenterology, Vol. II. Philadelphia, London: Saunders 1964.
2. Classen, M.: Epikritische Studie zur Colitis ulcerosa. In: Dünndarm-Dickdarm. (Boecker, W., Ed.). Stuttgart: Thieme 1969.
3. Counsell, P.B., Dukes, C.E.: The association of chronic ulcerative colitis and carcinoma of the rectum and colon. Brit. J. Surg. **39**, 485 (1952).
4. Fuchs, H.-F.: Die Röntgenuntersuchung des Dickdarms, insbesondere bei Colitis ulcerosa und granulomatosa (Crohn). Fortschr. Med. **89**, 1330 (1971).
5. Koch, H., Classen, H.: Colitis ulcerosa. Fortschr. Med. **87**, 1199 (1969).
6. Krauspe, C., Müller-Wieland, K., Stelzner, F.: Colitis ulcerosa und granulomatosa. München, Berlin, Wien: Urban u. Schwarzenberg 1972.

Crohn's Disease of the Colon (Granulomatous Colitis)

This disease of unknown etiology (8–20 percent of all cases of colitis [8]) typically involves isolated segments of the gastrointestinal tract (skip areas). Genetic influences are suggested by the increased incidence in certain families and races [9]. Possible causes are bacterial or viral infection and autoimmune mechanisms [10]. The site most commonly affected is the terminal ileum. Simultaneous or isolated involvement of other segments of the gastrointestinal tract, from esophagus to anus, is frequently observed. Simultaneous disease of the colon (Fig. XXIII a–c) is identified in about 50 percent of cases [6] (Table 13a). Conversely, involvement of the terminal ileum will be found in 60–90 percent of patients with Crohn's colitis [20]. Several authors have reported an increase in newly diagnosed cases, especially in Europe [1–3, 5, 7, 13, 14, 18, 19, 21–23].

Differences from idiopathic ulcerative colitis include a more chronic course with a tendency to formation of fistulas and abscesses (Fig. 248), no increased incidence of carcinoma with terminal ileitis [11], the rare occurrence of a fulminating course with toxic dilatation [12] and the histologic changes present in biopsies. A positive histologic diagnosis can only be made when the biopsy contains accumulations of epitheloid cells, or fistulous tracts of the mucosa. Typical granulomata in the colon wall or mesen-

Table 13a Crohn's Disease

Oesophagus	1	(0,75%)
Stomach	1	(0,75%)
Stomach/Duodenum	4	(3,00%)
Duodenum	1	(0,75%)
Jejunum	1	(0,75%)
Ileum	60	(45,0%)
Ileum/Colon	65	(49,0%)
	133	(100,0%)

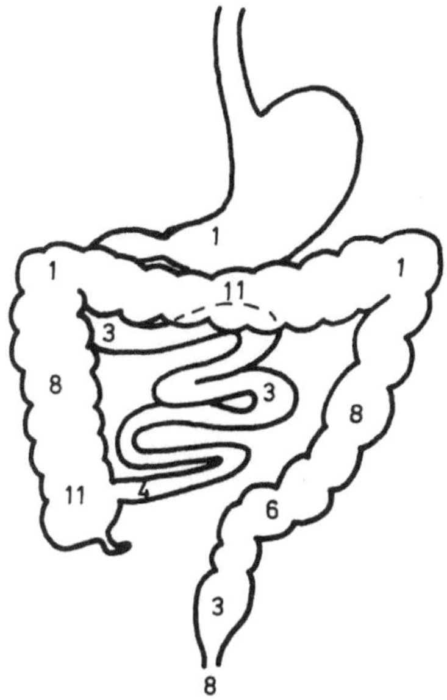

Fig. XXIIIa

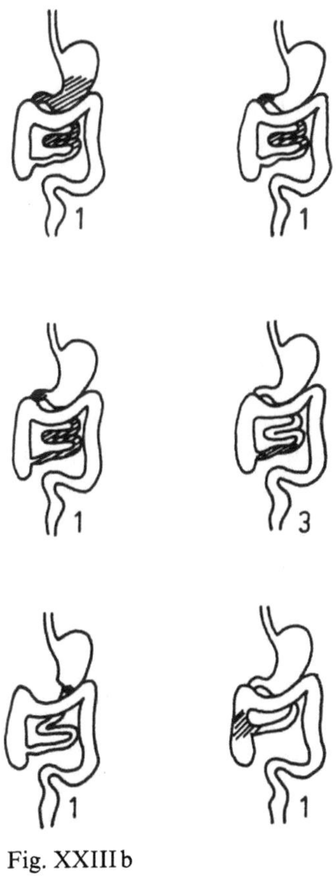

Fig. XXIIIb

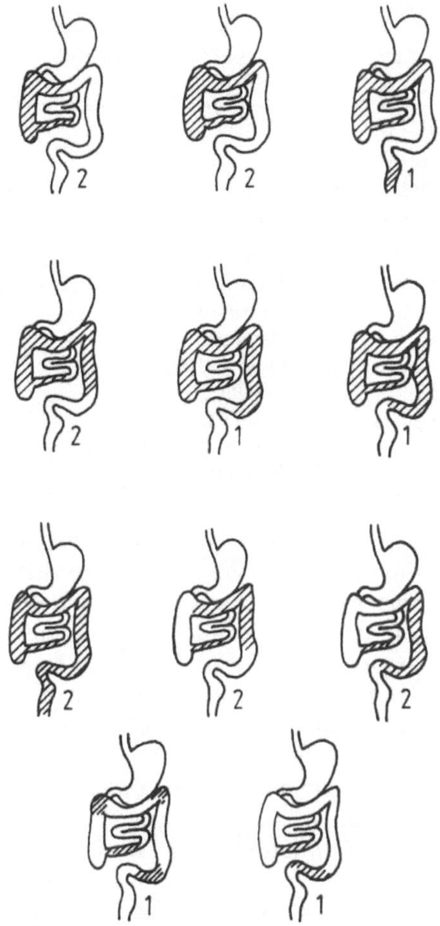

Fig. XXIIIc

teric lymph nodes are found in only 75–80 percent of surgical specimens [15, 16].

The endoscopic-bioptic examination has greatly improved the capability for recognition and differential diagnosis of idiopathic inflammatory colitis [4]. Idiopathic ulcerative colitis and Crohn's disease of the colon can be distinguished on morphological grounds (Table 14). Ulcerative colitis can be diagnosed by proctoscopy in more than 90 percent of cases. Crohn's disease of the colon, localized in more proximal parts of the colon, requires coloscopy to reveal its characteristic gross appearance. Extensive mucosal ulcerations may arise late during the course of the disease. Their presence

Table 14

Endoscopy	Idiopathic ulcerative colitis	Crohn's colitis
Manifest in		
Rectum	34/35	4/32
Terminal ileum	1/35	29/32
Colon lumen	Normal/Dilated	Normal/Narrowed
Distribution	Continuous	Discontinuous
Mucosa	Ulcers No fissures Hyperemia Granulation Friable	Solitary ulcers Fissures Normal areas Cobblestone pattern Edema
Healing phase	Mucosal atrophy Absent haustrations Pseudopolyps	Deformed by scars Stenoses Cobblestone pattern

makes the macroscopic differential diagnosis during acute exacerbations more difficult. This situation is rarely encountered and represents a contraindication to coloscopy anyway. In Crohn's colitis, areas of normal appearing mucosa always can be found, even when the entire colon appears to be involved.

The histologic and macroscopic appearance of Crohn's disease is characteristic but not specific. Granulomata, the most reliable finding, could be demonstrated in only 18/67=27 percent of biopsies and in 84 percent of surgical specimens of our patients. According to Morson [16, 17], however, the diagnosis may be made when the histologist identifies fissures, lymphocytic aggregates with germinal centers and transmural or submucosal inflammation beneath normal mucosa in the presence of a corresponding clinical and endoscopic picture. This approach has led to an increase in the rate of histological confirmation of endoscopically diagnosed Crohn's disease to 44/67=66 percent in biopsy material and to 12/13=92 percent in surgically resected specimens (Table 15).

In 7 out of 74 (9.5 percent) patients with clinical or radiologic signs suggesting inflammatory bowel disease, such disease could be excluded by coloscopy with biopsy (Table 16).

Coloscopy has been particularly helpful for postoperative follow-up and for early diagnosis of postoperative recurrences of Crohn's colitis (Table 17; Figs. 259–261).

Endoscopic findings include mucosal edema, pronounced segmental rigidity and

Table 15

Histology	Crohn's disease		Ulcerative Colitis
	Biopsy	Surgical Specimen	Biopsy
Granulomas	18	11	
No granulomas, but consistent with clinical diagnosis	26	1	
Nonspecific inflammation	15	1	78
Normal mucosa	8	0	3
Total	67	13	81

Table 16

Colitis	Crohn's colitis	Ulcerative colitis
Diagnosis ($n=67$)		
Coloscopy	24	35
Enteroscopy	8	—
Exclusion (7/74=9.5%)		
Coloscopy	3	3
Ileoscopy	1	—

Table 17

Crohn's disease	n	Recurrence	
		Endoscopy	Radiology
Ileocolostomy	8	7	4
Gastrojejunostomy	1	1	1
Ileal resection	1	1	0
Total	10	9	5

contraction, stenoses and superficial ulcerations which lead to undermining of the mucosa and to intramural abscess formation (Figs. 252–256). Irregularities of the lumen due to scarring and cobblestone appearance of the mucosa may develop during the chronic stage (Figs. 257, 258). While the course of both diseases is one of remissions and exacerbations, ulcerative colitis primarily affects the mucosa and Crohn's disease is a transmural process. Typical findings are islands of normal mucosa within abnormal areas (skip areas) and solitary, superficial ulcers in grossly normal regions (skip lesions) [16] (Figs. 249, 256). The earliest stage, which may precede clinical manifestations for some time, is characterized by an "aphthoid" mucosal lesion a few millimeters in diameter (Fig. 261).

Therapy should be conservative as long as possible. Surgical intervention is indicated only when complications arise or when medical therapy fails. The recurrence rate after resections and bypass procedures is up to 50 percent; postoperative fistulas may also develop. Anal fistulas as well as fissures (Fig. 248) frequently coexist and may precede the clinical manifestations and intestinal involvement.

In situations where the history, clinical and radiologic findings do not allow a differentiation from ulcerative colitis, coloscopy with biopsy should be employed to settle the issue. This will help in planning a therapeutic regimen and in assessing the prognosis.

Complications: gastrointestinal bleeding, perforations, stenoses, ileus, fistulas, abscesses.

Diagnosis: clinical findings, proctoscopy, radiologic studies, coloscopy with biopsy.

Differential diagnosis: idiopathic ulcerative colitis, diverticulitis, carcinoma; rarely intestinal tuberculosis and radiation colitis.

References

1. Cooke, W.T., Brooke, B.N.: Non-specific enterocolitis. Quart. J. Med. **24**, 1 (1955).
2. Crohn, B.B., Yarnis, H.: Regional ileitis. New York: Grune and Stratton 1958.
3. Demling, L.: Entzündliche Erkrankungen des Dickdarmes. Langenbecks Arch. Chir. **319**, 326 (1967).
4. Frühmorgen, P.: Diagnosis of inflammatory diseases of the colon by coloscopy. Acta gastro-ent. belg. **37**, 154 (1974).
5. Gjone, E., Orning, O.M., Myren, J.: Crohn's disease in Norway 1956–1963. Gut **7**, 372 (1966).
6. Goligher, J.F., de Dombal, F.T., Burton, I.: Crohn's disease with special reference to surgical management. In: Progress in surgery, Vol. 10. Basel: Karger 1972.
7. Grözinger, K.-H., Wenz, W., Krupka, I.: Ileitis terminalis und Colitis ulcerosa Münch. med. Wschr. **12**, 649 (1967).
8. Hafter, E.: Praktische Gastroenterologie, 4. Aufl. Stuttgart: Thieme 1970.
9. Hinslop, J.G., Grant, A.K.: Genetic tendency in Crohn's disease. Gut **10**, 994 (1969).
10. Janowitz, H.D., Present, D.H.: Granulomatous colitis, pathogenetic concepts. Gastroenterology **51**, 779 (1966).
11. Johnes, J.H.: Colonic cancer and Crohn's disease. Gut **10**, 651 (1969).
12. Kasper, H.: Klinik und Therapie der Enteritis regionalis (M. Crohn). Dtsch. med. Wschr. **87**, 811 (1972).
13. Krauspe, C., Müller-Wieland, K., Stelzner, F.: Colitis ulcerosa und granulomatosa. München, Berlin, Wien: Urban u. Schwarzenberg 1972.

14. Kümmerle, F., Schier, J.: Enteritis regionalis und Proktocolitis. Chirurg **10**, 437 (1968).
15. Lockhart-Mummery, H.E., Morson, B.C.: Crohn's disease of the large intestine. Gut **5**, 493 (1964).
16. Morson, B.C.: Pathologisch-anatomische Veränderungen des Dickdarmes und der Analregion bei Crohn'scher Erkrankung. Z. Gastroent. **2**, 255 (1964).
17. Morson, B.C.: Histopathology of Crohn's disease. Scand. J. Gastroent. **6**, 573 (1971).
18. Norlen, B.J., Krause, U., Bergman, L.: An epidemiological study of Crohns disease. Scand. J. Gastroent. **5**, 385 (1970).
19. Patter, W.N., van, Bargen, J.A., Dokkerty, M.B., Feldmann, W.H., Mayr, C.W., Wangh, J.M.: Regional enteritis. Gastroenterology **26**, 347 (1954).
20. Vandenbroucke, J., Vantrappen, G., Tytgat, G., Ruttgerts, L., Ponette, E.: Die Ileocolitis Crohn. Internist (Berl.) **9**, 335 (1968).
21. Widmaier, F., Heinkel, K.: Enteritis regionalis (Morbus Crohn). Z. Gastroent. **7**, 174 (1969).
22. Yamase, K., Masuda, K., Shimada, S.: Regional enteritis in Japan. A review of 548 cases. Int. Surg. **47**, 497 (1967).
23. Zeitler, H., Classen, M.: Morbus Crohn: Verlauf und Prognose. Fortschr. Med. **89**, 1333 (1971).

Rare Diseases

On rare occasions, decrease in the arterial blood supply leads to the clinical picture of *Ischemic Colitis*. This disease affects mainly elderly females and is manifested by acute abdominal pain, bleeding per rectum and diarrhea and, occasionally, by nausea and vomiting. The colon segment involved, usually the splenic flexure or the sigmoid, shows hemorrhagic mucosa with extensive pseudomembranes. The necrosis may be transmural in which case impending perforation dictates segemental resection. Lesser degrees of necrosis are more common and will go on to spontaneous healing with or without development of a fibrous stenosis. Coloscopy is contraindicated during the acute stage.

Radiation Proctitis following radiation therapy especially of pelvic cancer and abdominal lymphoma is rarely seen in the setting of an internist's practice. Early changes are mucosal edema and epithelial alterations; mucosal bleeding, increasing fibrosis with stricture formation (Fig. 262) and fistulization occur later. Radiation colitis, frequently with coexistent radiation ileitis and multiple fistulas, can become life-threatening and may require extensive resections. The involved tissue is very friable and coloscopy should probably be avoided.

Tuberculosis of the Colon has become extremely rare in the wake of the introduction of tuberculostatic medications and the elimination of bovine tuberculosis. We observed one patient who displayed ulcerating and hyperplastic alterations of the mucosa in the ileocoecal area.

Actinomycosis, Lues, and Lymphogranuloma Inguinale of the colon are equally rare and will not be discussed further.

4.8.4 Diverticula

Diverticula are pouches of the intestinal wall. The wall of true diverticula contains all layers of the colonic wall. More frequent are the so-called false or acquired diverticula where the muscular layer is absent (mucosal hernias) (Figs. 264, 265). The incidence rises with advancing age. Most diverticula are found in the sigmoid but they may arise anywhere in the colon. Acquired diverticula are the result of raised intraluminal pressure pushing the mucosa through the muscle layer in areas where mechanical resistance is diminished due to penetrating blood vessels.

Diverticula with narrow necks can easily be missed endoscopically and need to be demonstrated by the radiologist. In cases where diverticula and polyps coexist, differentiation frequently becomes difficult because some diverticula cannot be projected in profile to demonstrate their extraluminal location (Fig. 210c). Coloscopy can resolve this issue and is further indicated in situations where subacute or chronic diverticulitis with narrowing of the lumen is suspected.

Diverticulosis *per se* is not a disease. Its

complications, however, such as diverticulitis, bleeding, perforation, penetration, peritonitis, obstruction and fistulization may be life-threatening [3]. The degree of symptoms rarely correlates with the extent of involvement.

Active diverticulitis occurs in 12–17 percent of patients with diverticulosis [1, 2] and is a contraindication to coloscopy because of the danger of perforation. After the acute symptoms have subsided under appropriate therapy, coloscopy may underestimate the extent of the acute disease. The endoscopist can only report thickening and rigidity of the segments involved by the inflammatory process (Fig. 265). In cases where diagnostic clarification is urgent, the patient should be minimally prepared and residual fecal matter can be irrigated away during the coloscopic procedure.

Chronic diverticulits results in thickening of the colonic wall and, frequently, in marked stenosis and obstruction which may be very difficult to differentiate from a stenosing carcinoma and from Crohn's disease [4]. Coloscopic biopsies of affected areas are hard to obtain when the instrument tip cannot be advanced into progressively stenosed areas. Nonetheless, preoperative diagnosis by endoscopic biopsy is particularly important in this situation because carcinoma of the colon and chronic diverticulitis may produce identical symptoms, can rarely be differentiated with certainty by the radiologist and because both diseases may be present in the same patient.

Differential diagnosis: Carcinoma, Crohn's colitis, ulcerative colitis, tuberculosis of the colon, nonspecific inflammatory stenosis; during acute involvement of the cecal area by Crohn's disease, differentiate from acute appendicitis.

Referenes

1. Hafter, E.: Sigmadivertikulose medizinisches oder chirurgisches Problem? Helv. chir. Acta **24**, 476 (1957).
2. Horner, J.L.: Natural history of the diverticulosis of the colon. Amer. J. dig. Dis. **3**, 343 (1958).
3. Pross, E.: Die rezidivierende Diverticulitis coli Indikation zur Operation. Z. Gastroent. **9**, 594 (1971).
4. Schmidt, G.T., Lennard-Jones, J.E., Morson, B.C., Young, A.C.: Crohn's disease of the colon and its distinction from diverticulitis. Gut **9**, 7 (1968).

4.8.5 Endometriosis

Endometriosis affects the colon in 10–25 percent of cases [1, 2]. Aside from the occasional periodicity of symptoms (pain, intestinal bleeding), this disease frequently cannot be differentiated from a malignant colon tumor on clinical grounds alone. Barium enema reveals polypoid lesions which, again, do not allow the exclusion of carcinoma or inflammatory stenosis. Endoscopic biopsy of the submucosal lesions, performed shortly before, during or after the menses, is the diagnostic method of choice. The lesions of endometriosis should not, however, be removed endoscopically but rather be excised by the surgeon [3, 4].

In cases where the lesions are located deep in the colonic wall, biopsies will be negative and the endoscopist only sees a deformation of the mucosal surface.

References

1. Erdi, A., Köves, I., Földvari, G., Baranyai, L., Lövey, G.: Endometriosis in the large intestine. Recent progress in the study of disorders of the colon and rectum. Edited by S.S. Drobni and M. Fehér, Budapest 1970.
2. Röhrer, H.D., Grözinger, K.H.: Endometriosis of the rectum. Recent progress in the study of disorders of the colon and rectum. Edited by S. Drobni and M. Fehér. Budapest 1970.
3. Röher, H.-D.: Diagnostik der Dickdarm-Endometriose. Dtsch. med. Wschr. **98**, 1408 (1973).
4. Röher. H.-D., Grözinger, K.H.: Zur Klinik, Diagnostik und Therapie der Dickdarm-Endometriose. Med. Welt Stuttg. N.F. **24**, 534 (1973).

4.8.6 Melanosis coli

Melanosis coli (Fig. 263) is a noninflammatory mucosal alteration without direct clinical significance. It occurs in patients who are chronic users of anthraquinone-containing laxatives. Clumps of brown pigment (melanin) are deposited in histiocytes and in the extracellular spaces of the submucosa. The intensity of this reticular pigmentation differs in the various segments of the colon. We have gained the impression that it is particularly heavy in the proximal colon where the mucosa may show a diffusely dark-brown to black discoloration.

4.8.7 Megacolon

Megacolon represents congenital or acquired dilatation affecting parts of or the entire colon.

Congenital megacolon, first described by HIRSCHSPRUNG in 1887 [1, 2], manifests itself at birth or shortly thereafter by obstipation and abdominal distention. The pathologic substrate is the absence of parasympathetic ganglion cells in Auerbach's and Meissner's plexus. The aganglionic segment is usually limited to the rectum and distal sigmoid. The diagnosis rests on clinical and radiologic findings and on the results of rectal biopsy; coloscopy, especially in newborns, is rarely necessary.

Symptomatic or organic megacolon is the result of incomplete mechanical obstruction. It usually is caused by slowly developing benign strictures but may occur with obstructing carcinomas.

The etiology of the idiopathic or functional megacolon is heterogeneous. No stenosis or aganglionic segment is present.

References

1. HIRSCHSPRUNG, H.: Stuhlträgheit Neugeborener infolge von Dilatation und Hypertrophie des Kolons. Jb. Kinderheilk. **27**, 1 (1887).
2. HIRSCHSPRUNG, H.: Erweiterung und Hypertrophie des Dickdarms. Berl. klin. Wschr. **36**, 977 (1899).

4.8.8 Enteric Parasites

Worm infestations play no important role in coloscopy.

Trichiuris trichiura was detected accidentally in the cecum of two patients (Fig. 266a). While ova had already been found in the stool of one patient, none were detected on three occasions in the stool of the other, who suffered from vague abdominal distress. The clinical relevance of this parasitosis is debated and appears to depend on the intensity of the infestation. The worms are up to 50 mm long and 1–2 mm wide and reside in the distal small intestine and proximal colon. A filiform whip, roughly two-thirds as long as the entire parasite, lends it a characteristic appearance. This structure penetrates the mucosa and serves to feed the parasite (Fig. 266b). The whiplashtype motions which were observed by us are not caused by this filiform structure but rather by the thickened posterior part of the worm which protrudes into the lumen. Massive infestation may lead to inflammatory tumors of the cecum and the symptoms of colitis with diarrhea and anemia. The parasite is acquired in tropical and subtropical regions by swallowing egg-containing larvae. Mixed infestations by several parasites are frequent.

4.8.9 Appendix

Direct inspection of the appendiceal lumen is not yet possible for technical reasons. Indirect visualization has to be resorted to when indicated. Even the normal appendix is not regularly demonstrated during barium enema examination. We have, therefore, attempted to fill the appendix selectively through a teflon catheter introduced through the coloscope (Figs. 185–187). The rare indications for this approach consist of suspected carcinoid, carcinoma, foreign body or endometriosis of the appendix.

4.9 Complications

Isolated reports of complications of coloscopy have appeared although none have occurred in our personal experience.

Perforation

Perforations [2] may occur in the presence of a diseased colon (ulcerations, malignant tumors, diverticulitis, colitis), during blind introduction of the instrument, especially in the sigmoid and the colon flexures, and with forced air insufflation into diseased areas. It follows that all manipulations of the instrument tip should be performed under constant visual control. When the lumen is not in view, blanching of the mucosa sliding past the lens is a signal of impending perforation. When mucosal tears are encountered, water-soluble contrast material may be injected under fluoroscopic control but plain films of the abdomen should be obtained in any case in search of free intraabdominal air. Therapy consists of immediate surgical repair.

Bleeding

Bleeding may result from polypectomy, biopsy, or iatrogenic injury of friable mucosa. Minor bleeding after forceps biopsy is of no significance. We have not observed severe bleeding because the commercially available biopsy forceps do not allow penetration beyond the submucosal layer. Polypectomy will be followed by bleeding when the stalk is partly or completely severed by mechanical force without effective electrocoagulation. Most of these bleeding episodes subside spontaneously. Therapy limited to the instillation of vasoconstricting agents on the bleeding surface is thwarted by the fact that the agent is washed away by the emerging blood. Electrocoagulation of bleeding sites is currently under investigation and cannot yet be recommended for general use. Operative intervention is indicated when bleeding persist.

Gas Explosion

Isolated reports exist of gas explosions during polypectomy with high frequency diathermy current [1, 3, 4, 5]. This risk can be eliminated by replacing the methane-oxygen mixture present in the colon by insufflation of an inert gas such as carbon dioxide. Thorough cleansing of the colon alone will reduce this risk considerably.

References

1. BECKER, G.L.: Prevention of gas explosions in the large bowel during electrosurgery. Surg. Gynec. Obstet. **97**, 463 (1953).
2. FIELDING, J.F., LUMSDEN, K.: Large-bowel perforations in patients underjoing sigmoidoscopy and barium enema Brit. Med. J. **1**, 471 (1973).
3. GALLEY, A.H.: Combustible gases generated in alimentary tract and other hollow viscera and their relationship to explosions occurring during anesthesia. Brit. J. Anaesth. **26**, 189 (1954).
4. LEVY, E.I.: Explosions during lower bowel electrosurgery: method of prevention. Amer. Surg. **88**, 754 (1954).
5. TURELL, R., HALLER, J.D.: Adenomas of the colon and rectum. In: Diseases of the colon and anorectum (TURELL, R., Ed.), Vol. I. Philadelphia, London, Toronto: Saunders 1969.

5. Illustrations

Endoscopic Orientation in the Duodenum

1 Normal duodenal bulb

2 Superior duodenal flexure

3 Descending duodenum

4 Descending duodenum with papilla of Vater

Duodenal Peptic Lesions and Their Sequelae

5 Round duodenal ulcer

6 2 large duodenal ulcers (kissing ulcers)

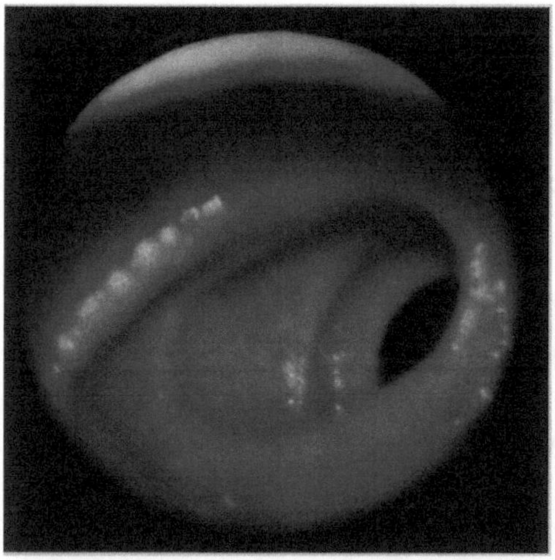

1

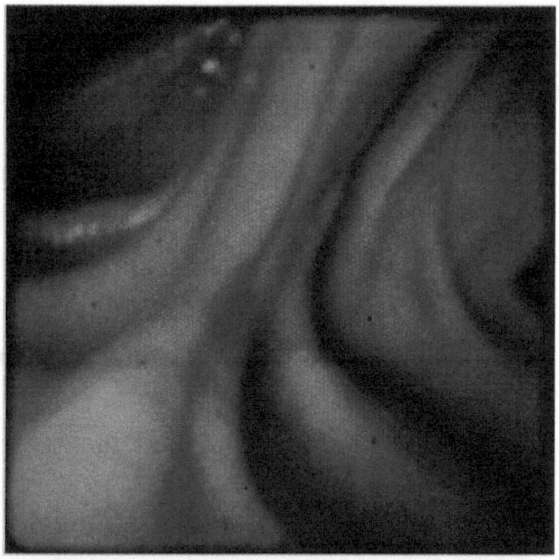

2

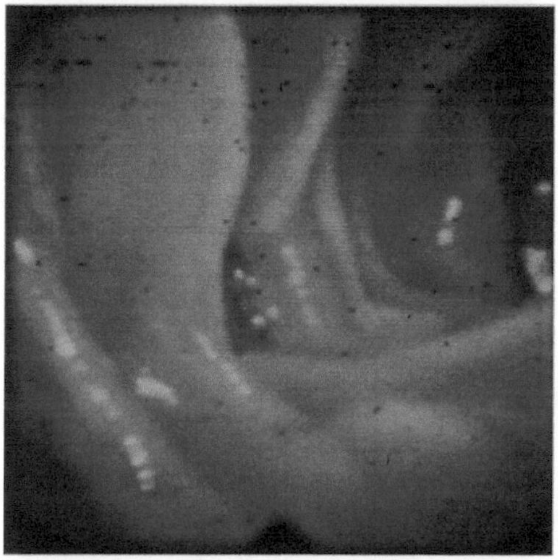

3

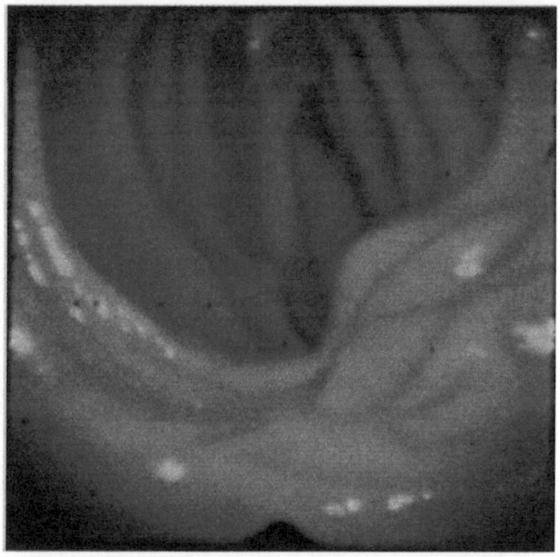

4

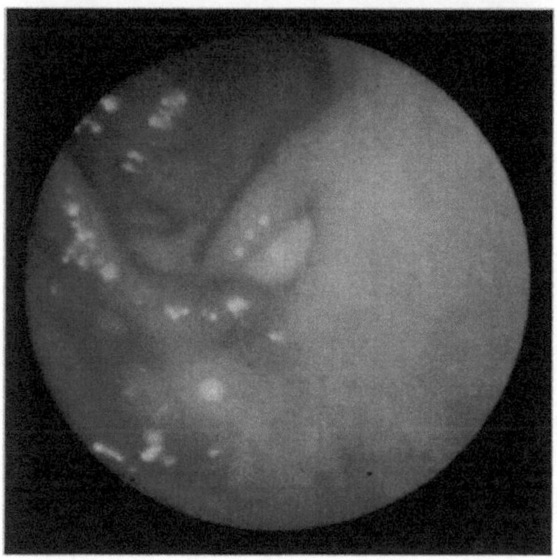

5

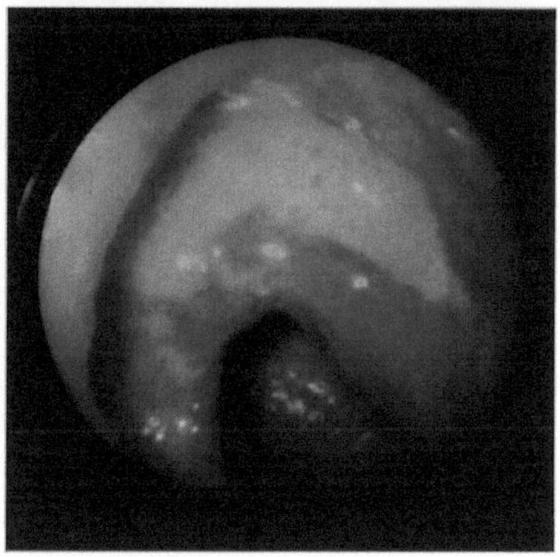

6

Duodenal Peptic Lesions and Their Sequelae (Continuation)

7 Florid duodenal ulcer with erythematous margin

8 Linear duodenal ulcer

9 "Salami" ulcer (healing duodenal ulcer)

10 Active duodenal ulcer in a scarred bulb

11 Healing duodenal ulcer

12 Bleeding duodenal ulcer

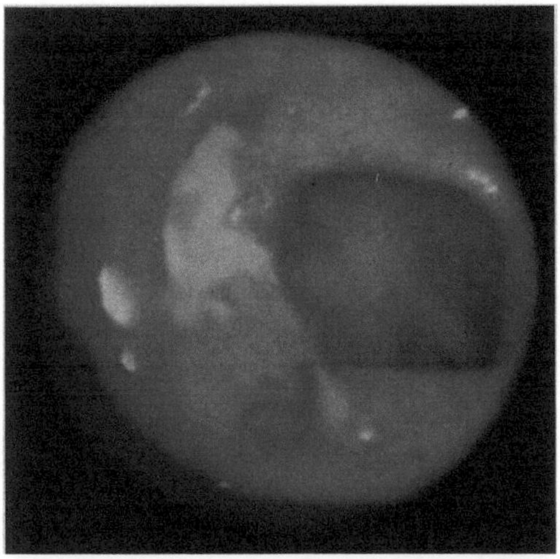
7

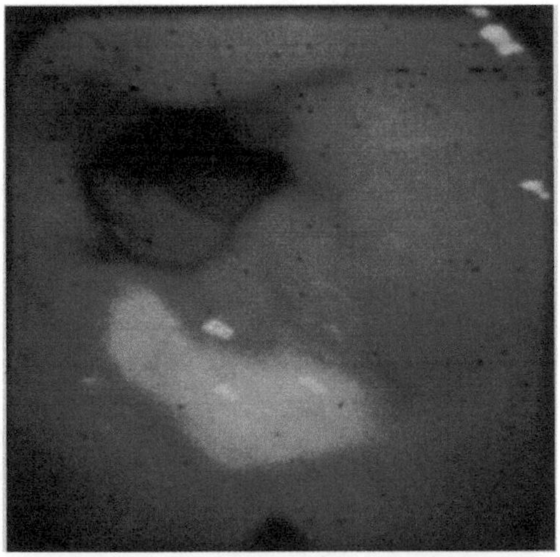
8

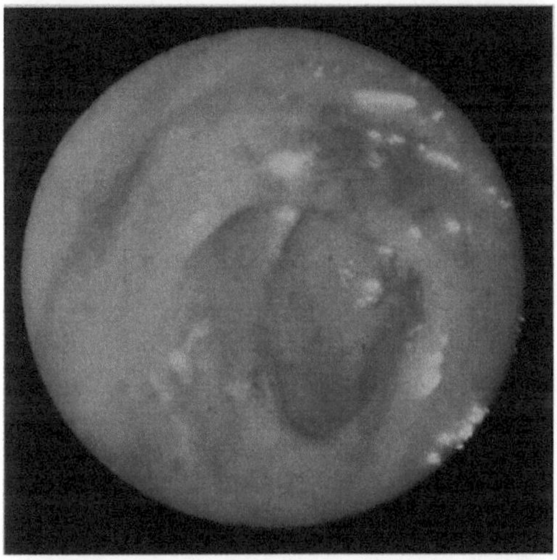
9

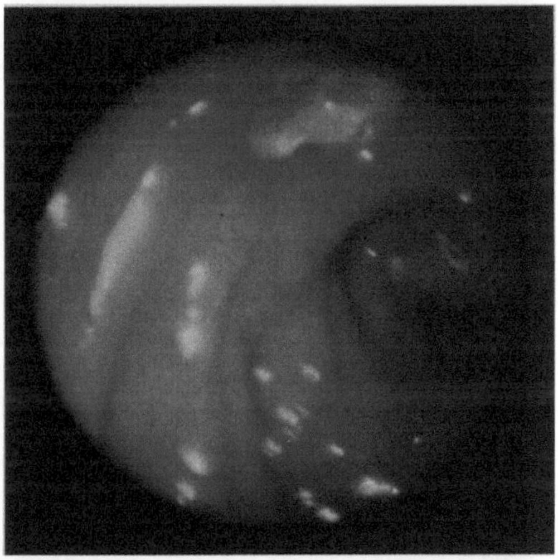
10

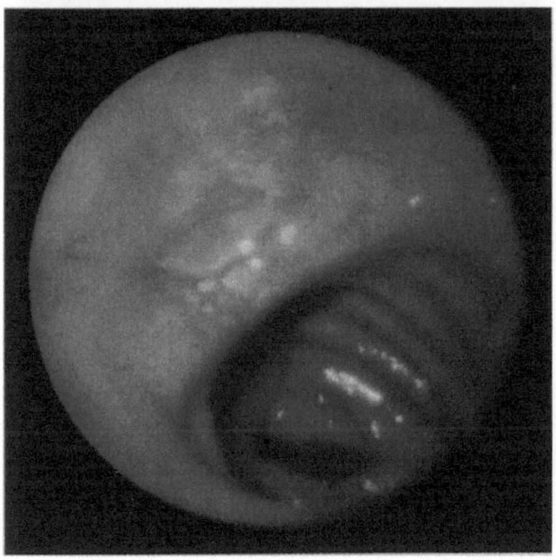
11

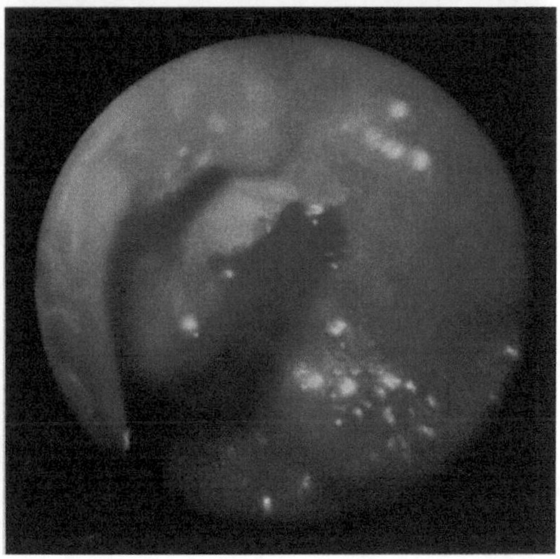
12

Duodenal Peptic Lesions and Their Sequelae (Continuation)

13 Bleeding duodenal ulcer

14 Erosions of the bulb

15 Erosions of the bulb

16 Scar of the bulb

17 Scarred bulb with scarred recesses and duodenal stenosis

Duodenitis

18 Hemorrhagic duodenitis

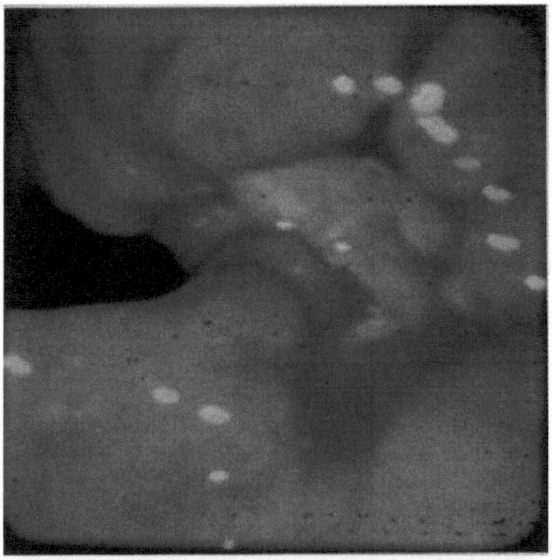

13

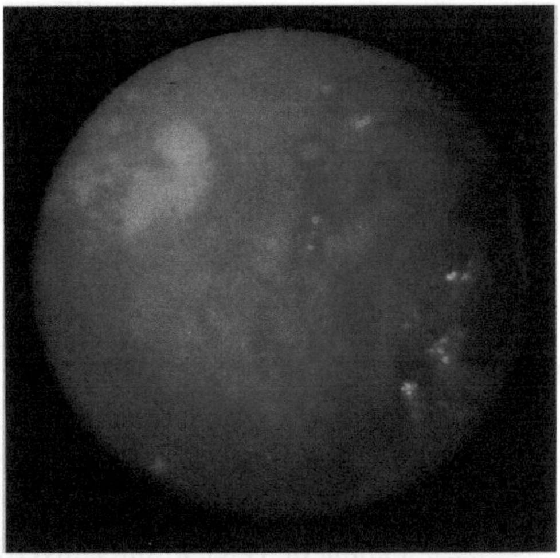

14

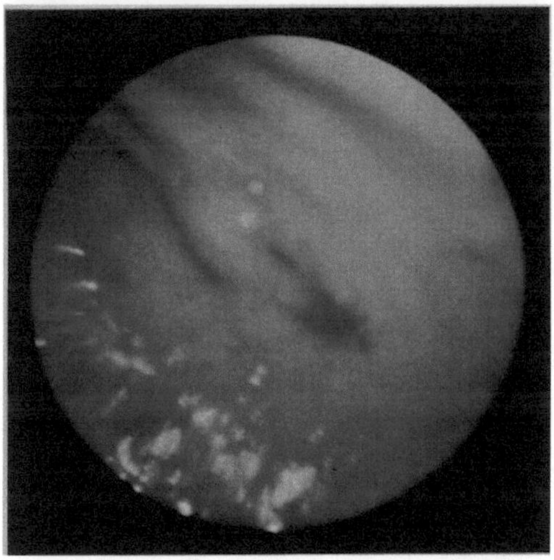

15

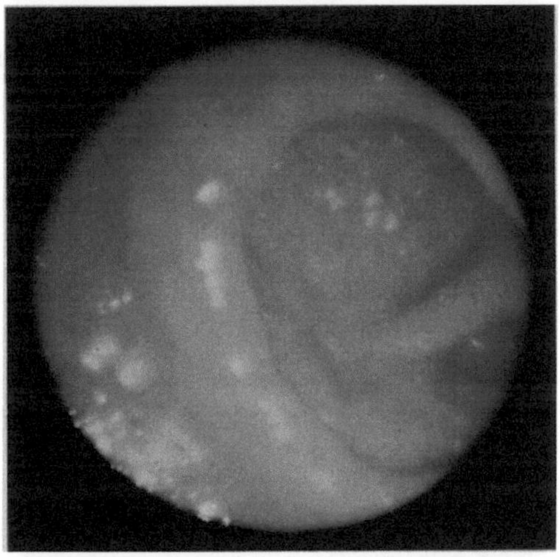

16

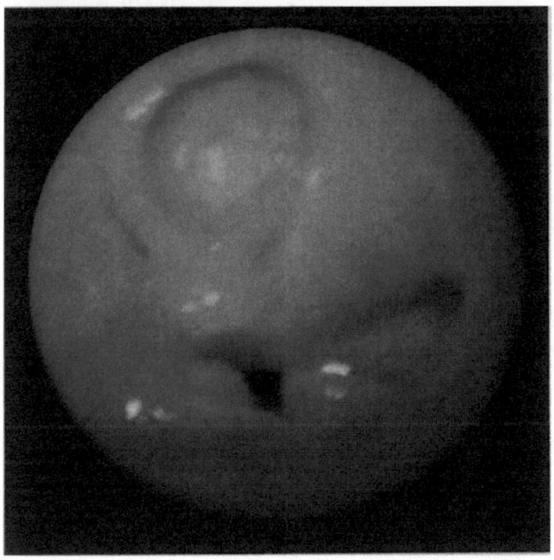

7

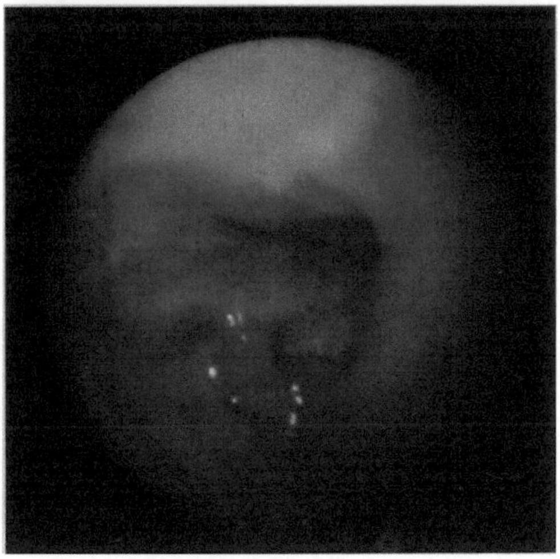

18

Duodenitis (Continuation)

19 Severe hemorrhagic duodenitis

20 Hemorrhagic duodenitis in the presence of mesenteric venous thrombosis

Diverticula

21 Duodenal diverticulum

22 Papilla of Vater within a diverticulum

23 Pancreatic and bile duct emptying into a diverticulum

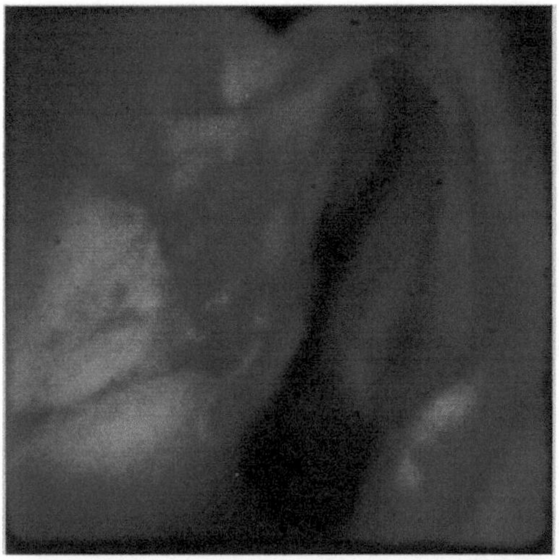
19

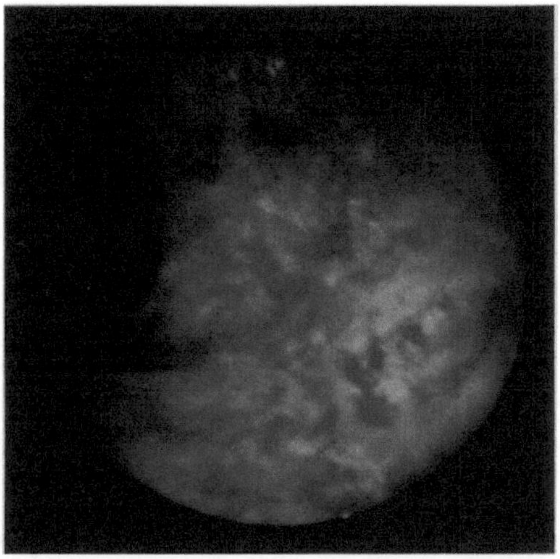
20

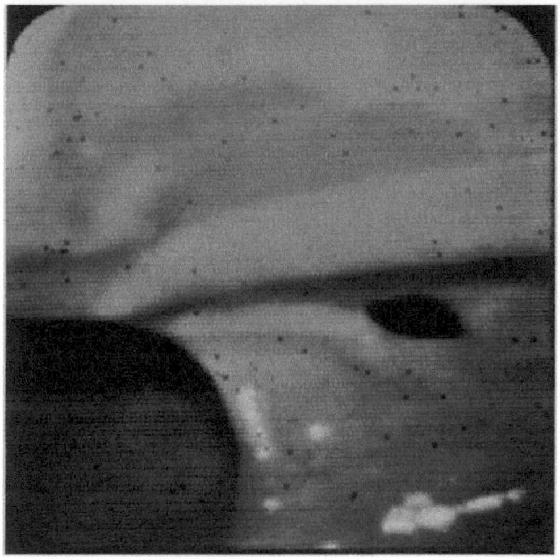
21

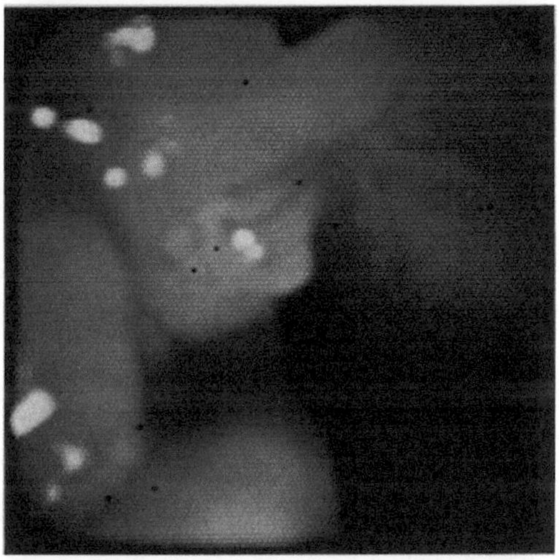
22

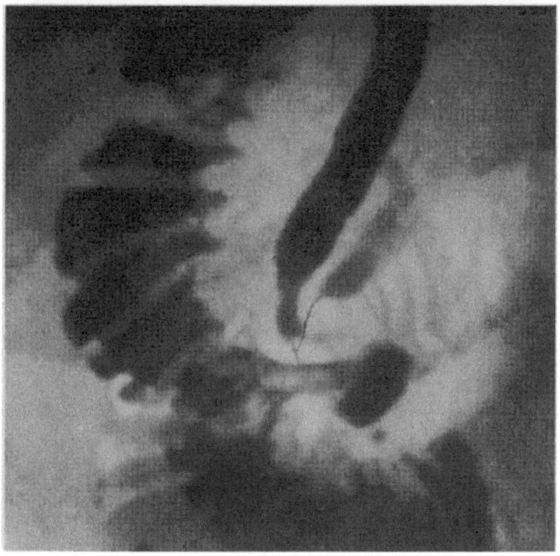
23

Tumors and Heterotopic Lesions

24 Radiologic appearance of adenomata of Brunner's glands

25 Endoscopic appearance of adenomata of Brunner's glands

26 Radiologic appearance of a duodenal polyp (lipoma)

27 Excised lipoma

28 Radiologic appearance of a duodenal tumor (neurofibroma)

29 Endoscopic appearance of the same tumor

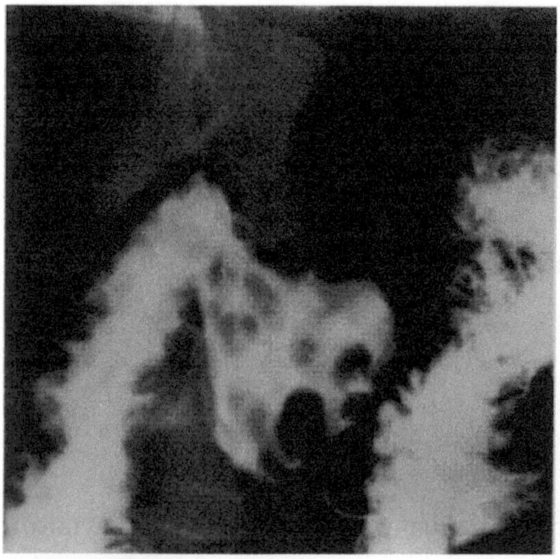
24

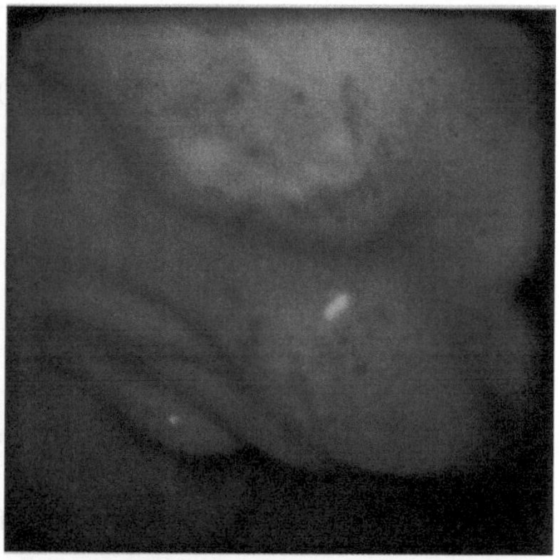
25

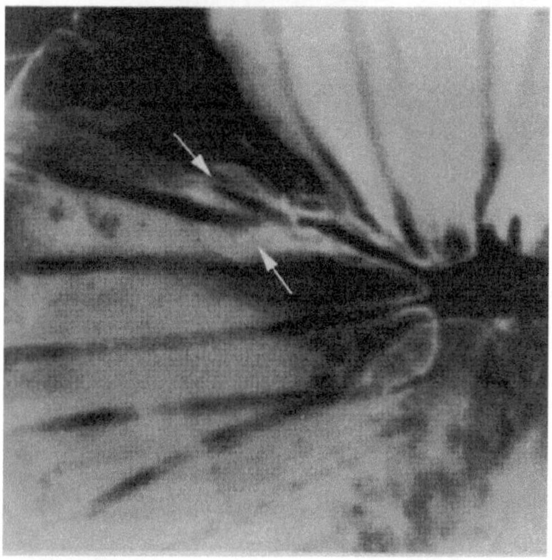
26

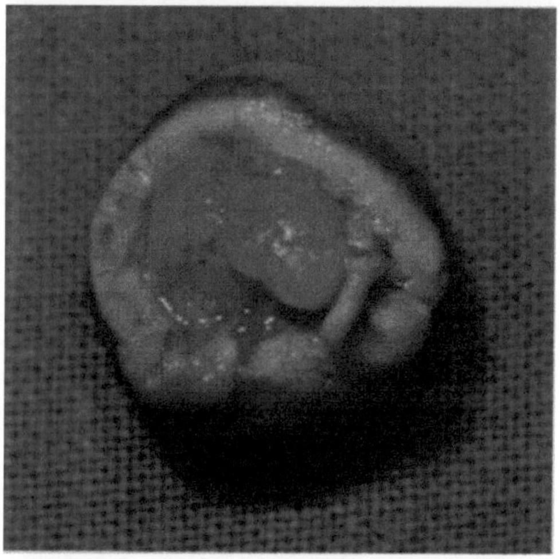
27

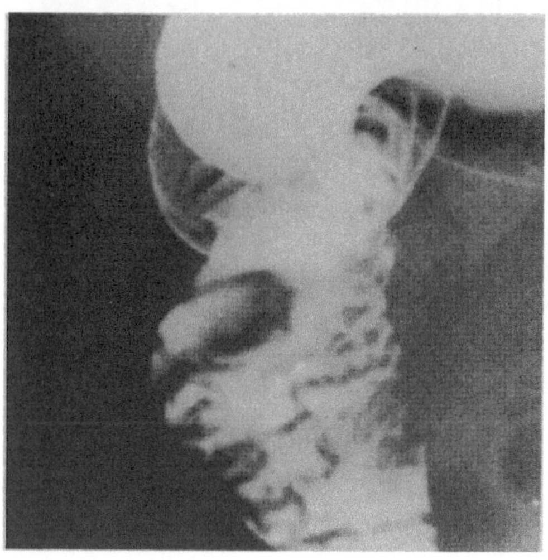
28

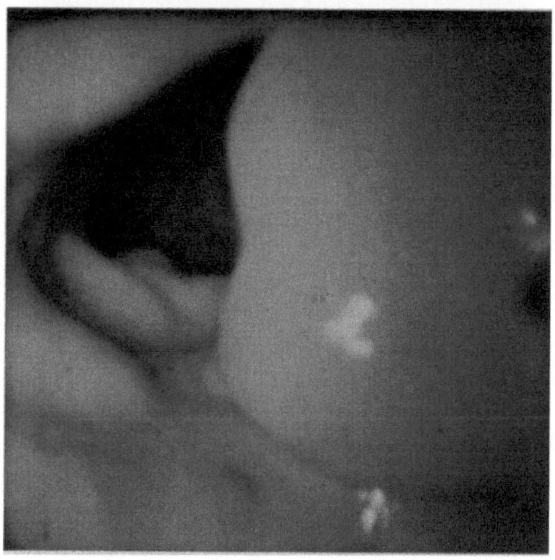
29

Tumors and Heterotopic Lesions (Continuation)

30 Duodenal polyp; Cronkhite-Canada syndrome

31 Histologic appearance of a Cronkhite-Canada polyp

32 Benign duodenal polyp

33 Retrieval of a duodenal polyp excised with the diathermy snare

34 Large duodenal polyp removed from a patient with the Peutz-Jeghers syndrome

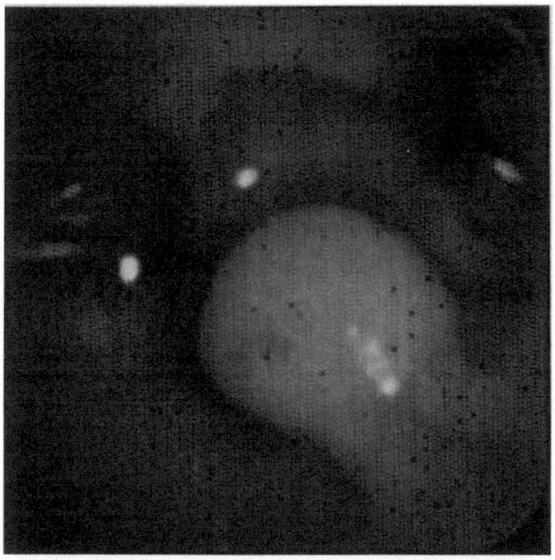
30

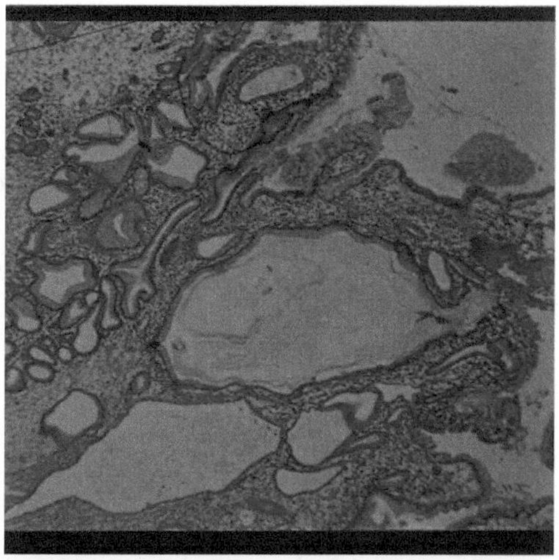
31

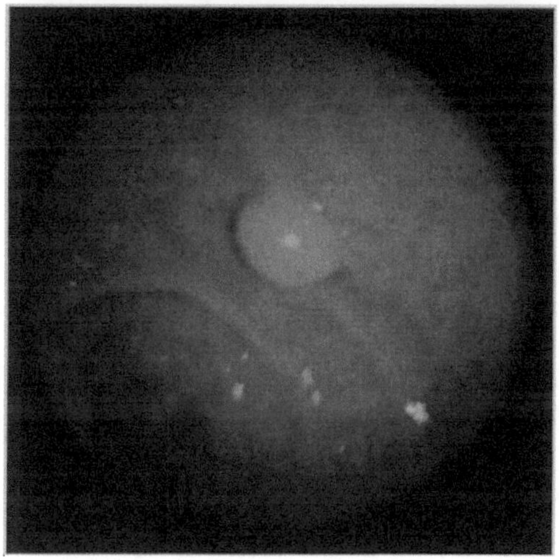
32

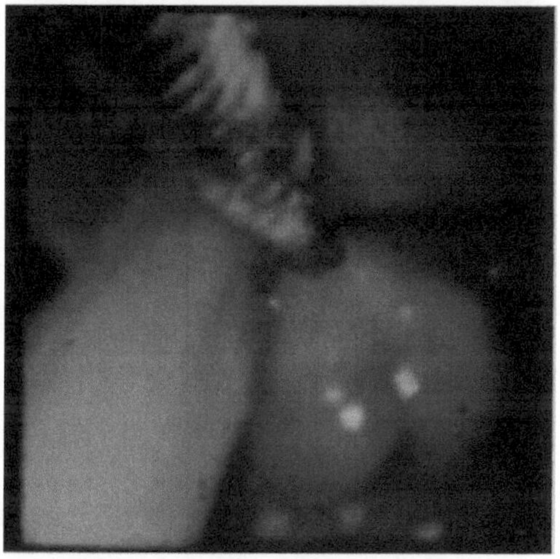
33

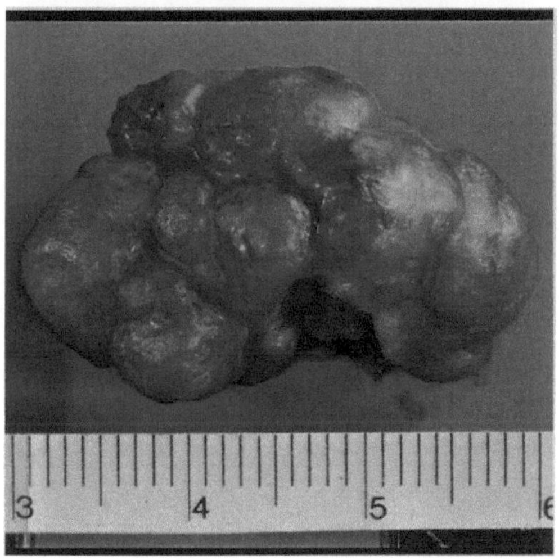

34

Tumors and Hetrotopic Lesions (Continuation)

35 Primary carcinoma of the duodenum

36 Penetrating carcinoma of the head of the pancreas

37 Duodenal sarcoma

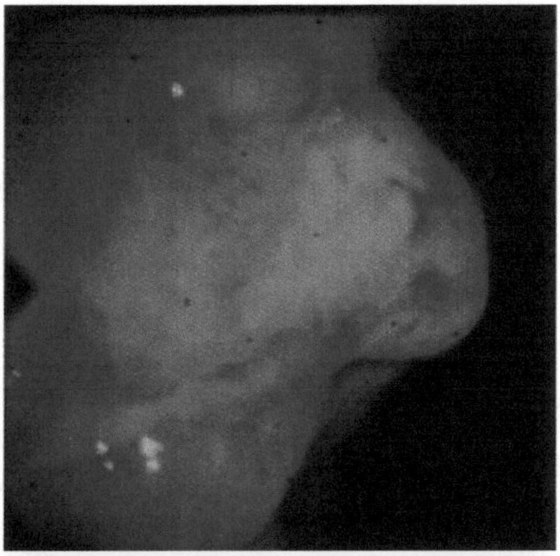

35

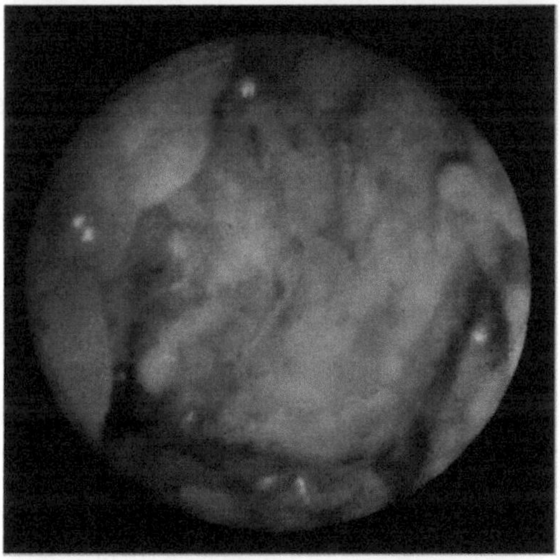

36

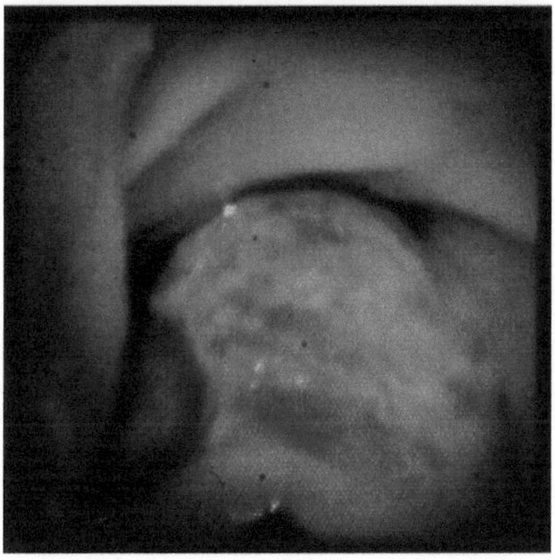

37

Afferent Loop Following Gastric Resection with Billroth II Anastomosis

38 Inverted suture line in an afferent loop following Billroth II anastomosis

39 Residual antral mucosa in the duodenal stump (courtesy of Professor ELSTER, Bayreuth, Germany)

Endoscopy of the Papilla of Vater

40 Demonstration of the papilla of Vater by double contrast method

41 Schematic drawing of the papilla of Vater (according to ELIAS)

42 Variations in the terminal course of the common bile and pancreatic ducts

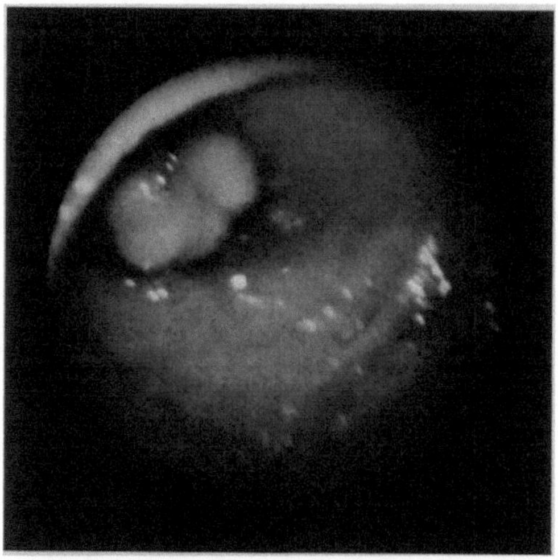

38

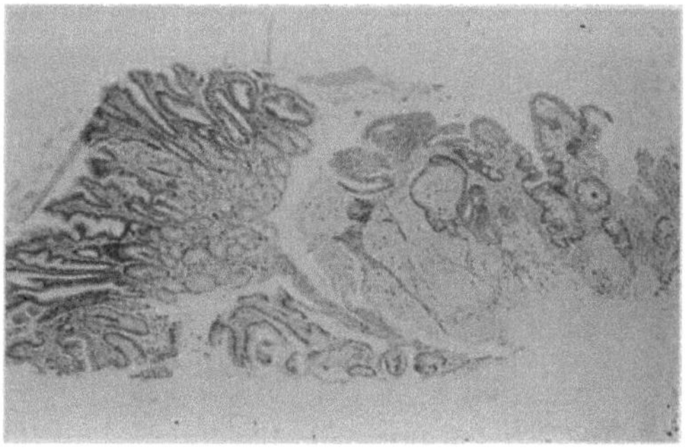

39

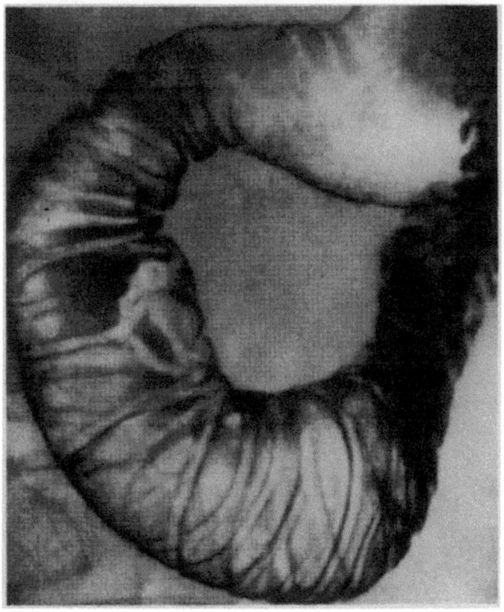

40

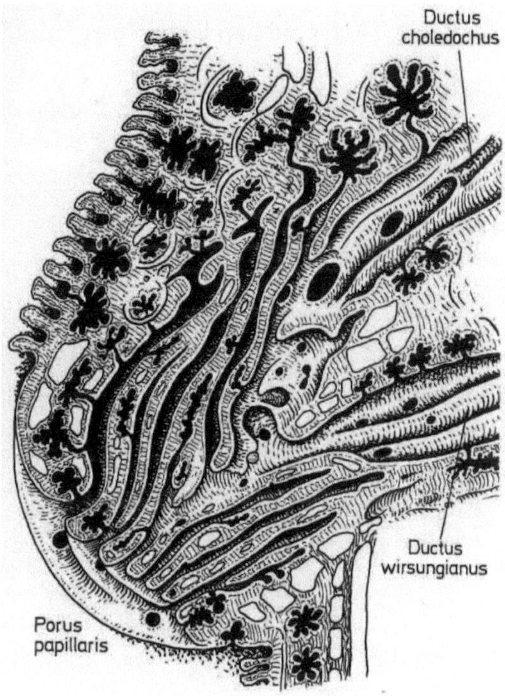
Ductus choledochus
Ductus wirsungianus
Porus papillaris

41

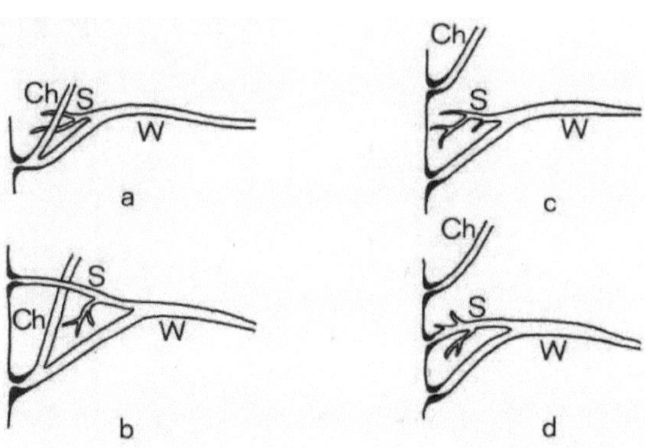
Ch
S
W
a
Ch
S
W
b
Ch
S
W
c
Ch
S
W
d

42

Endoscopy of the Papilla of Vater (Continuation)

43 Hemispheric papilla

44 Flat papilla

45 Prominent papilla located on the plica longitudinalis

46 Polypoid papilla of Vater

47 Papilla hidden behind folds

48 Papilla with 2 orifices

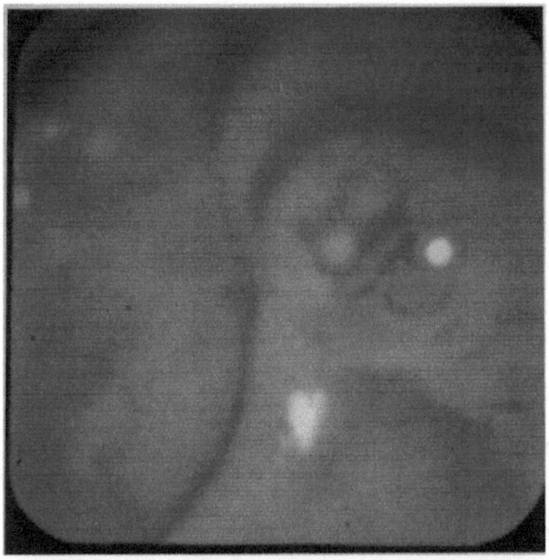
43

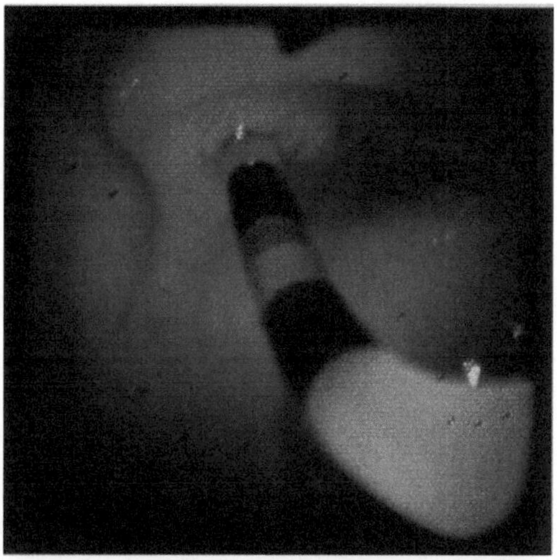
44

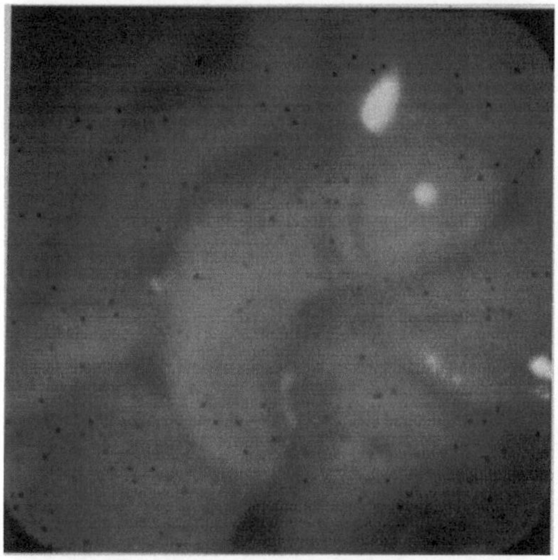
45

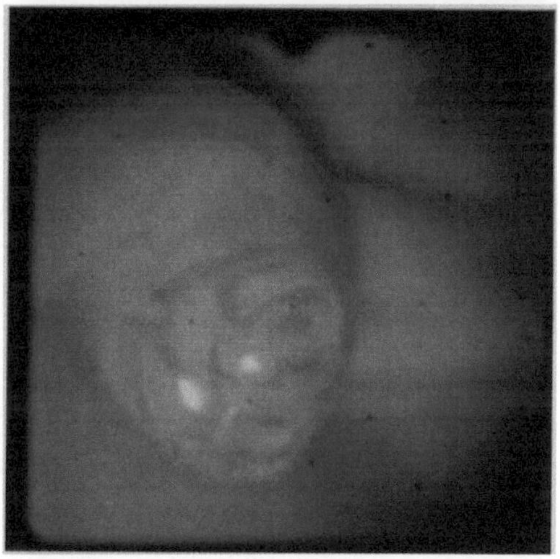
46

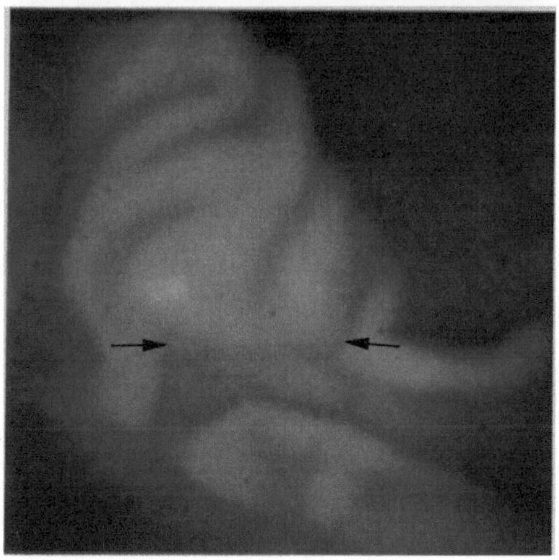
47

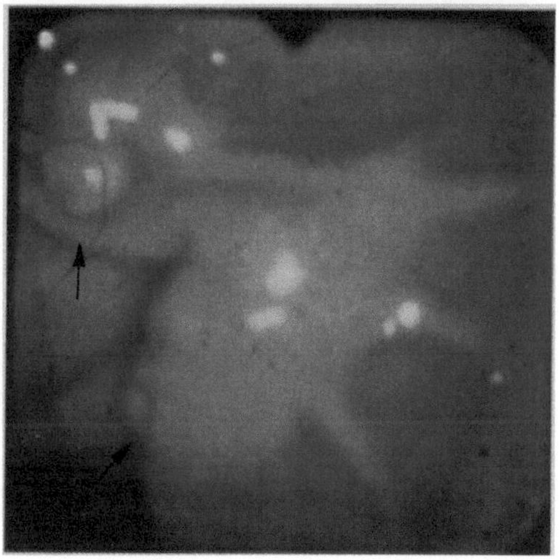
48

Endoscopy of the Papilla of Vater (Continuation)

49 Double papilla

50 Papilla major and minor

51 Papilla minor

52 Papilla of Vater distended by impacted concrement

53 Status post-papillotomy in the presence of 2 orifices

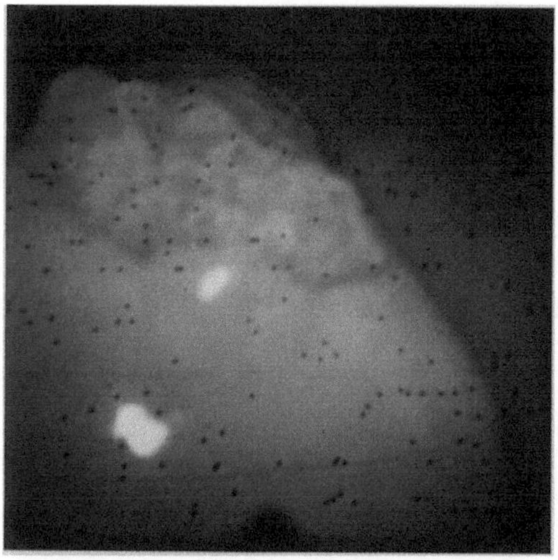

49

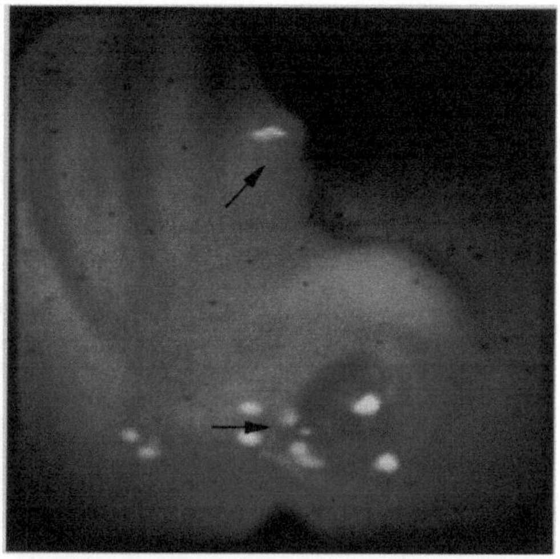

50

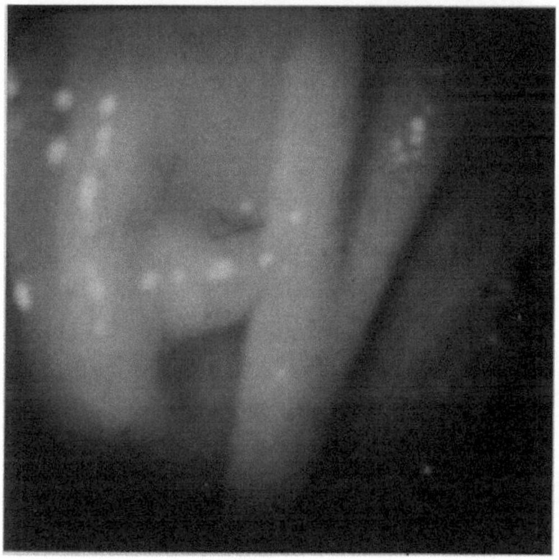

51

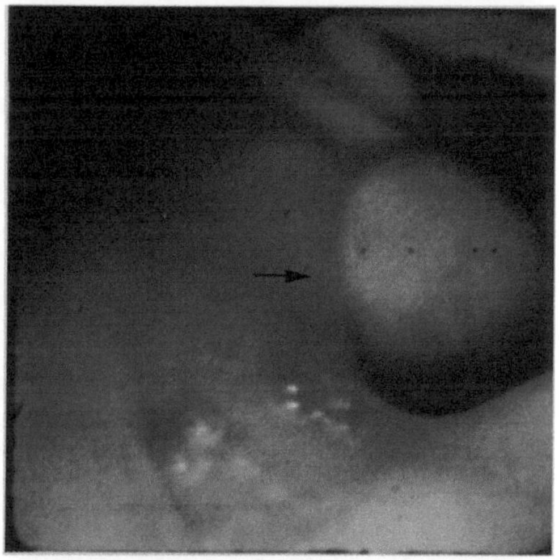

52

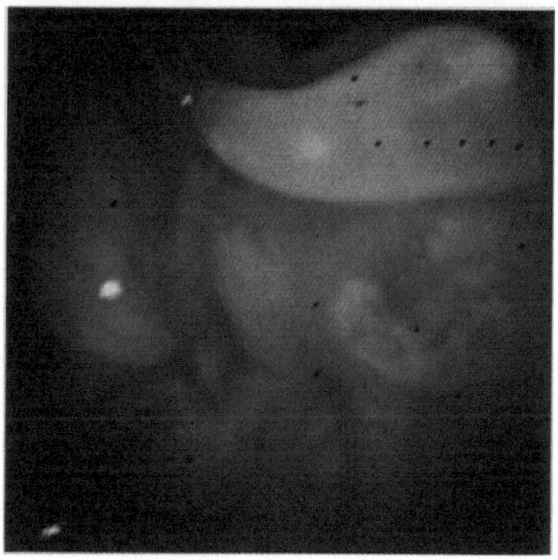

53

Endoscopy of the Papilla of Vater (Continuation)

54 Visualization of accessory pancreas and of choledochus in the presence of a pancreas divisum

55 Visualization of the main pancreas through the second orifice in the same patient (Fig. 54) with pancreas divisum

56 Papillary stenosis with prestenotic dilatation of the common bile ducts

57 Papillary stenosis with prestenotic dilatation of the common bile duct

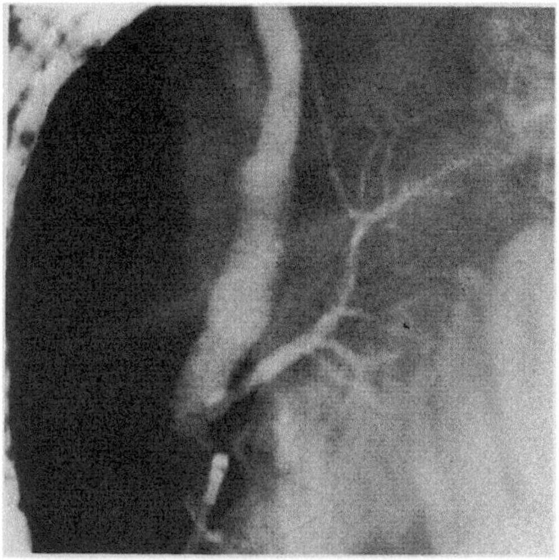
54

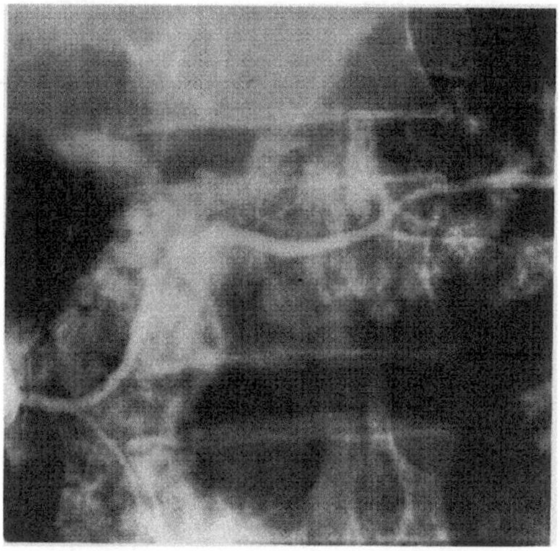
55

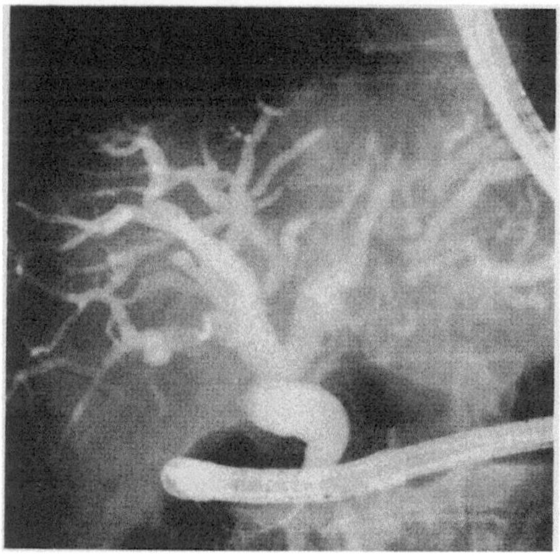
56

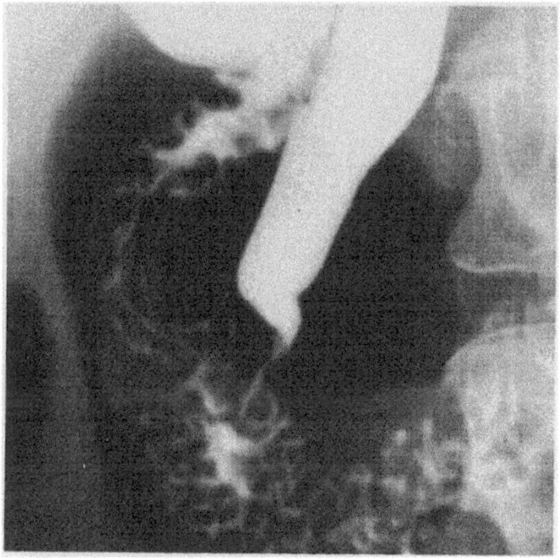
57

Endoscopy of the Papilla of Vater (Continuation)

58 Papillary stenosis with massive dilatation of the main pancreatic duct

59 Hydrops of the ampulla of Vater

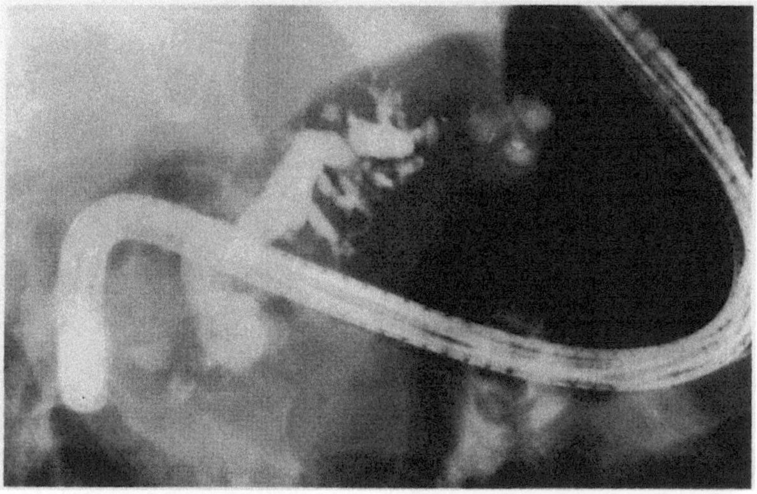
58

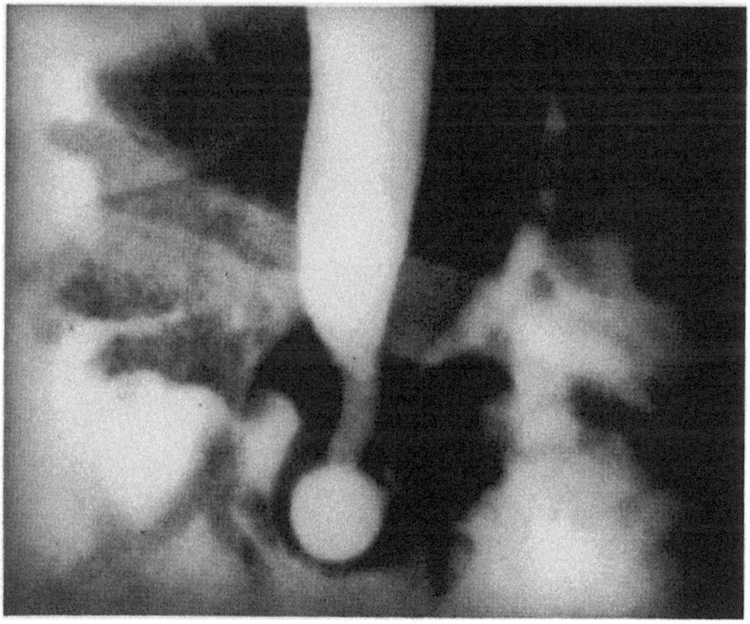
59

Endoscopy of the Papilla of Vater (Continuation)

60 Histologic appearance of sclerosis of the papilla

61 Histologic and endoscopic appearance of adenomyomatosis of the papilla of Vater

62 Histologic appearance of glandular hyperplasia of the papilla of Vater

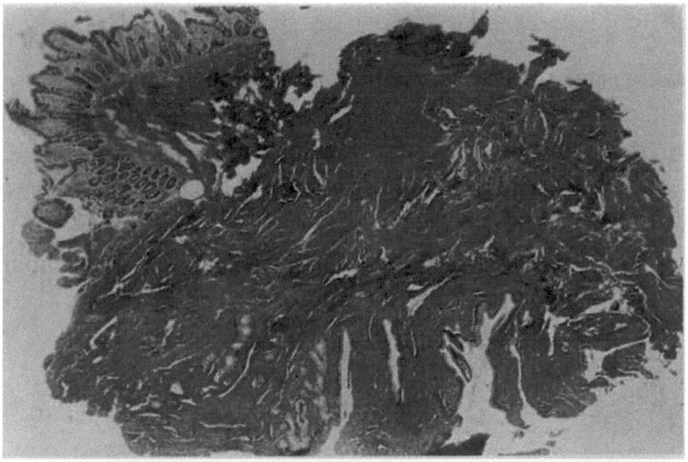
60

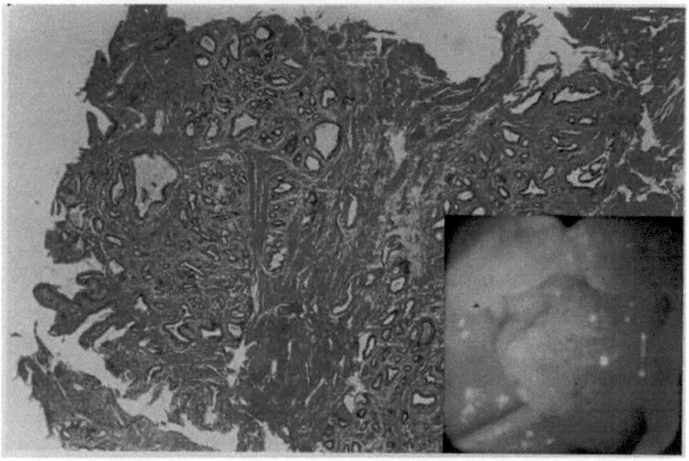
61

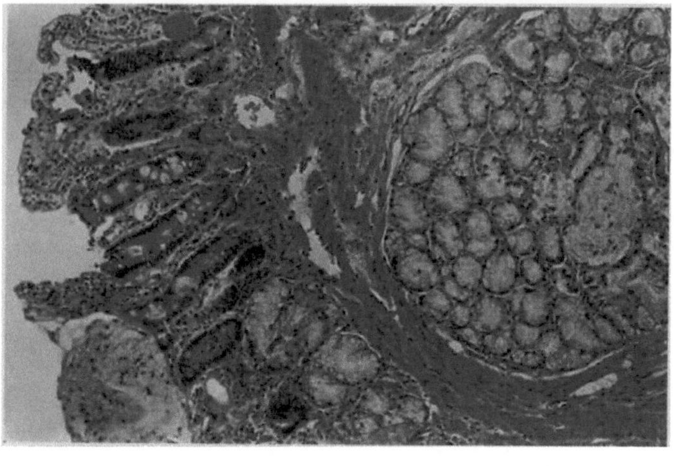
62

63 Massive dilatation of pancreatic duct system and moderate enlargement of bile ducts due to carcinoma of the ampulla of Vater

64 Histologic and endoscopic appearance of carcinoma of the papilla

65 Surgical specimen of carcinoma of the papilla

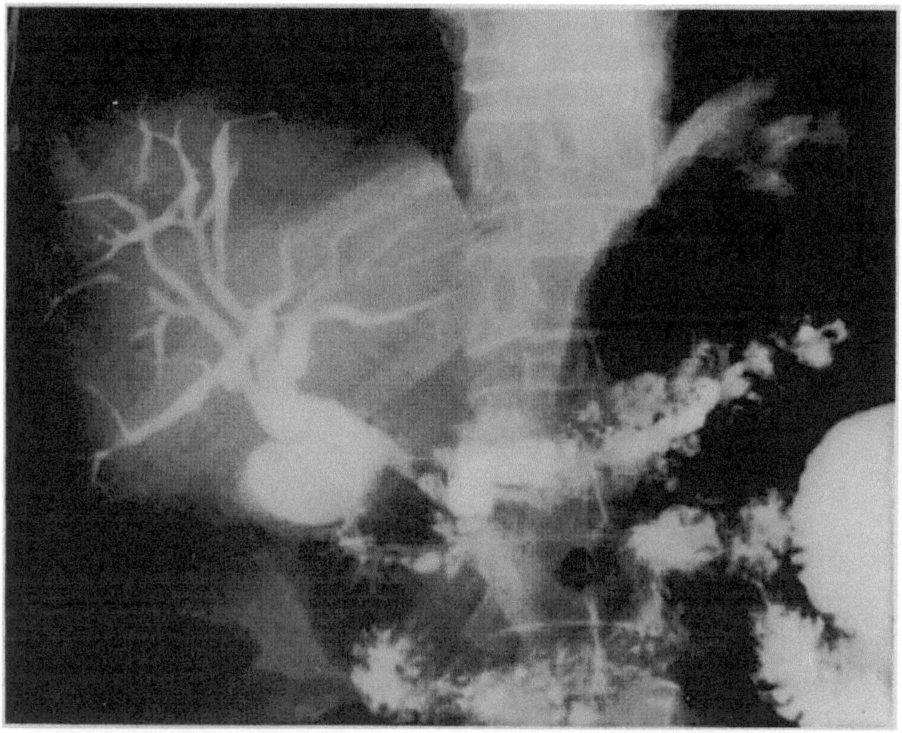
63

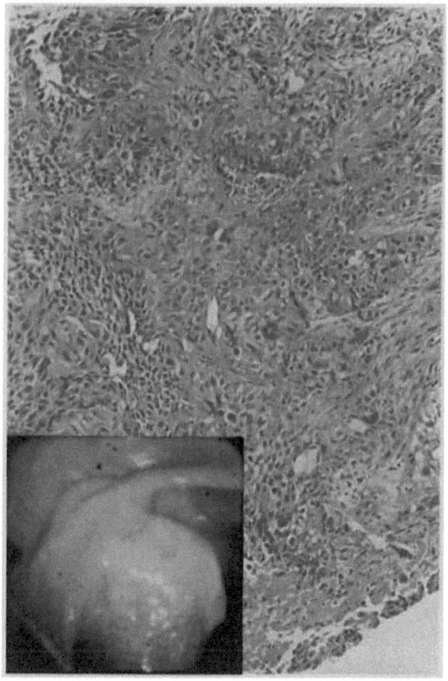
64

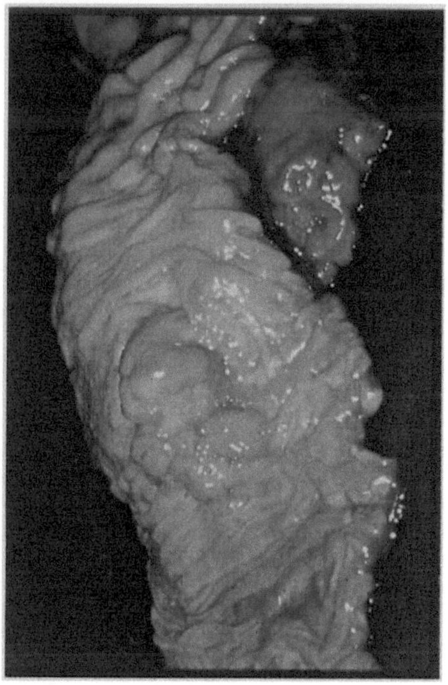
65

Retrograde Cholangiography

66 Normal cholangiopancreatogram

67 Cholelithiasis

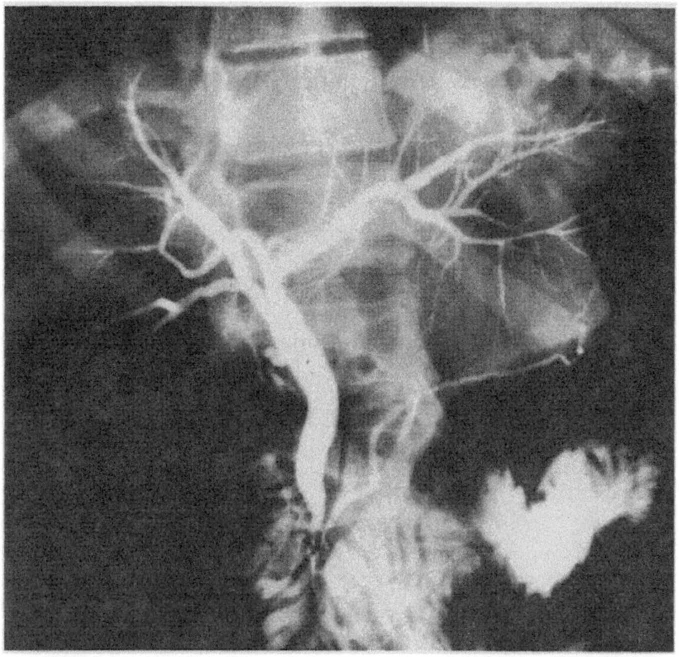

66

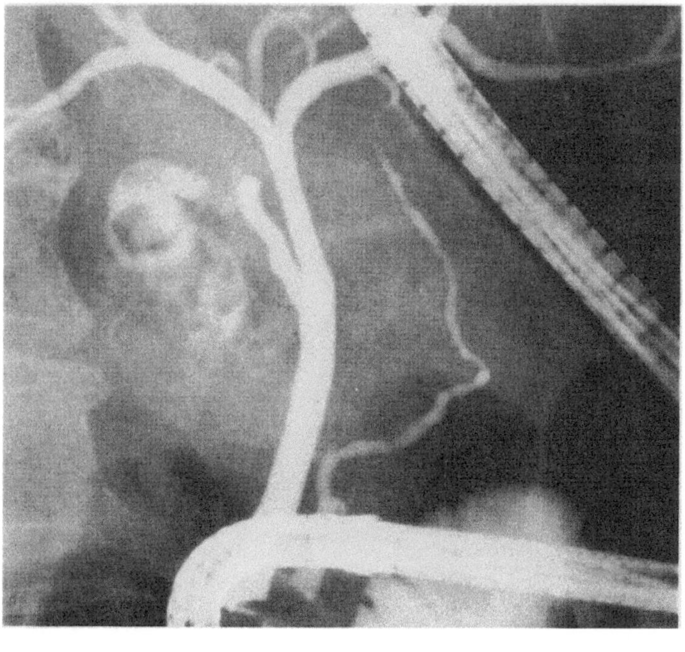

67

Retrograde Cholangiography (Continuation)

68 Cholelithiasis with choledocholithiasis

69 Cholelithiasis in the presence of stenosis of the papilla of Vater (abdominal position)

70 Large concrements and dilatation of the common bile duct

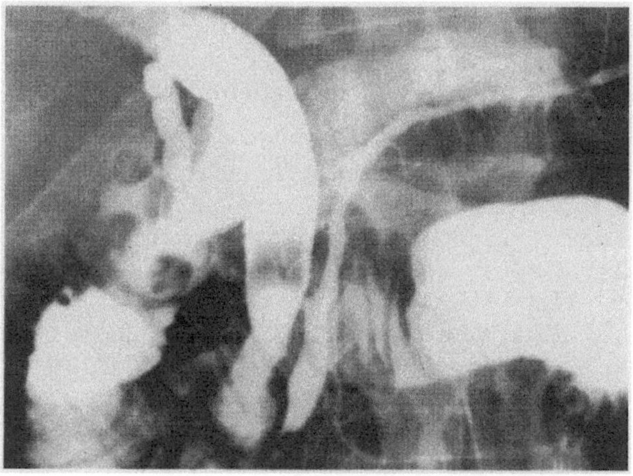

68

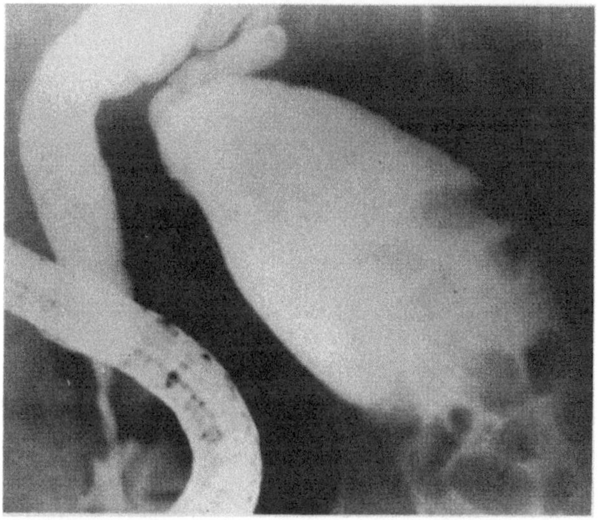

69

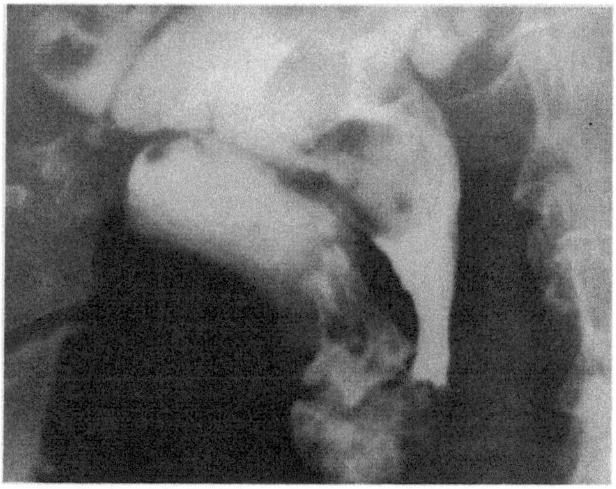

70

Retrograde Cholangiography (Continuation)

71 Multiple concrements in the common bile duct

72 Multiple concrements in the common bile duct

73 Porcelain gallbladder; concrement in the common bile duct

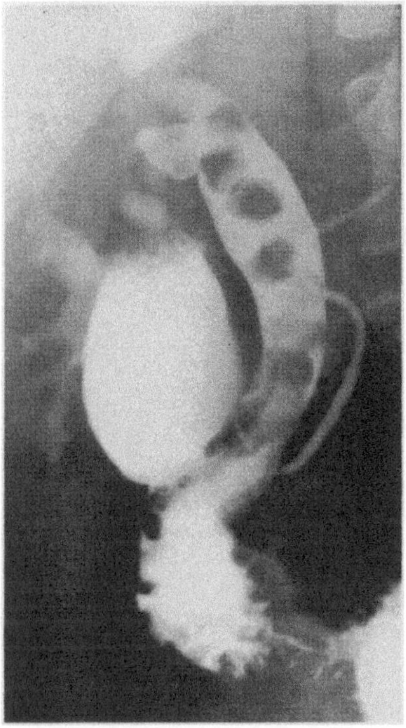

71

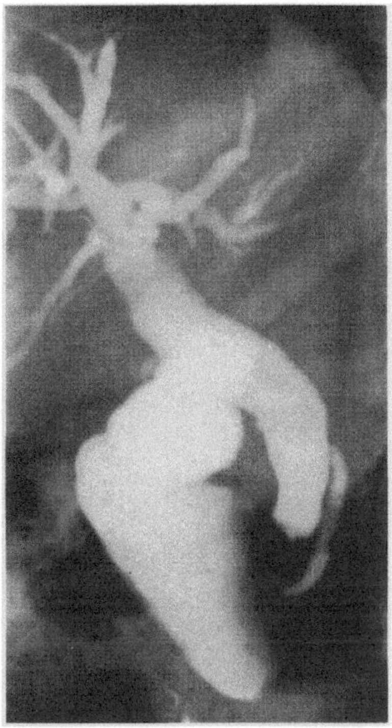

72

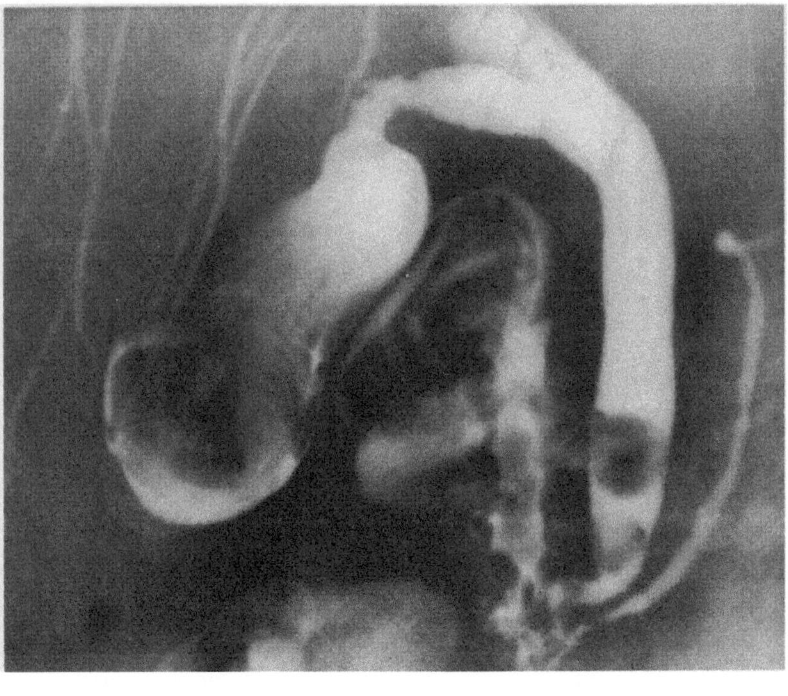

73

Retrograde Cholangiography (Continuation)

74 Primary sclerosing cholangitis

75 Secondary sclerosing cholangitis in a patient with ulcerative colitis

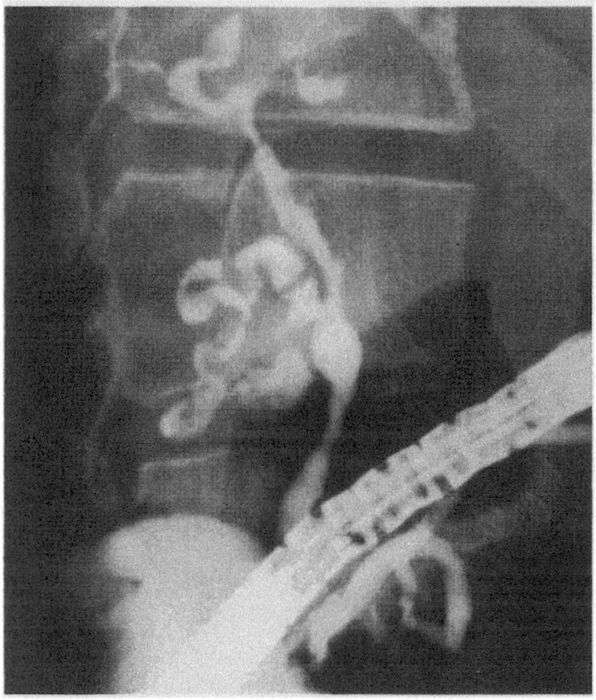
74

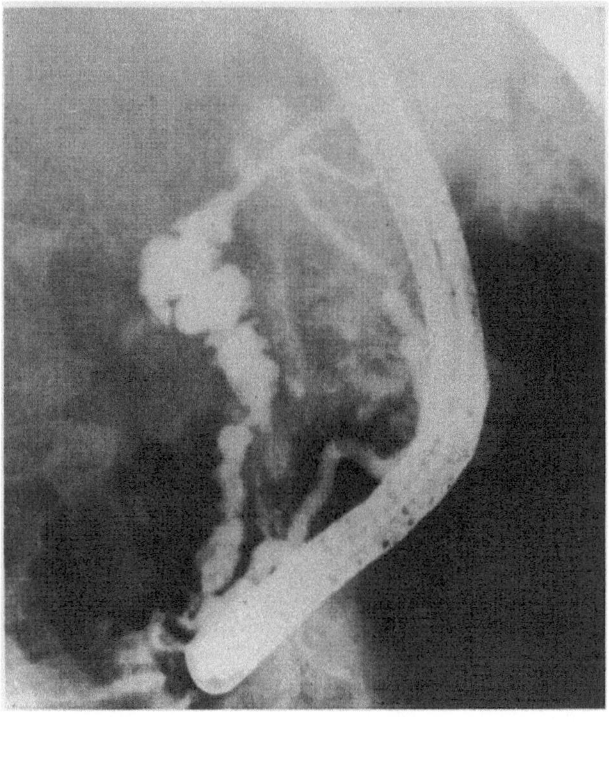
75

76 Changes of the common bile duct with hepatic involvement by Hodgkin's disease

77 Tuberculoma at the porta hepatis

78 Carcinoma of the common bile duct with severe stenosis and massive prestenotic dilatation of the intrahepatic bile ducts

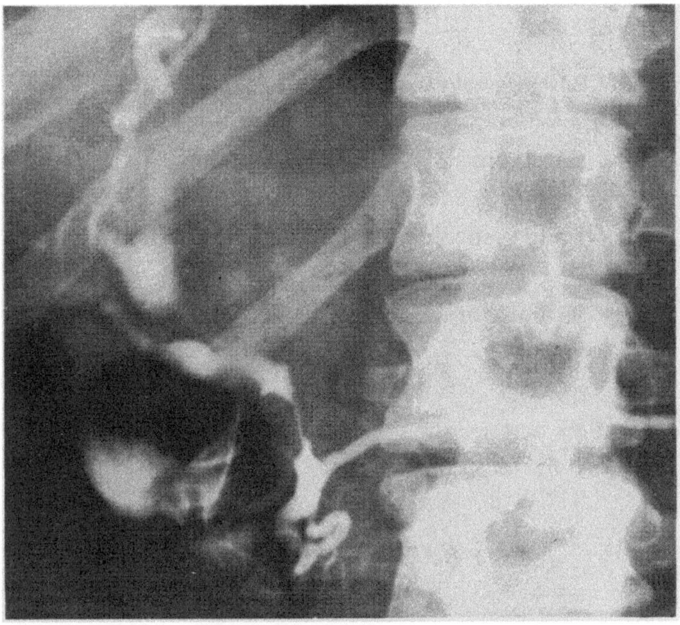

76

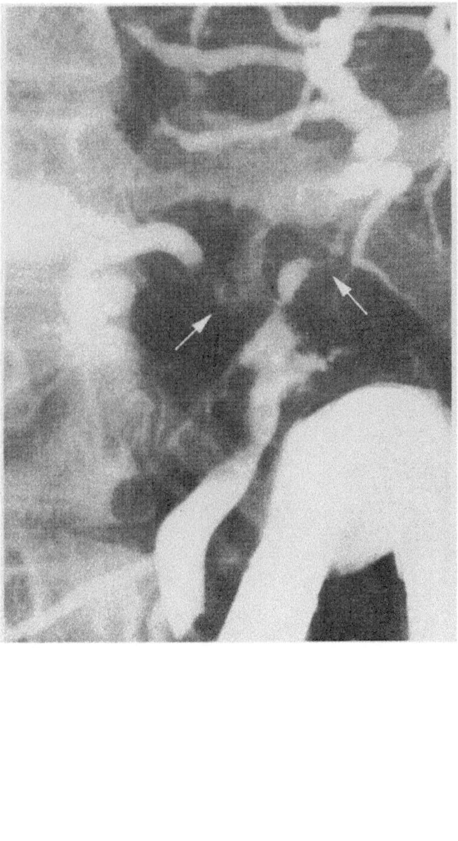

77

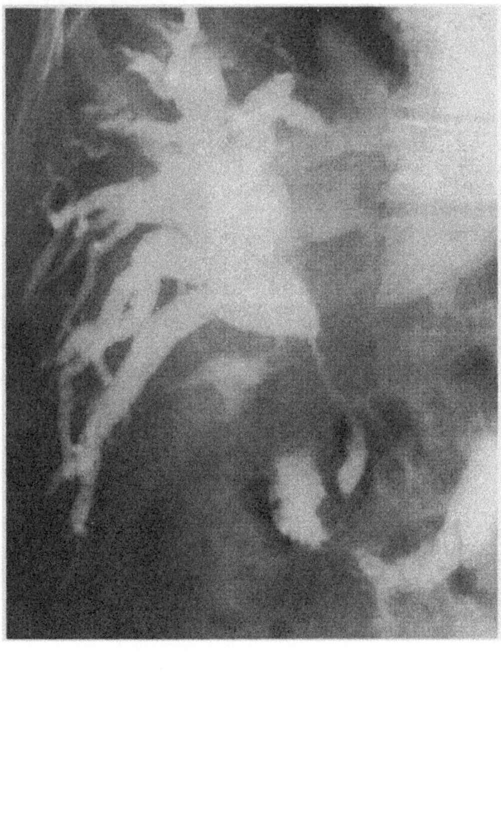

78

Retrograde Cholangiography (Continuation)

79 Carcinoma of the common bile duct (patient in left lateral supine position)

80 Long cystic duct stump after cholecystectomy

81 Stricture of the common bile duct after cholecystectomy

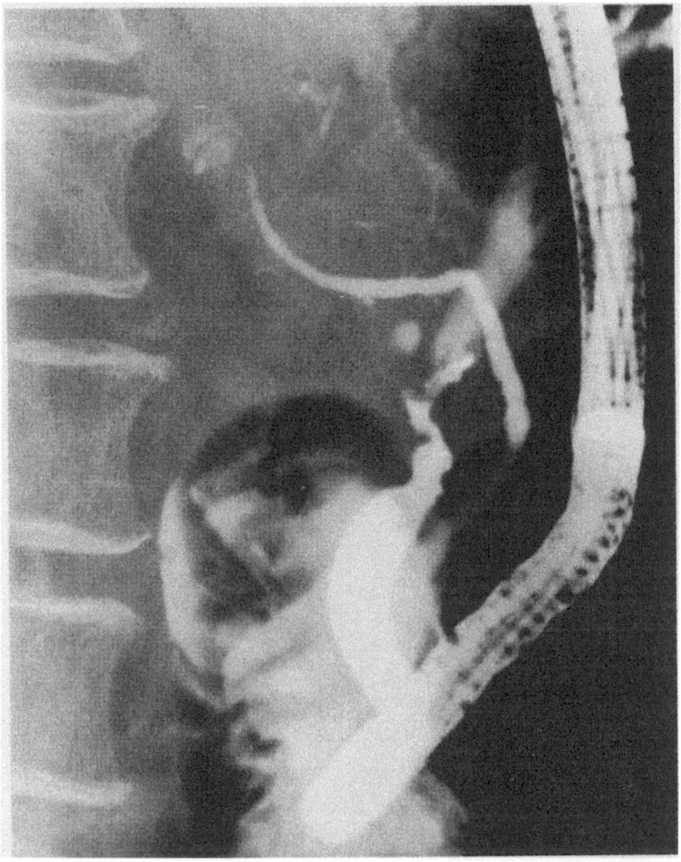

79

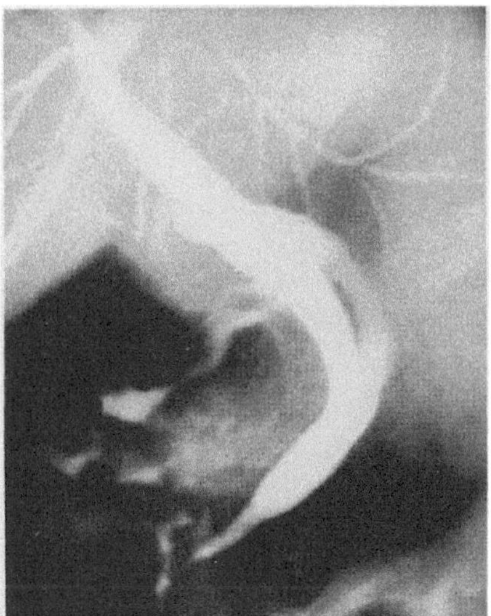

80

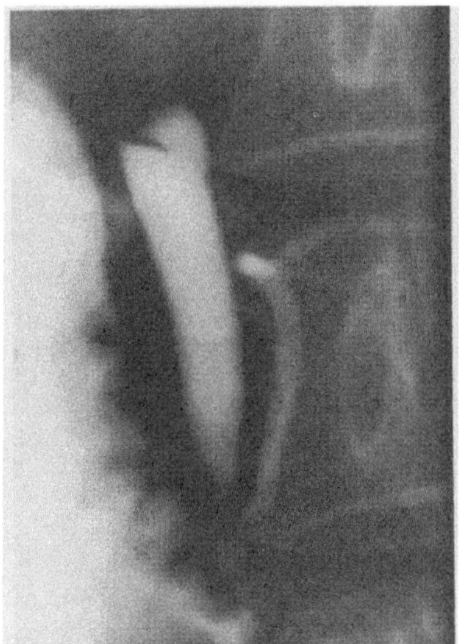

81

Retrograde Cholangiography (Continuation)

82 Status post choledochoduodenostomy. Massive dilatation of pancreatic and bile duct systems. Stenosis of the bypassed terminal portion of the common bile duct

83 Choledochoduodenostomy

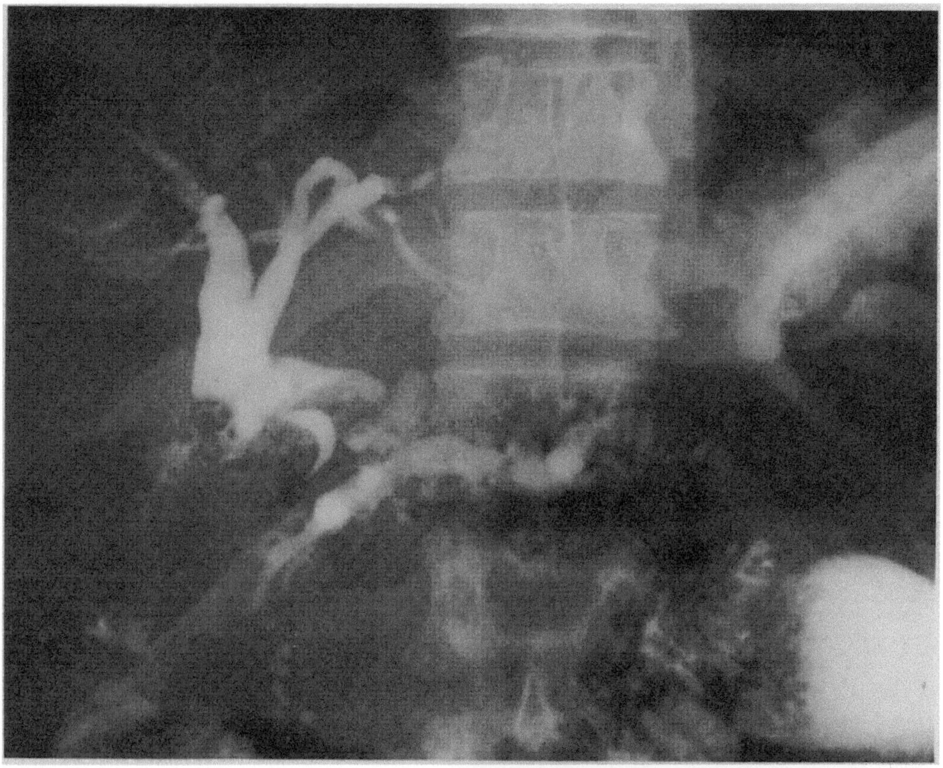
82

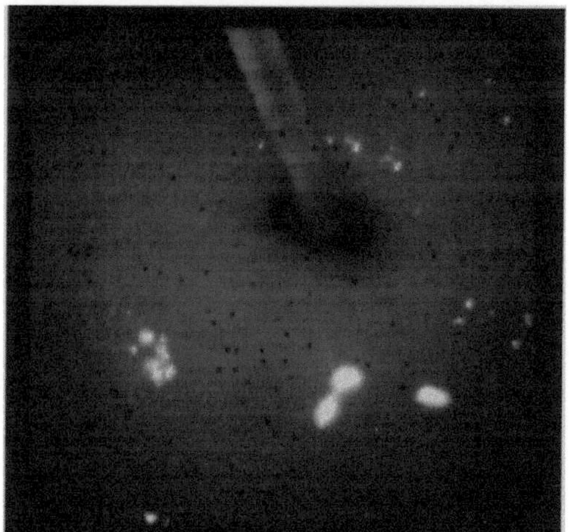
83

Retrograde Cholangiography (Continuation)

84 Cholecystoduodenostomy

85 Extraction of a drain which had slipped into the choledochus through the papilla

86 Drain within the papilla of Vater

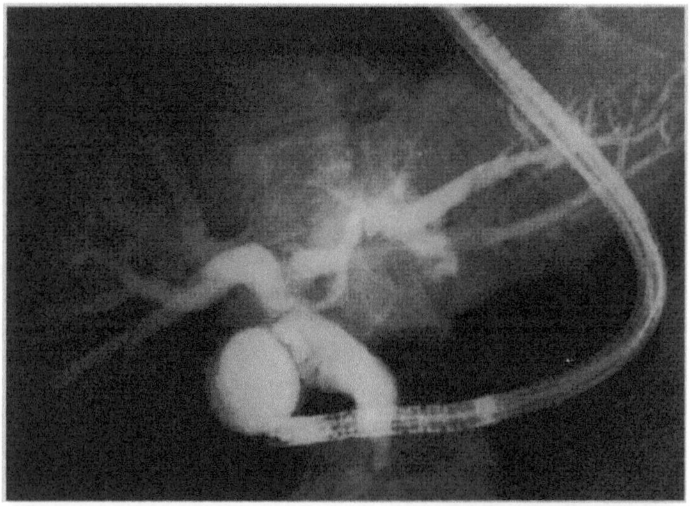
84

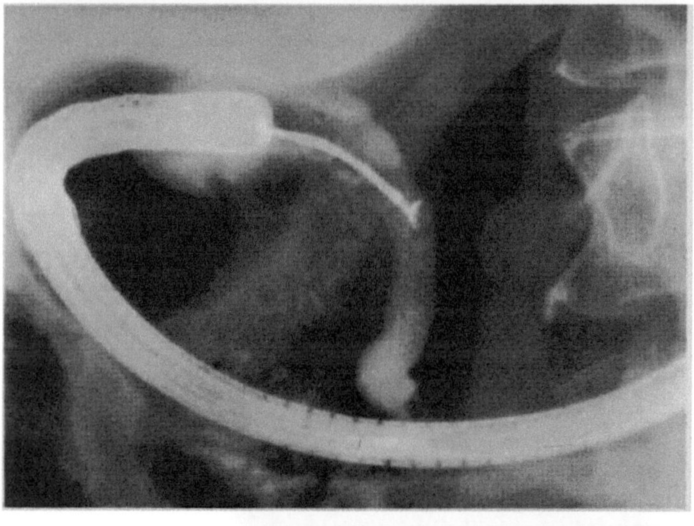
85

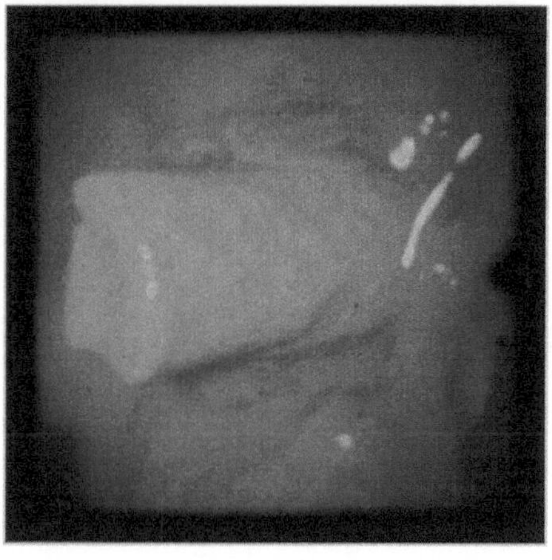
86

Retrograde Cholangiography (Continuation)

87 Hepatic abscess with duodenal fistula caused by primary cholangiocarcinoma

88 Biopsy of the abscess cavity in the same patient (Fig. 87)

89 Autopsy specimen of the liver abscess involving a primary cholangiocarcinoma

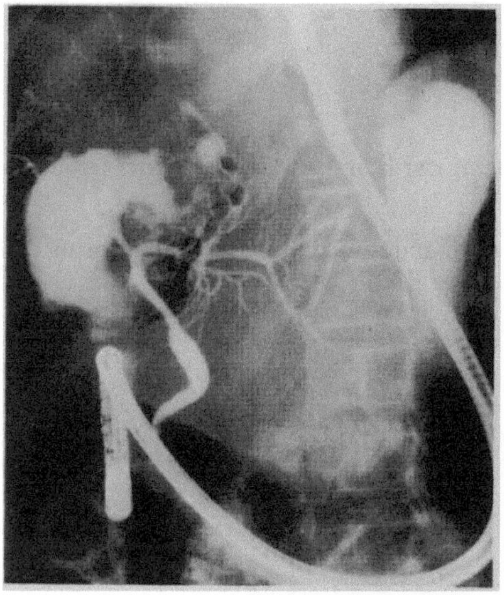
87

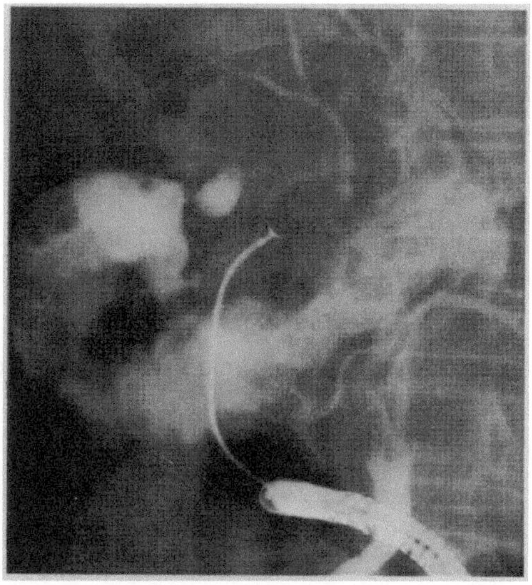
88

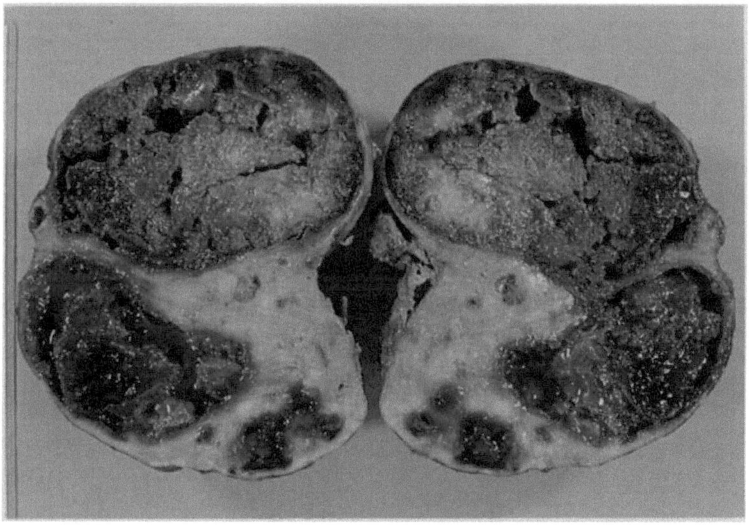
89

Retrograde Pancreatography

90 Normal major pancreatic duct (Wirsung) with first and second order tributaries

91 Major pancreatic duct (Wirsung) with narrow minor duct (Santorini) and Ramus capitis inferior

92 Large caliber main pancreatic duct

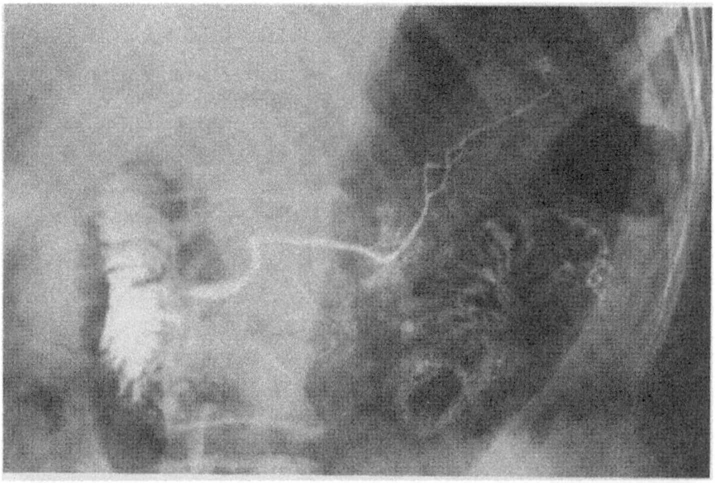

90

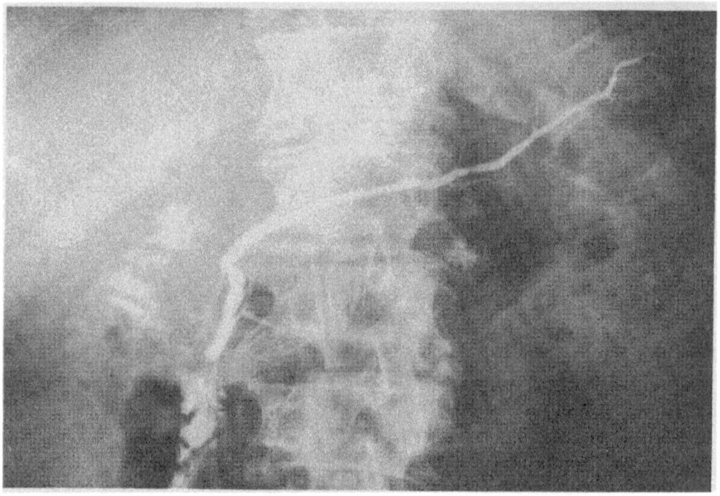

91

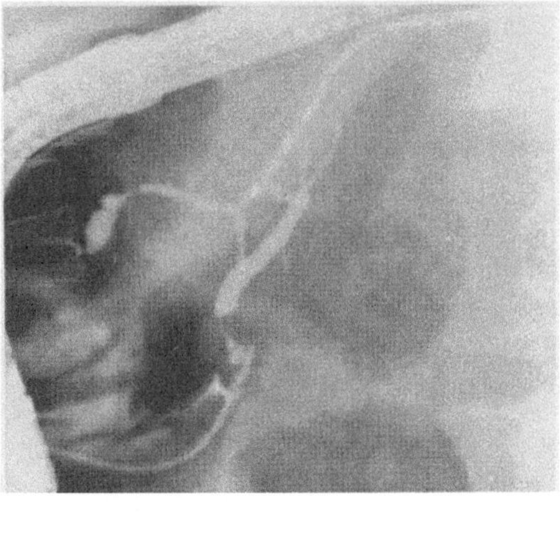

92

Retrograde Pancreatography (Continuation)

93 Double contrast radiograph of the duodenum with annular pancreas

94 Annular pancreas

95 Annular pancreas

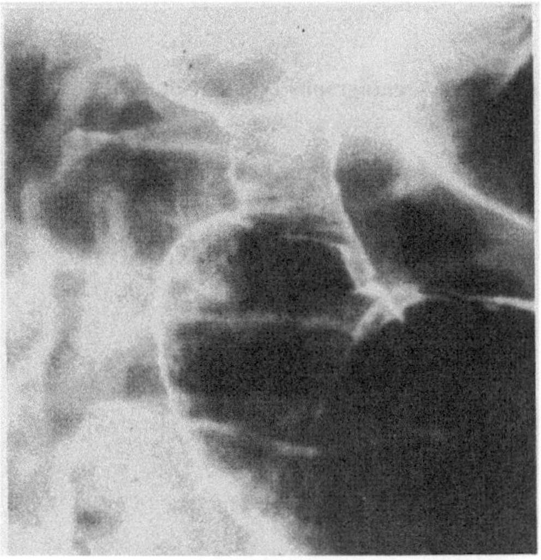
93

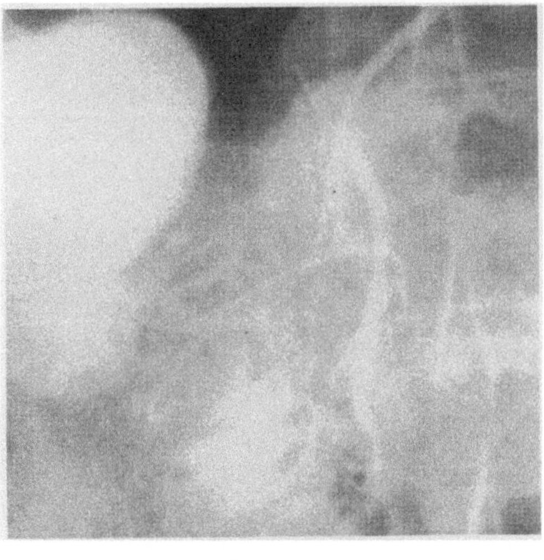
94

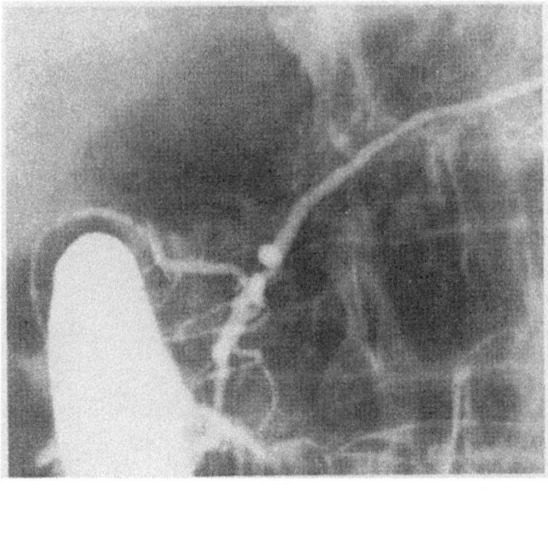
95

Retrograde Pancreatography (Continuation)

96 Multiple small pancreatic cysts

97 Cyst in the tail of the pancreas

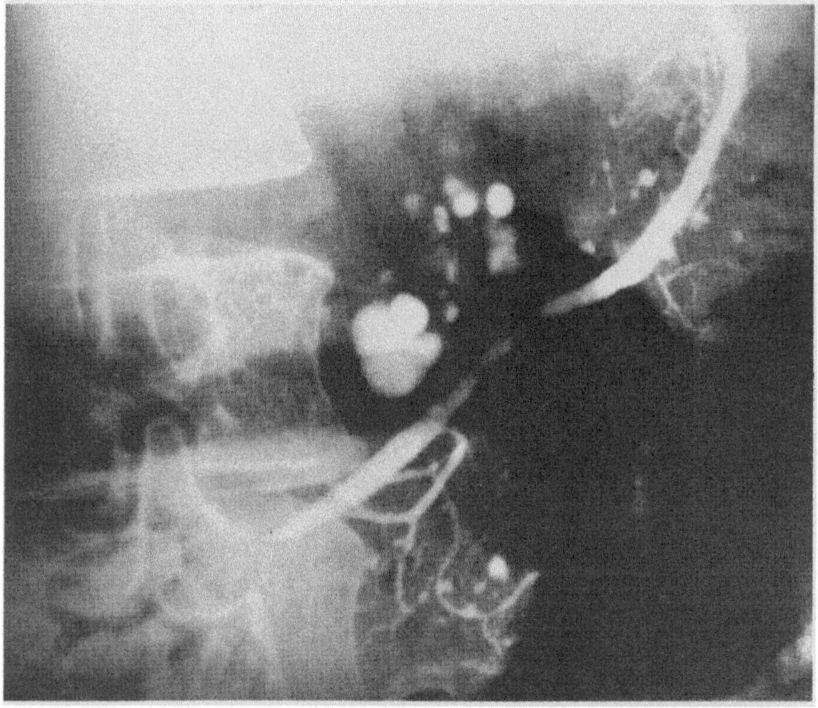

96

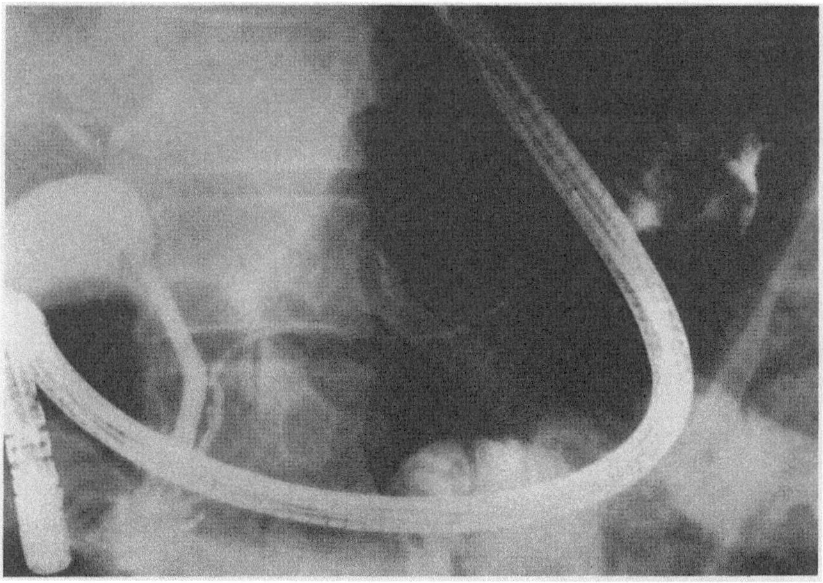

97

Retrograde Pancreatography (Continuation)

98 Cyst in the tail of the pancreas

99 Large cyst in the head of the pancreas, anastomosed to the duodenum

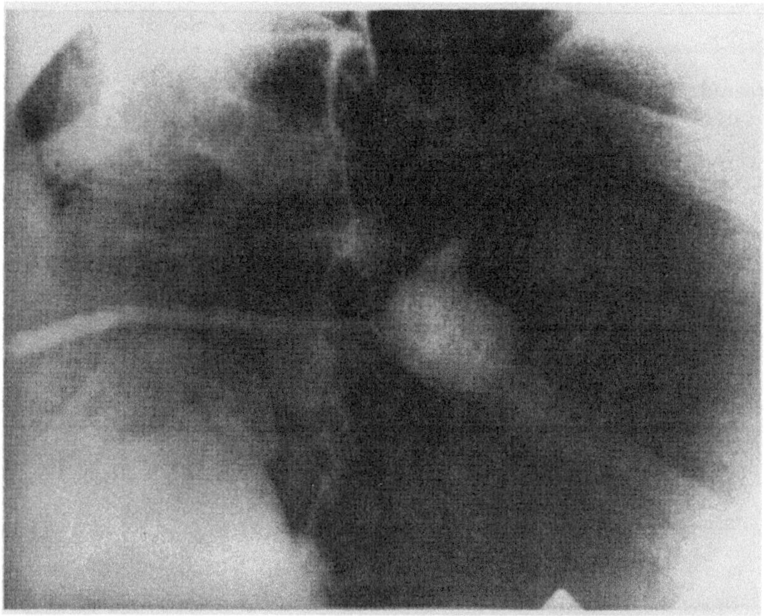

98

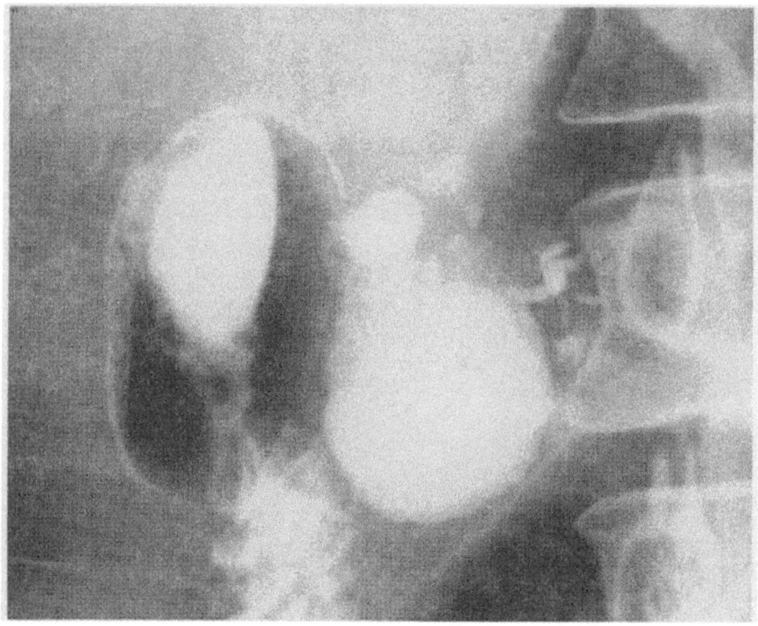

99

Retrograde Pancreatography (Continuation)

100 Large cyst in the head of the pancreas with definite signs of chronic pancreatitis

101 Cyst in the head of the pancreas draining via the minor pancreatic duct with normal major pancreatic duct

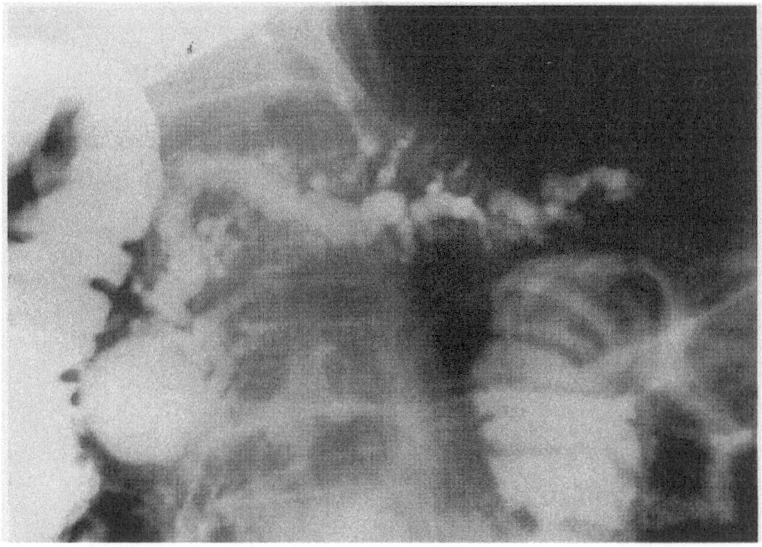
100

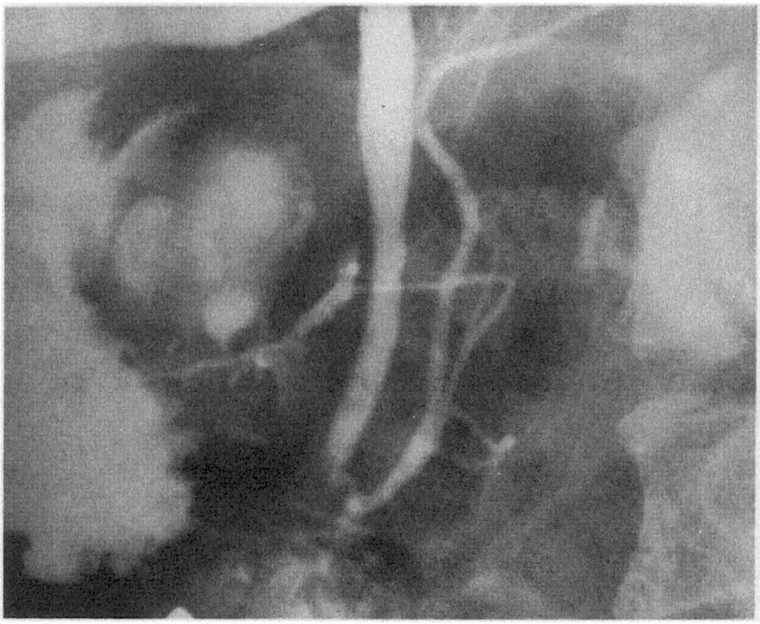
101

Retrograde Pancreatography (Continuation)

102 Break-off of the major pancreatic duct caused by a pancreatic cyst

103 Displacement of the tributaries of the main pancreatic duct within the tail of the pancreas by a cystadenoma

104 Surgical specimen of cystadenoma

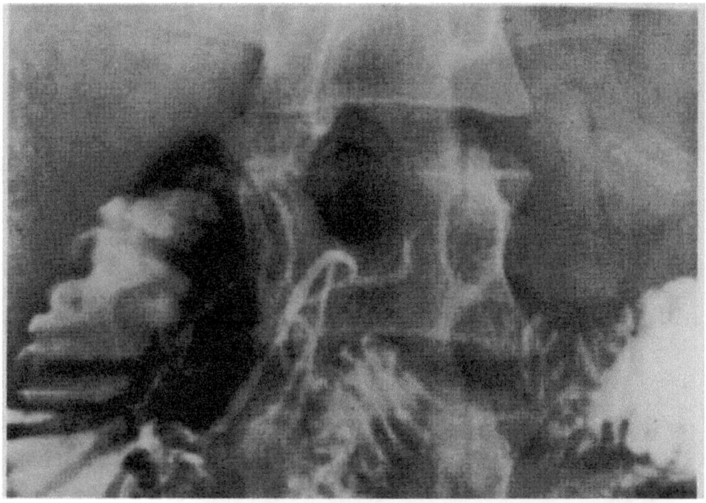

102

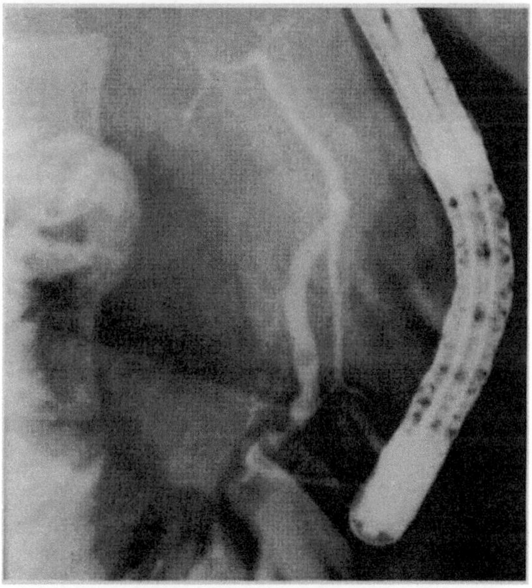

103

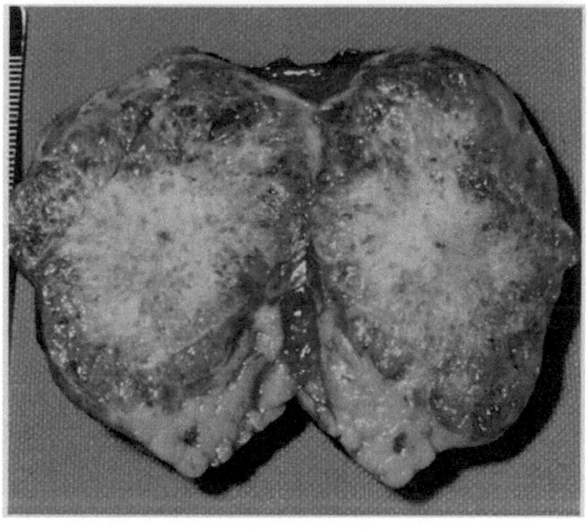

104

Retrograde Pancreatography (Continuation)

105 Massive pancreatic calcification with chronic pancreatitis

106 Corkscrew appearance of the major pancreatic duct in chronic pancreatitis

107 Dilatation of the major pancreatic duct with shortening and dilatation of its tributaries in chronic pancreatitis

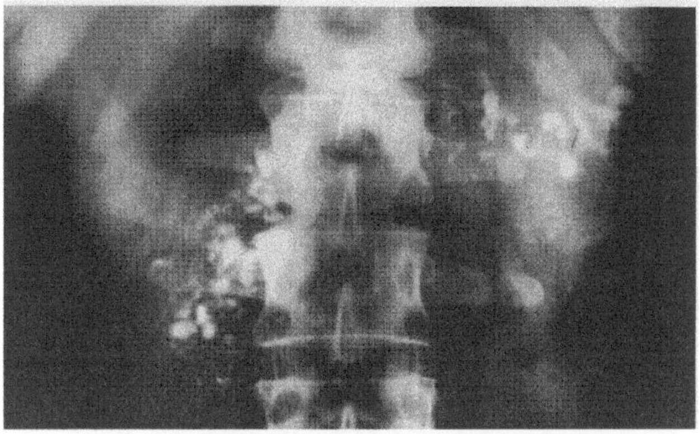

105

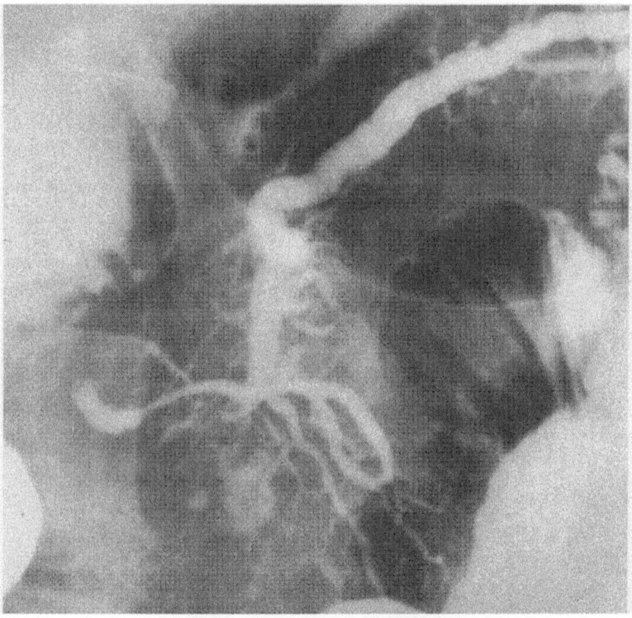

106

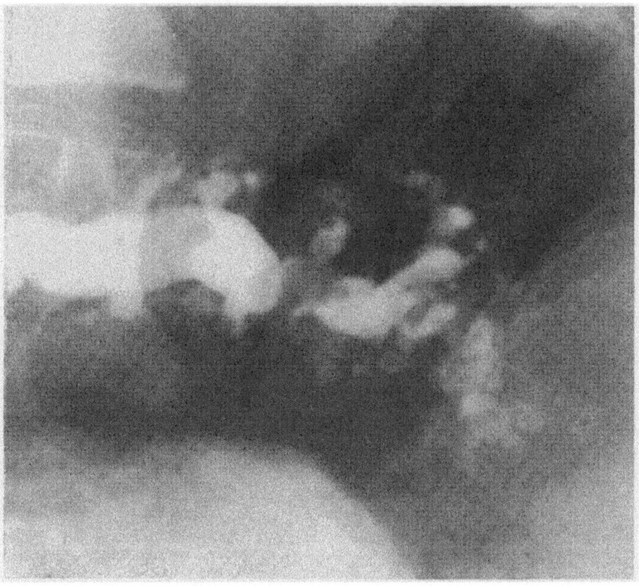

107

Retrograde Pancreatography (Continuation)

108 Severe chronic calcific pancreatitis with concrement in the major pancreatic duct

109 Severe chronic pancreatitis with concrements in the major pancreatic duct

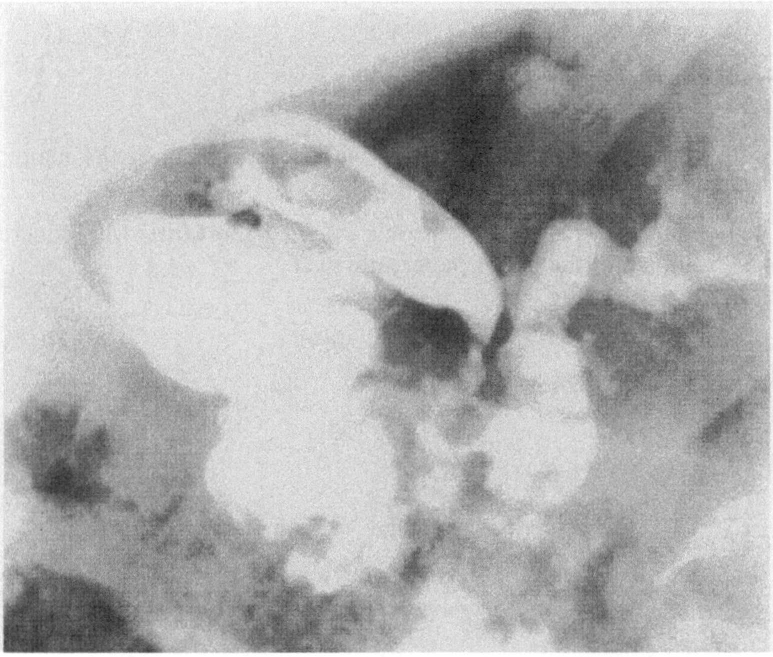
108

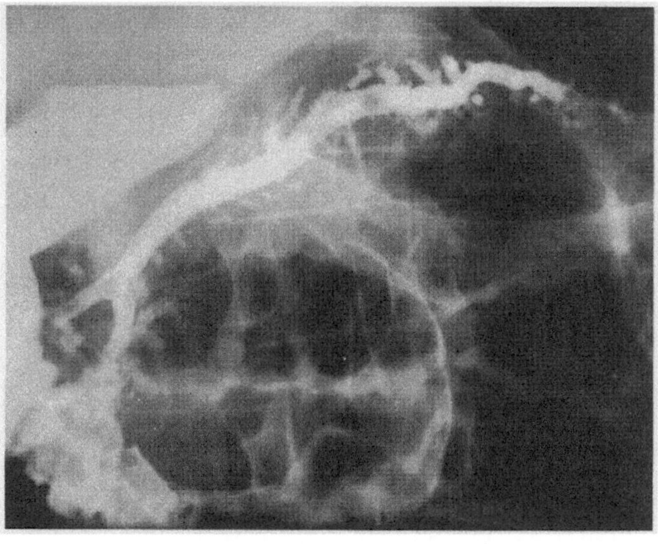
109

Retrograde Pancreatography (Continuation)

110 Severe chronic pancreatitis with concrements in the major pancreatic duct

111 Surgical specimen of chronic calcific pancreatitis with concrements filling the lumen of the major pancreatic duct

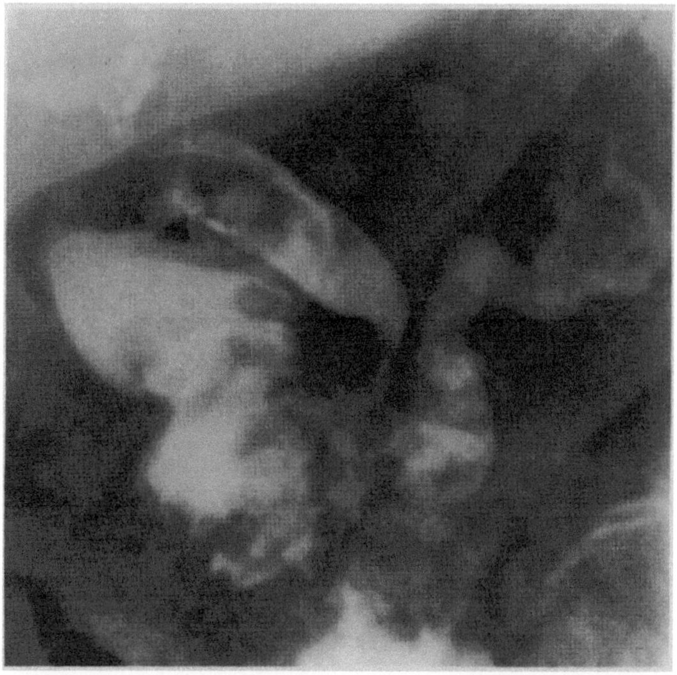

110

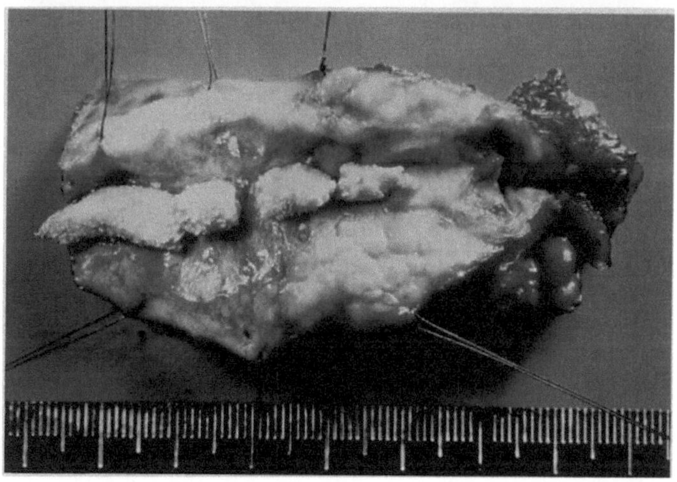

111

Retrograde Pancreatography (Continuation)

112 Advanced destruction of pancreatic ducts in chronic pancreatitis

113 Marked tubular stenosis of the terminal common bile duct in chronic pancreatitis

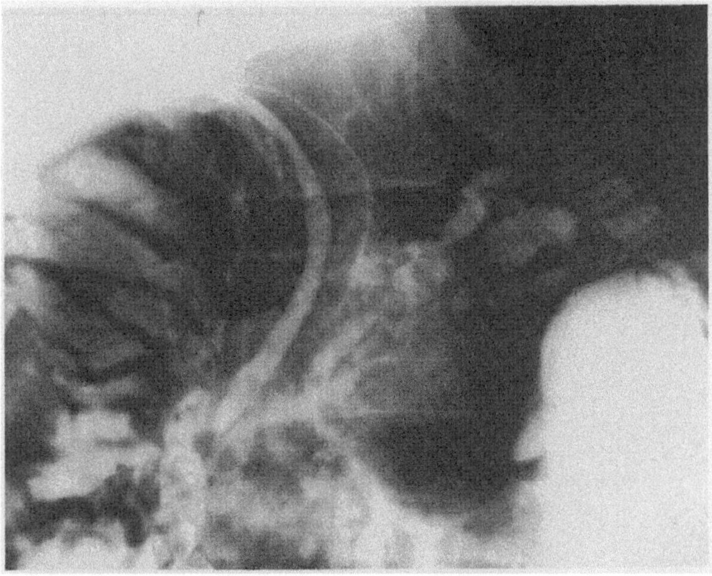
112

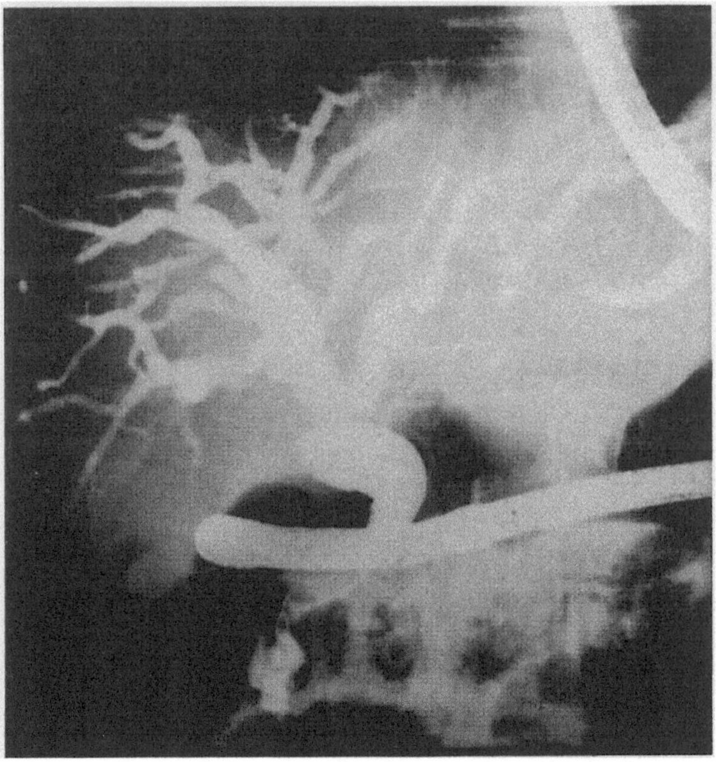
113

114 Marked tubular stenosis of the terminal common bile duct in chronic pancreatitis

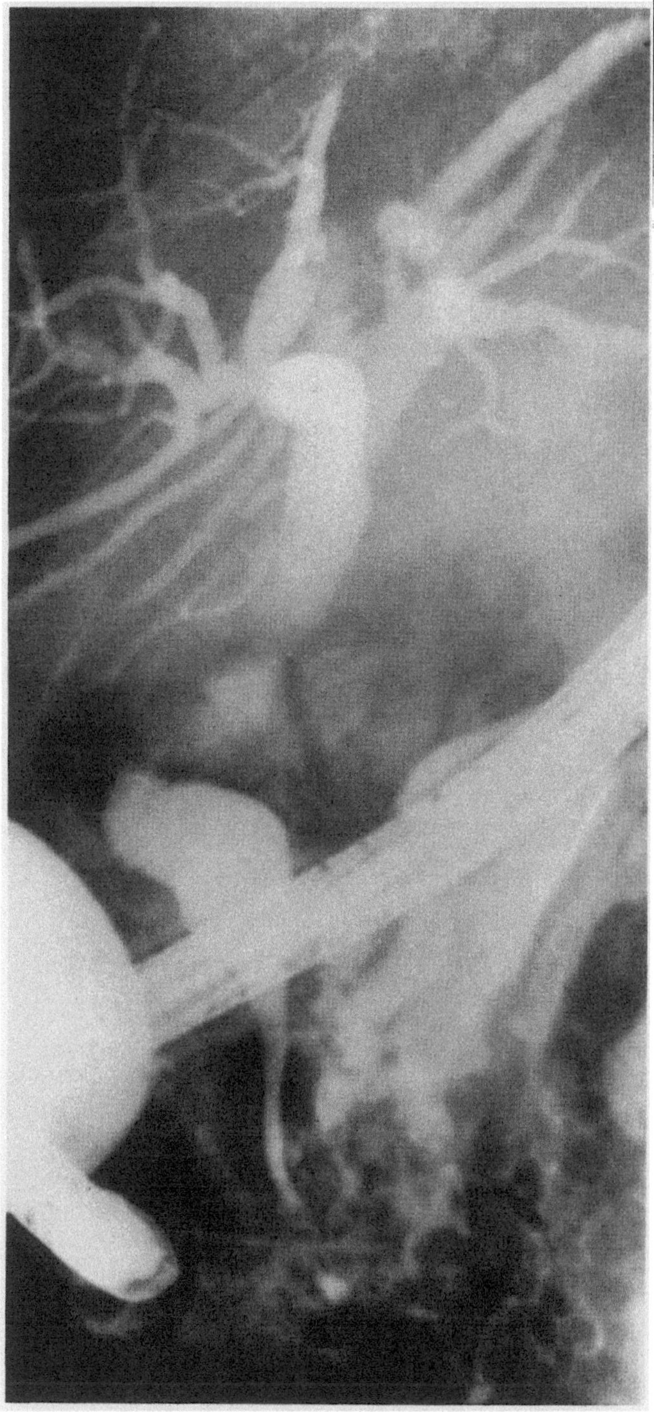

114

Retrograde Pancreatography (Continuation)

115 Filiform stenosis of the common bile duct in chronic pancreatitis

116 Involvement of the common bile duct in chronic pancreatitis

117 Bile duct carcinoma in chronic pancreatitis (courtesy of Dr. J.A. VENNES, Minneapolis, Minn.)

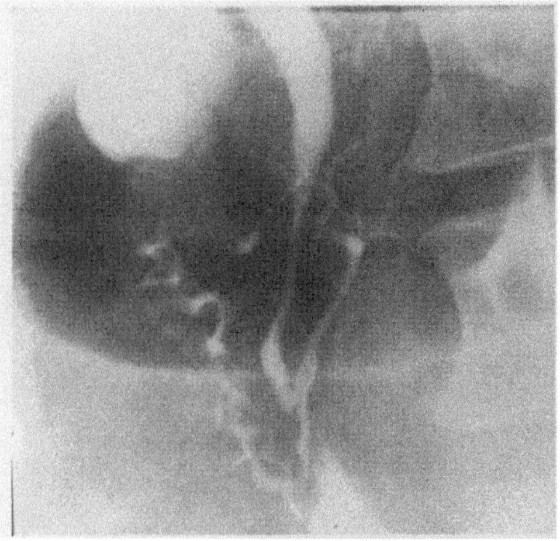
115

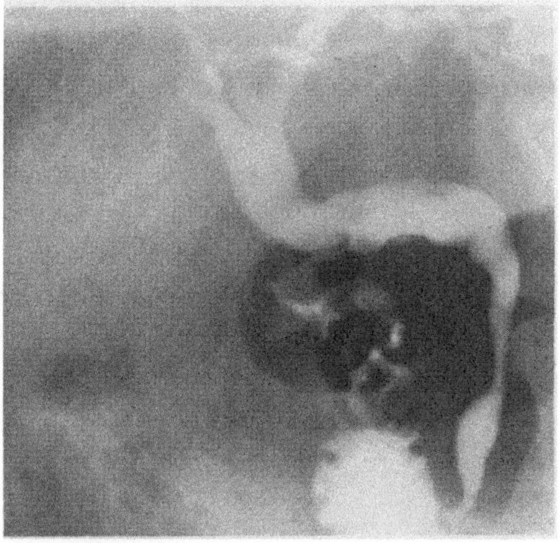
116

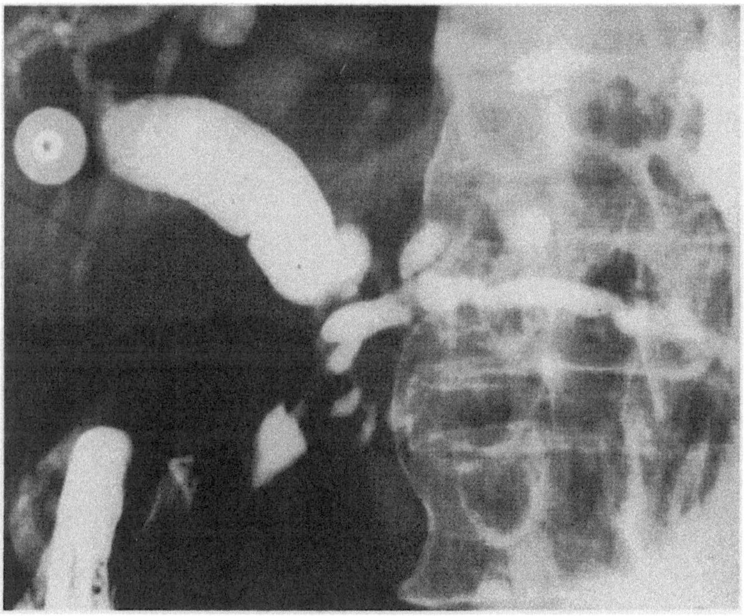
117

Retrograde Pancreatography (Continuation)

118 Bile duct carcinoma in chronic pancreatitis (courtesy of Dr. J.A. VENNES, Minneapolis, Minn.)

119 Break-off of the major pancreatic duct with carcinoma of the head of the pancreas

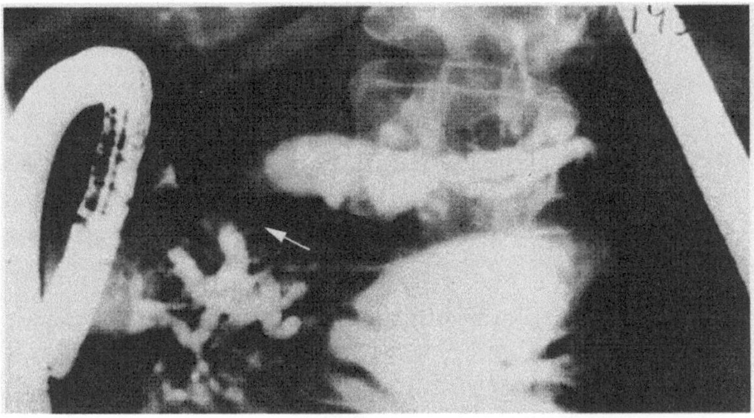

118

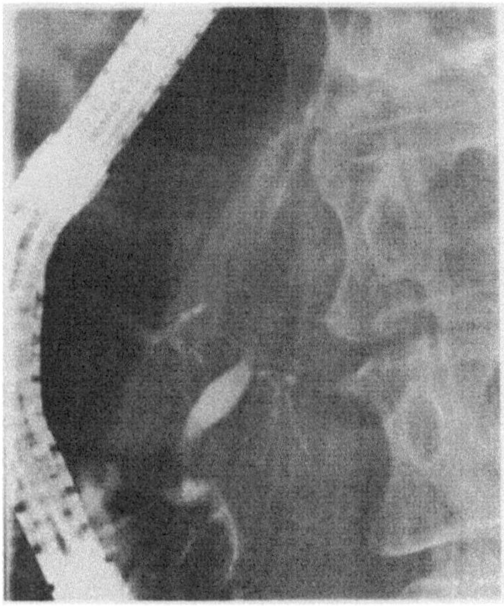

119

Retrograde Pancreatography (Continuation)

120 Stenosis of the major pancreatic duct with cancer of the head of the pancreas

121 Stenosis of the major pancreatic duct with cancer of the head of the pancreas

122 Cystic cavity formed by necrosis of pancreatic carcinoma

123 Massive destruction of major pancreatic duct by cancer of the head of the pancreas with extension to the prepapillary common bile duct

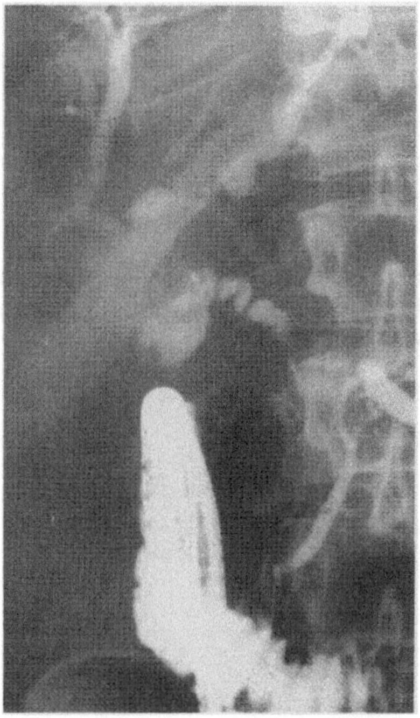
120

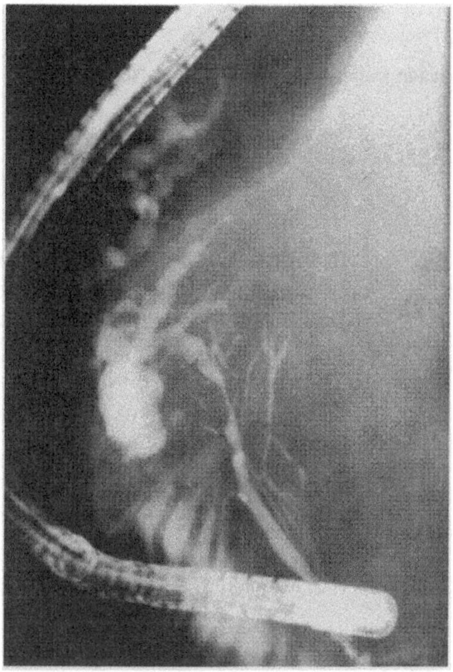
121

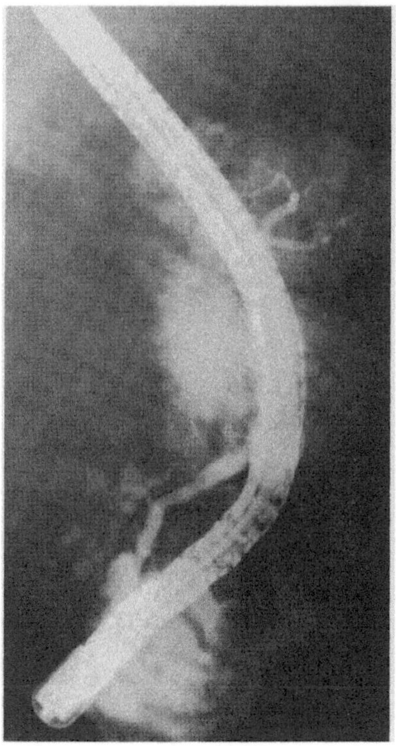
122

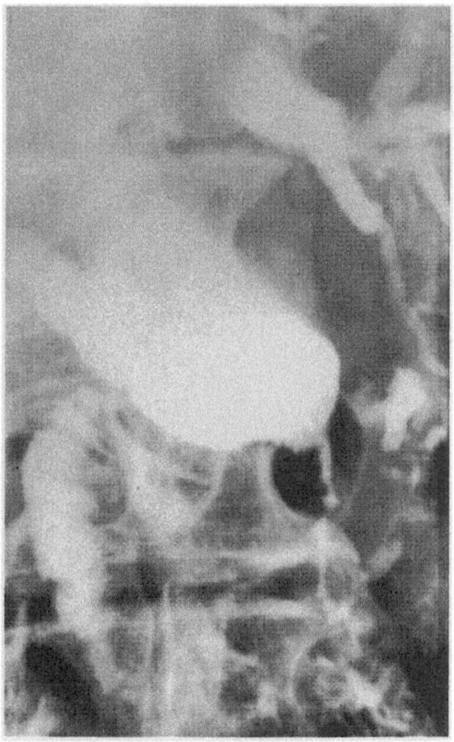
123

124 Stenosis of the major pancreatic duct caused by metastasis from a carcinoma of the sigmoid (prone position)

125 Carcinoma of the head of the pancreas causing prepapillary stenosis of the common bile duct with massive dilatation of intrahepatic bile ducts and hydrops of the gallbladder. Nonfilling of pancreatic duct system

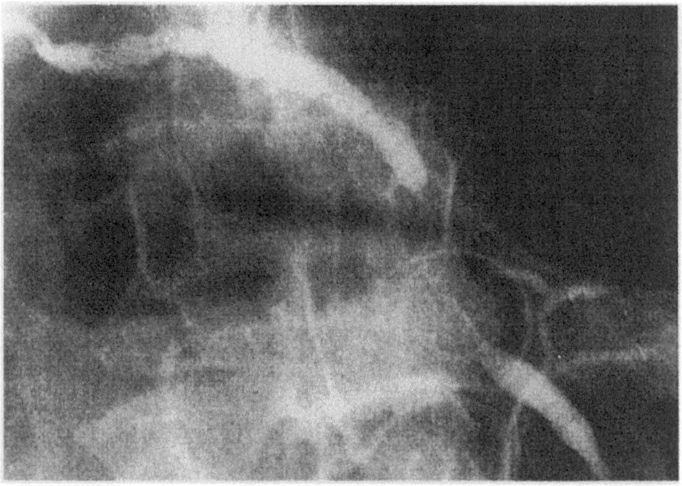
124

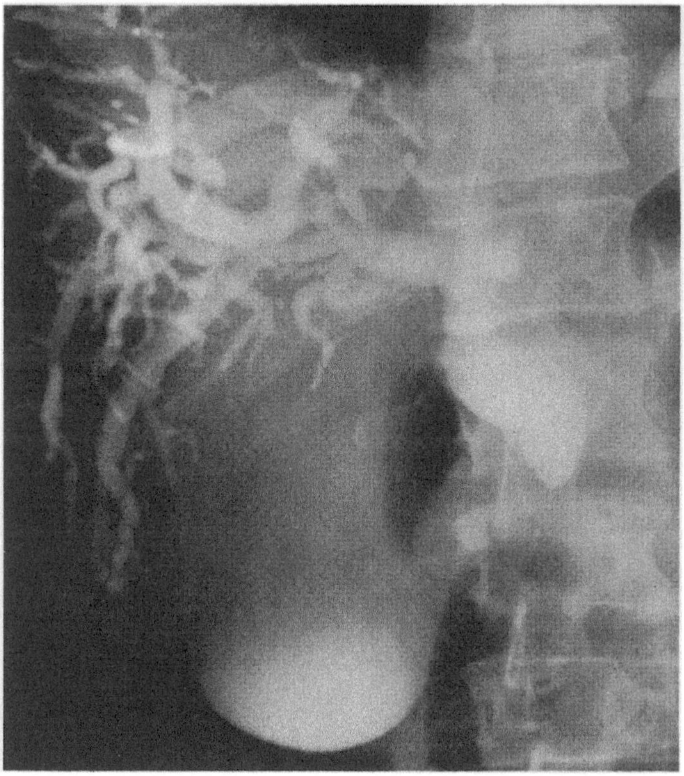
125

Retrograde Pancreatography (Continuation)

126 Fulminating pancreatitis with abscess formation following endoscopic retrograde pancreatography (ERP)

127 Large cyst in the tail of the pancreas following ERP

128 Surgical specimen of a carcinoma of the head of the pancreas

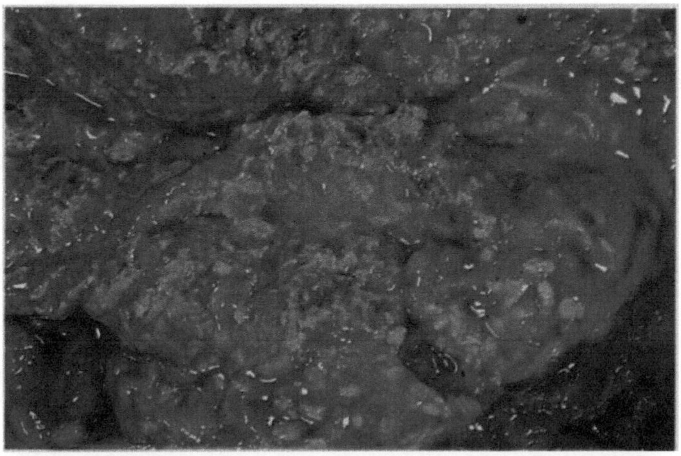

126

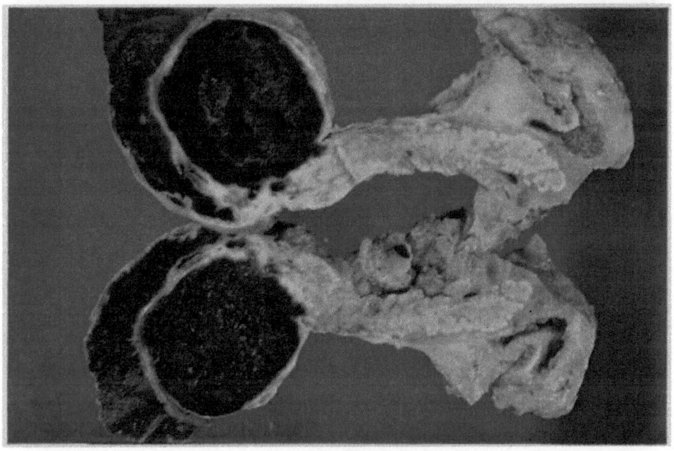

127

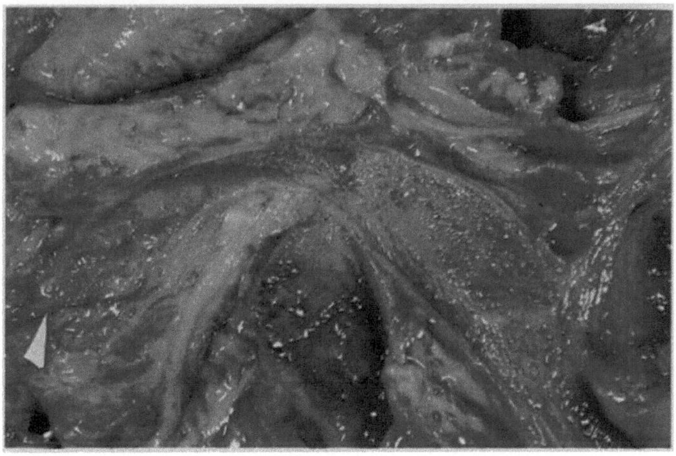

128

Retrograde Pancreatography (Continuation)

129 Severe experimental pancreatitis produced by instillation of contrast medium in the cat

130a Histologic appearance of experimental pancreatitis with marked parenchymal necrosis

130b Separation of pancreatic tissue architecture following instillation of contrast medium in the cat (left).
Right: normal cat pancreas

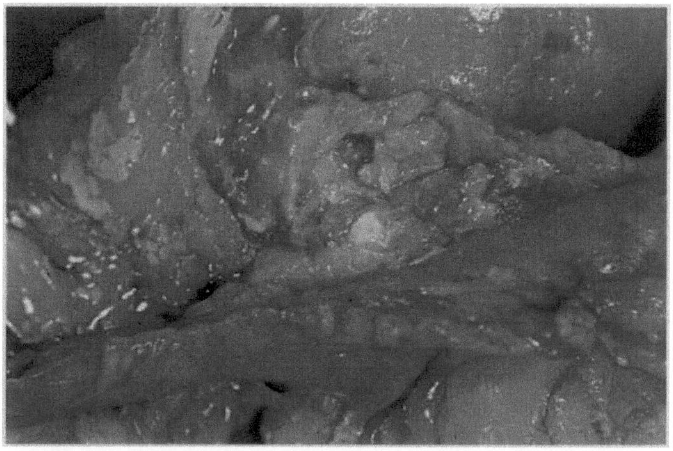

129

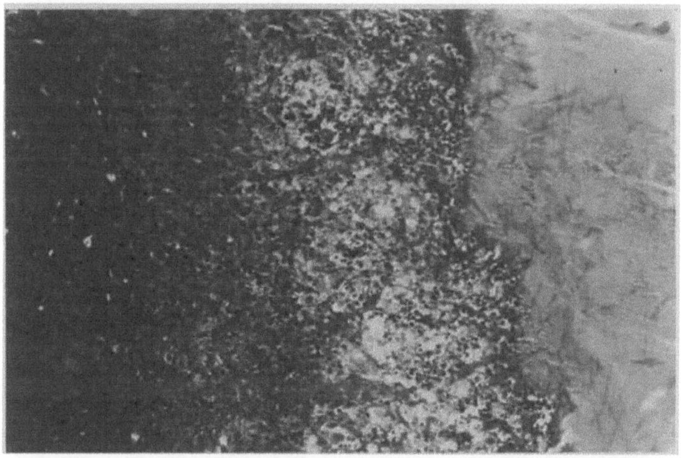

130a

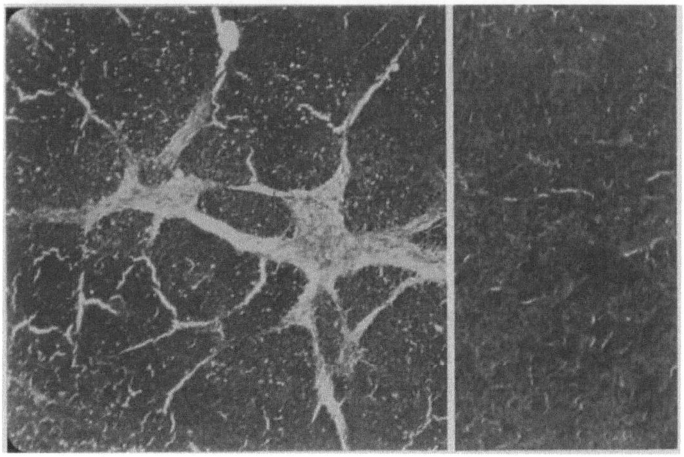

130b

Total Enteroscopy

131–136 Total enteroscopy. Passage of enteroscope through jejunum, ileum, and colon to the anus

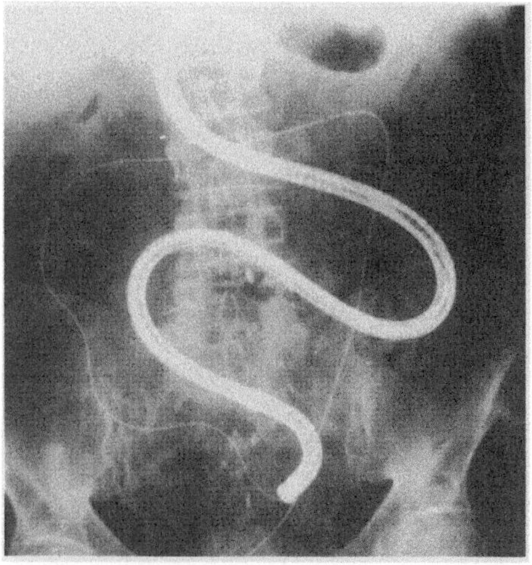
131

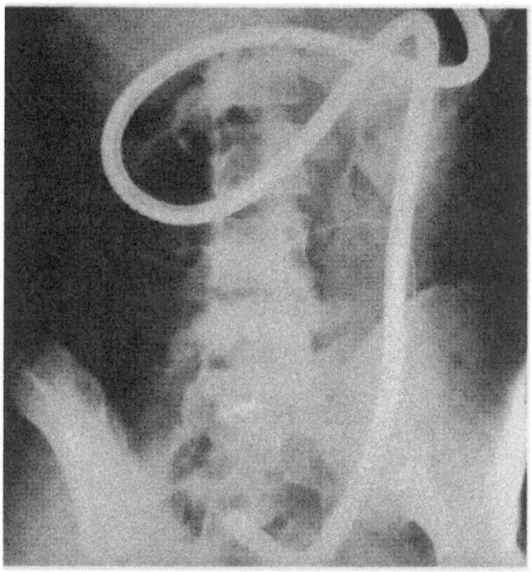
132

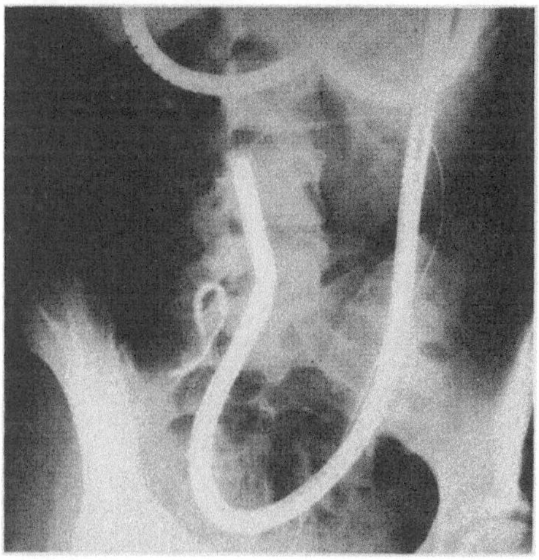
133

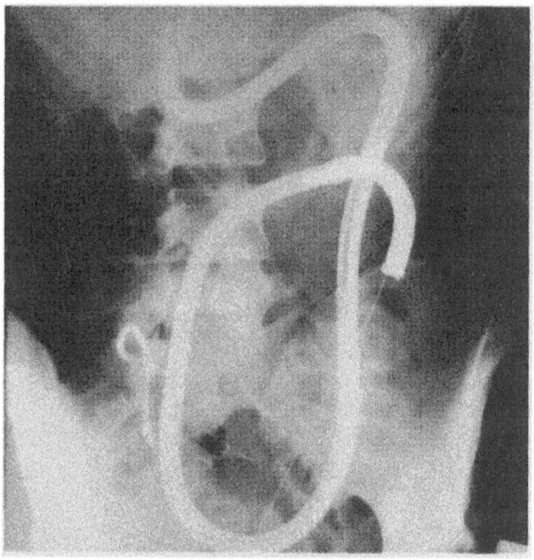
134

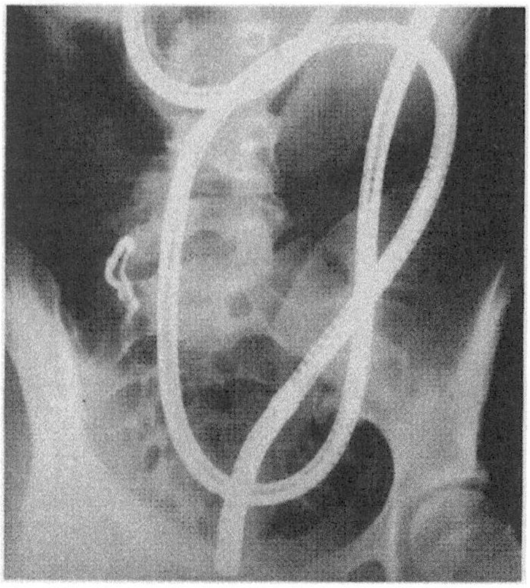
135

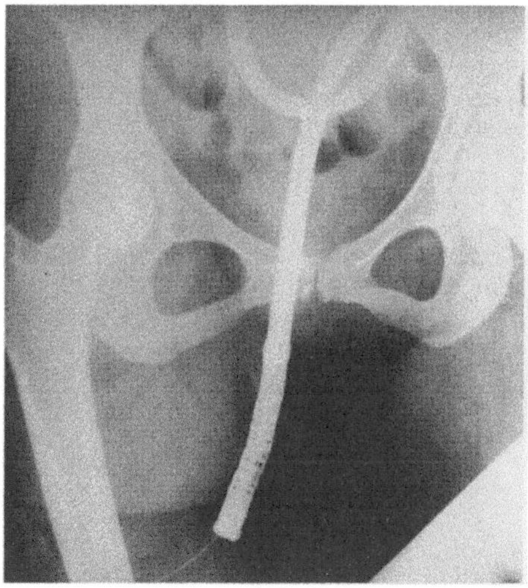
136

Enteroscopy

137 Follicular lymphoid hyperplasia of the duodenum

138 Sarcoma of the jejunum

139 a–b X-ray negative Crohn's disease of the terminal ileum

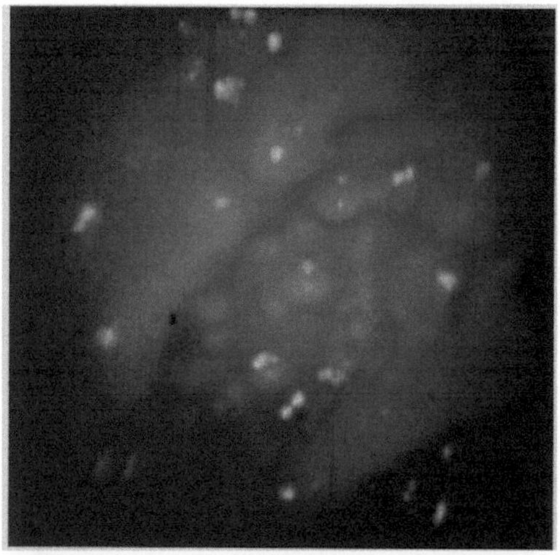

37

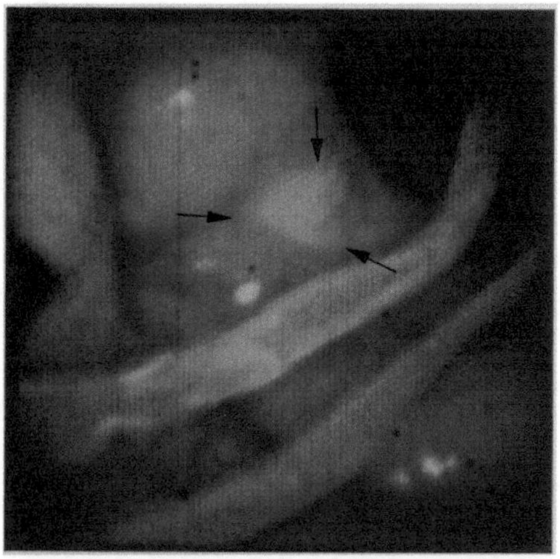

139 a

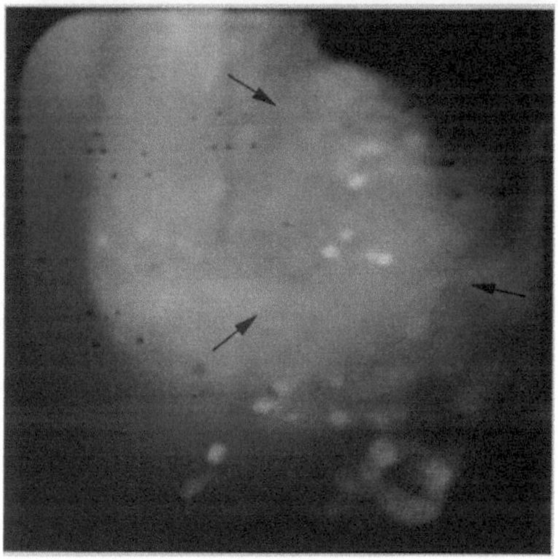

38

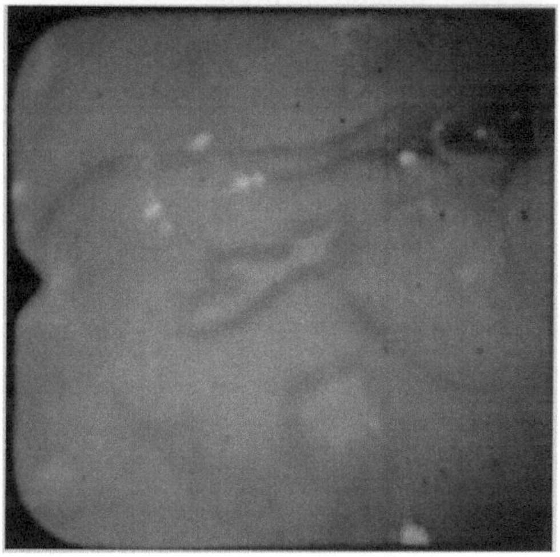

139 b

Coloscopy

1.Accessory Instruments

A variety of accessory instruments can be introduced into the colonic lumen through the instrumentation channel

140 Biopsy forceps with oval jaws

141 Thin Nylon brush for collection of material for cytology

142 Stabilizing probe

143 Measuring probe

144 High frequency diathermy snare of Deyhle and Seuberth (Fa. Storz, Tuttlingen, Germany)

145 Open, high frequency diathermy snare of Frühmorgen and Seuberth (Fa. Storz, Tuttlingen, Germany)

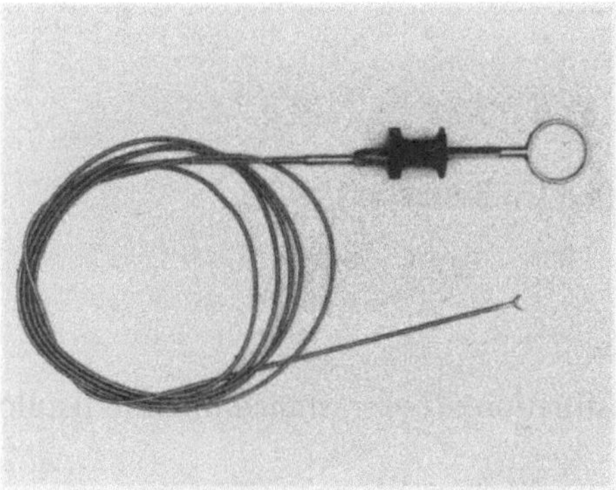

40

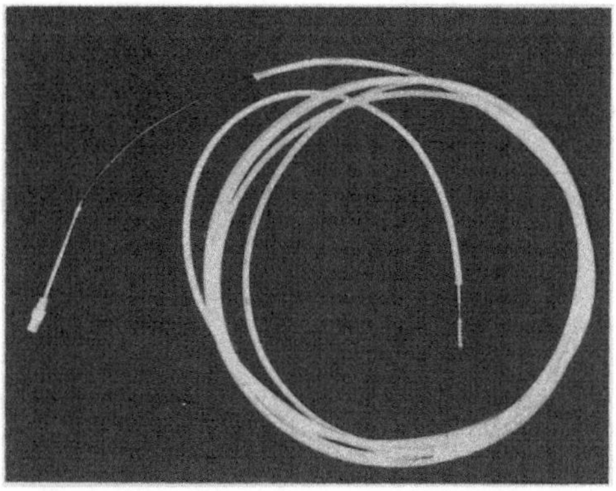

141

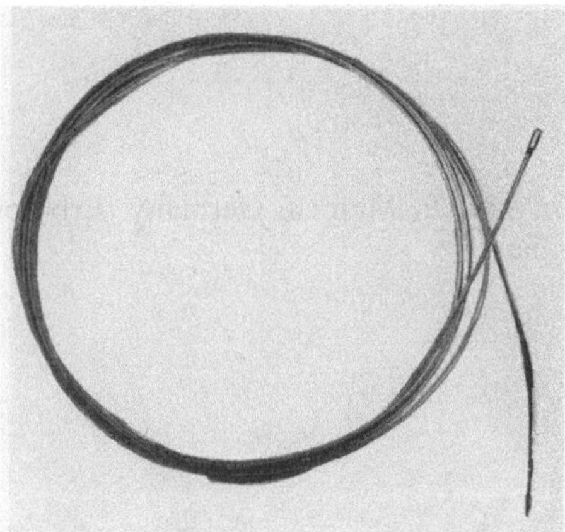

42

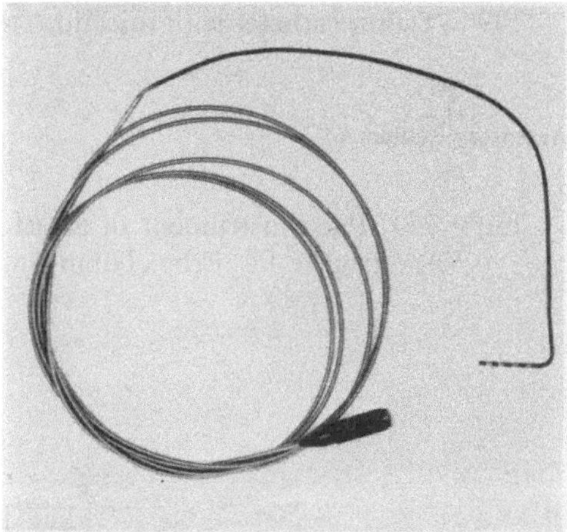

143

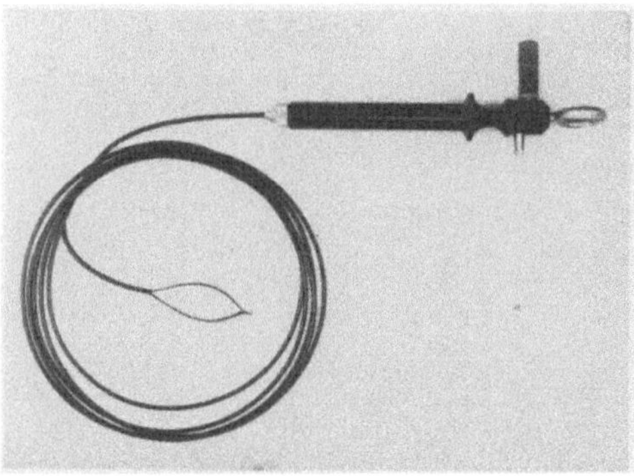

44

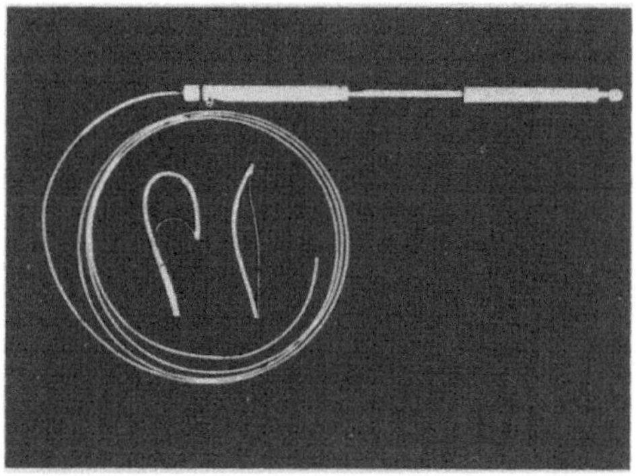

145

1. Accessory Instruments (Continuation)

146 Forceps for polyp extraction (modified from SEIFERT)

147 Coagulation probe

148 Teflon catheter for intubation and instillation of contrast medium into fistulous tracts and the appendix

149 Teflon catheter with injection needle and removable protective cap

2. Accessory Equipment

150 CO_2-Pneu instrument of SEMM (left), WISAP, Munich, Germany. Erbotom R 3 (right), Fa. Erbe, Tübingen, Germany

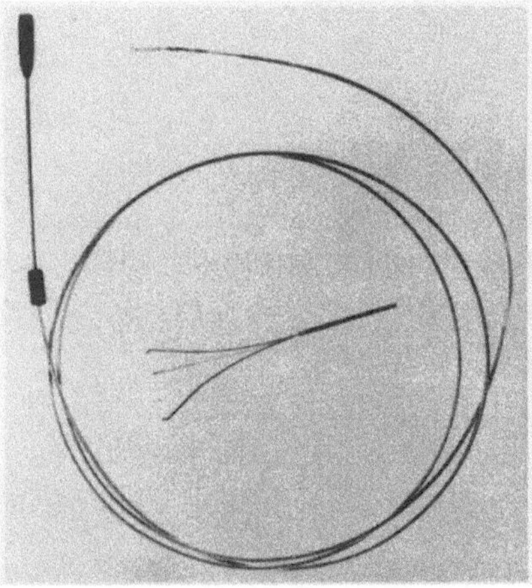

146

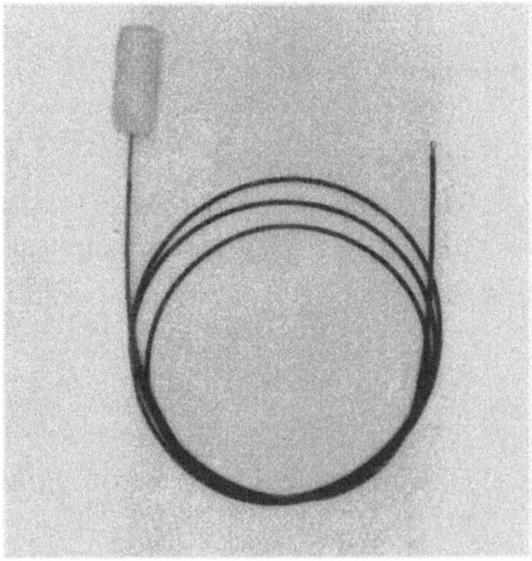

147

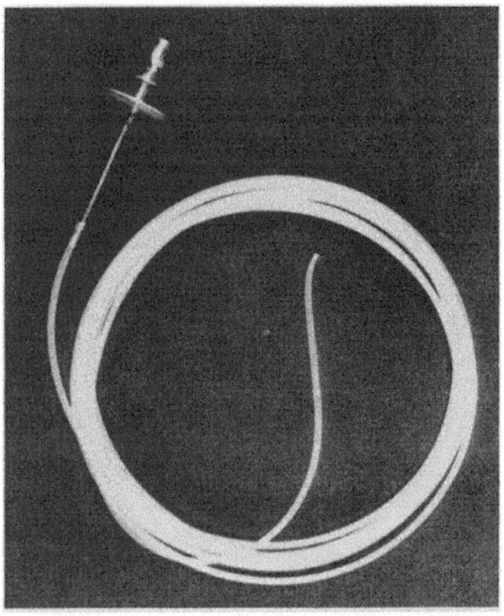

148

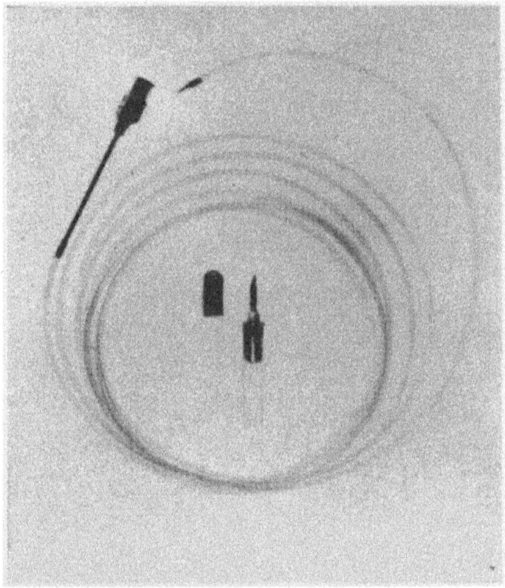

149

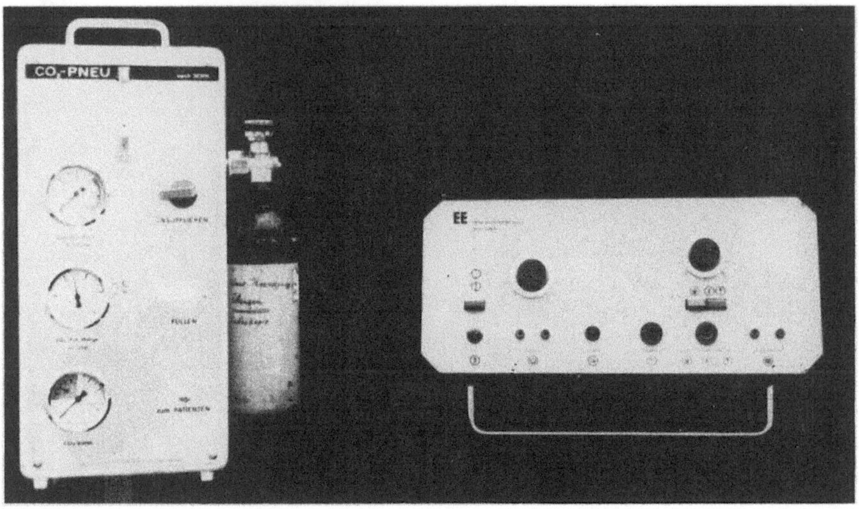

150

151 Biopsy forceps:
a) Forceps opened; normal vascular pattern of the colonic mucosa
b) Tentlike retraction of the mucosa; normal macroscopic and histologic appearance

152 Nylon brush for obtaining material for cytology

153 Objective measurement of sigmoid polyp by use of a graduated measuring probe

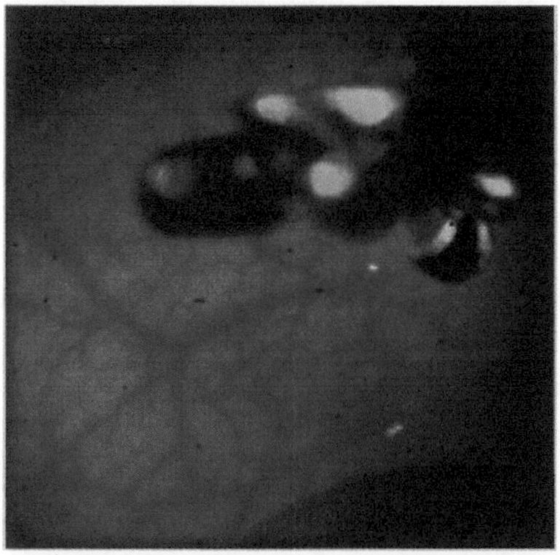
1a

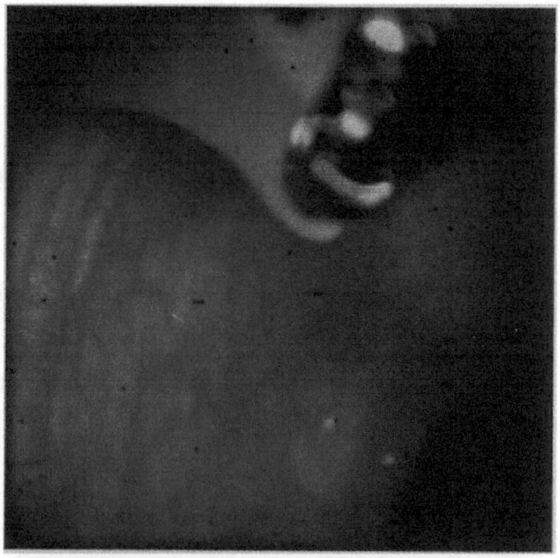
151b

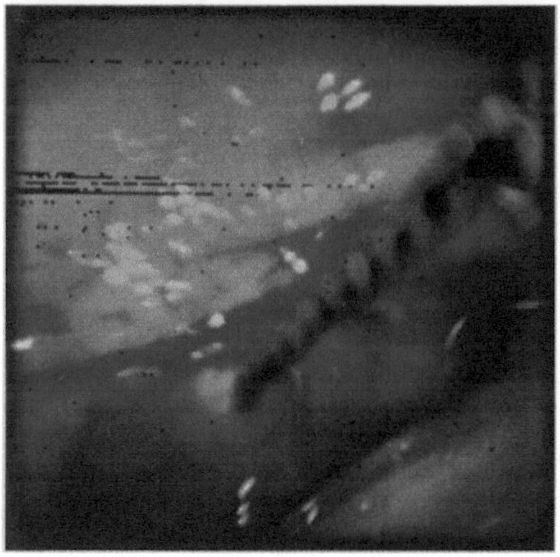
52

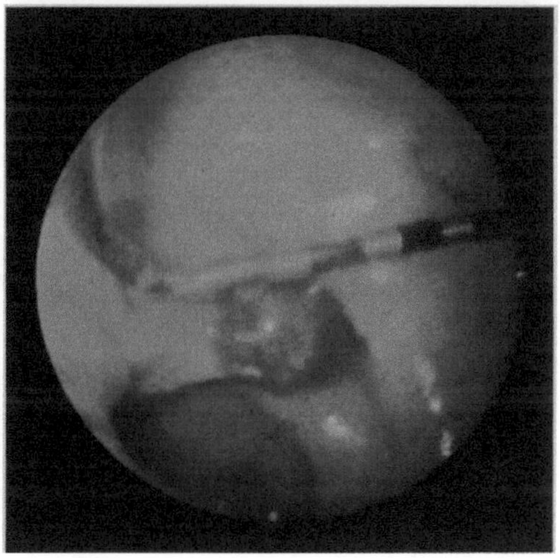
153

3. Use of Accessory Instruments (Continuation)

154 Ablation of a broadbased colon polyp with the high frequency diathermy snare

155 Retrieval of a colon polyp; line of excision is at the level of the mucosa

156 Electrocoagulation of a cecal hemagioma

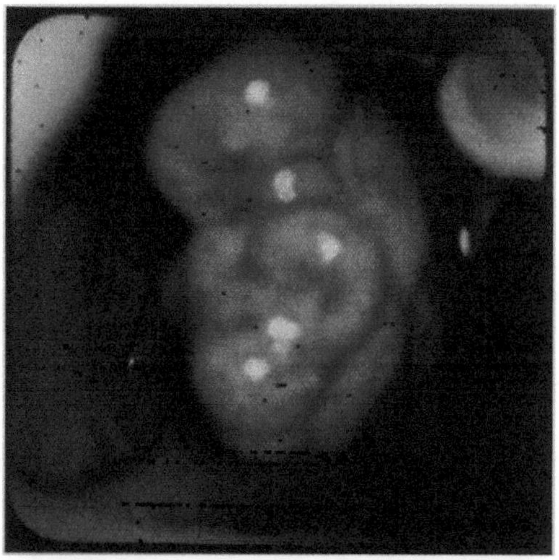

154

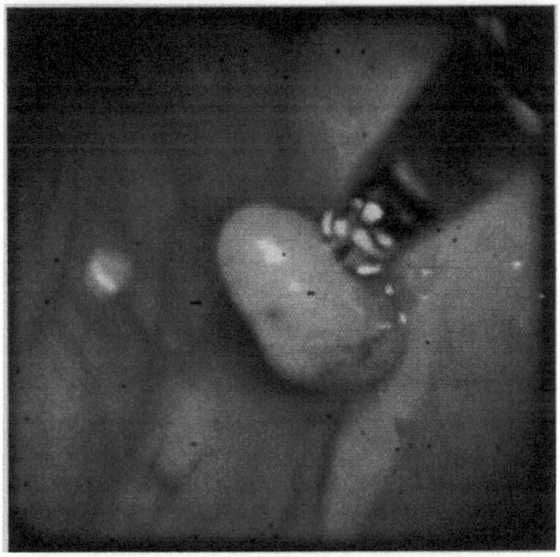

155

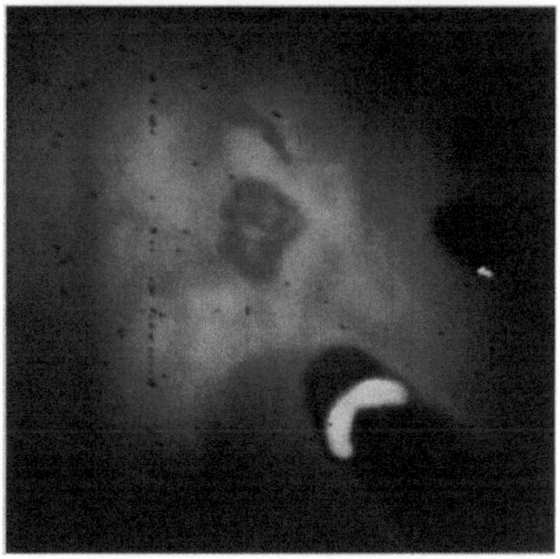

156

4. Anatomy

157 Topography of the colon

158 Cecum with ileocecal valve and appendiceal orifice

5. Technique

159 Schematic representation of the 2 sigmoid patterns; alterations induced during coloscopy

160 Partial stiffening of the coloscope with the stabilizing probe or tube after straightening of the sigmoid (schematic)

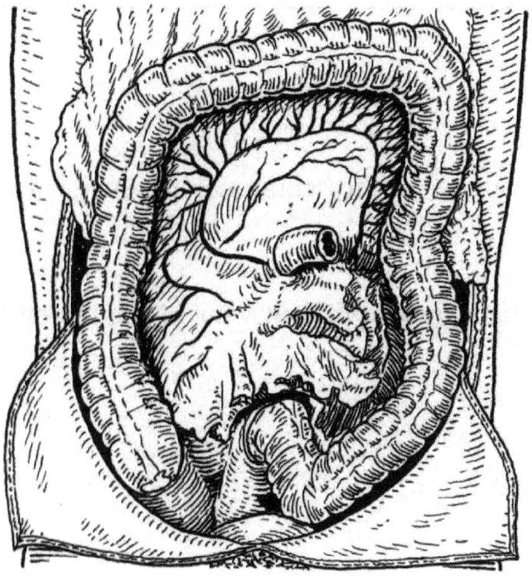

157

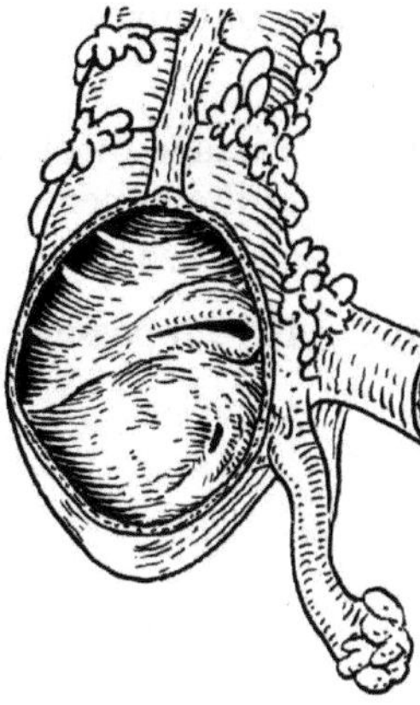

158

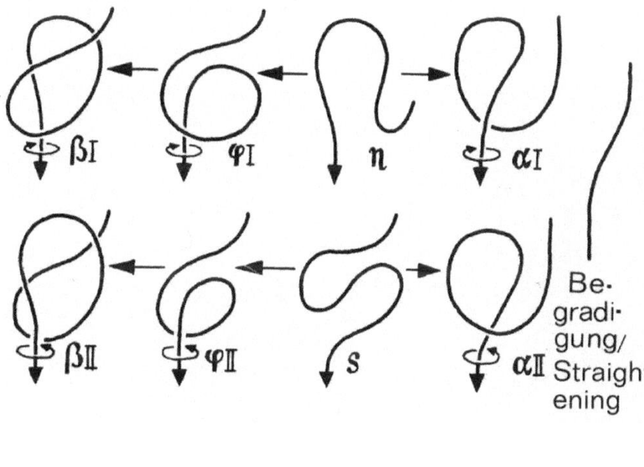

159

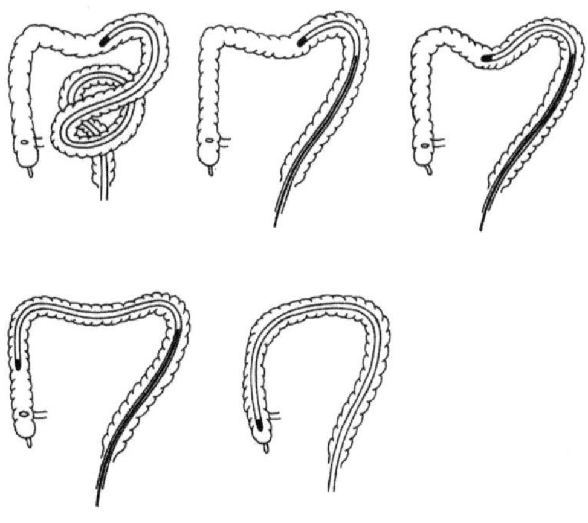

160

5. Technique (Continuation)

161 Passage through the transverse colon (triangular outline) with optimal view of the lumen

162 Partial passage through the sigmoid without view of the lumen

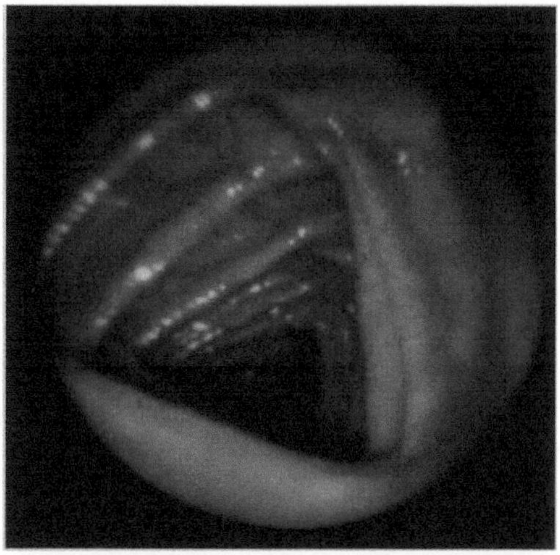
161

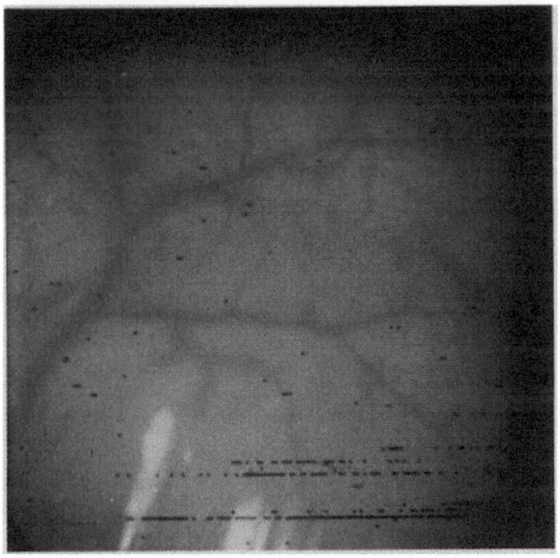
162

5.1 Sigmoid Colon

163a Alpha-shape prior to straightening

163b After straightening (fixation of the instrument tip in the splenic flexure)

163c Ideal position of the coloscope after complete introduction. Instrument tip in cecum

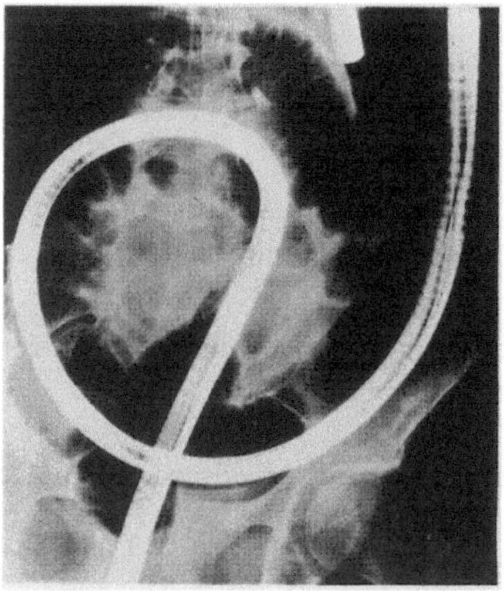

163a

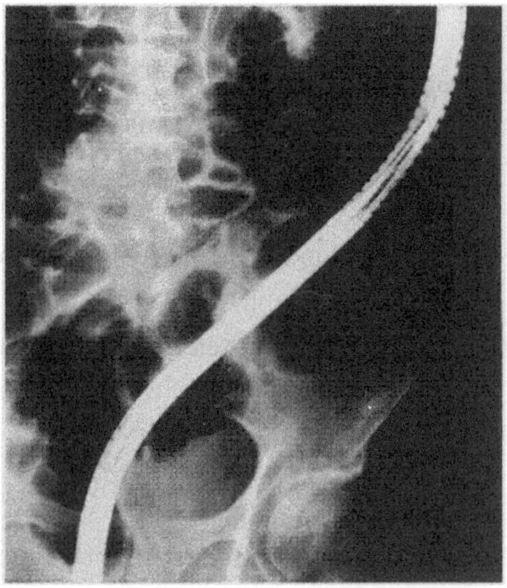

163b

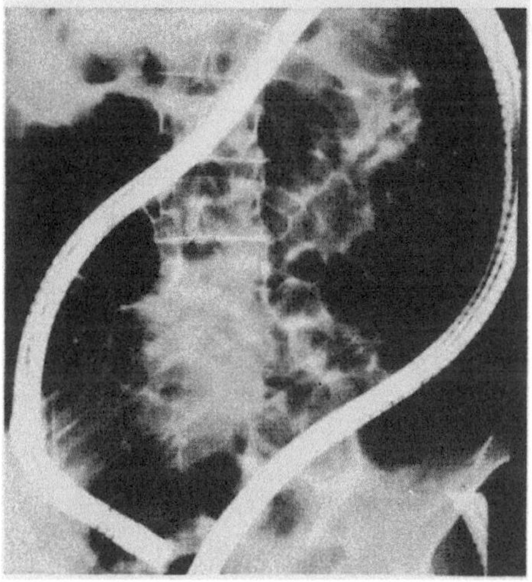

163c

5.1 Sigmoid Colon (Continuation)

164a Phi-shape

164b Hooking of the medially deflected coloscope tip at the splenic flexure

164c Partial straightening of the sigmoid by simultaneous withdrawal and rotation of the coloscope

164d Complete straightening of the sigmoid and further advance to the cecum

165a Beta-shape: bretzel-shaped sigmoid with long mesosigmoid

165b Coloscope reaching the cecum after straightening of the beta-shape and partial stiffening of the coloscope

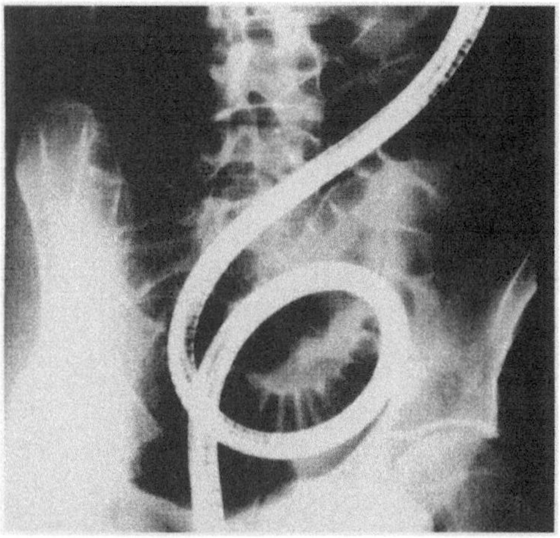
4a

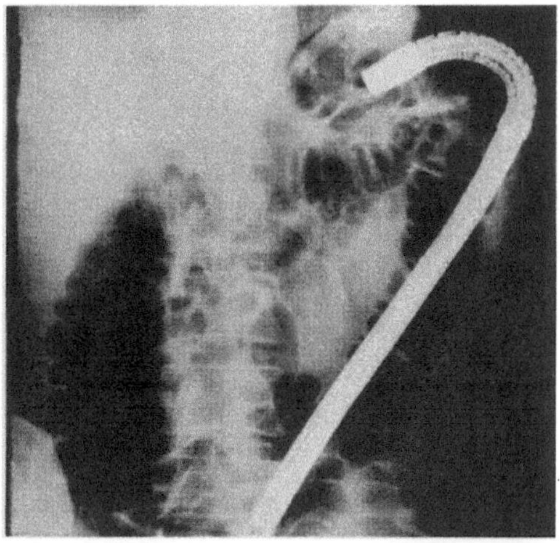
164b

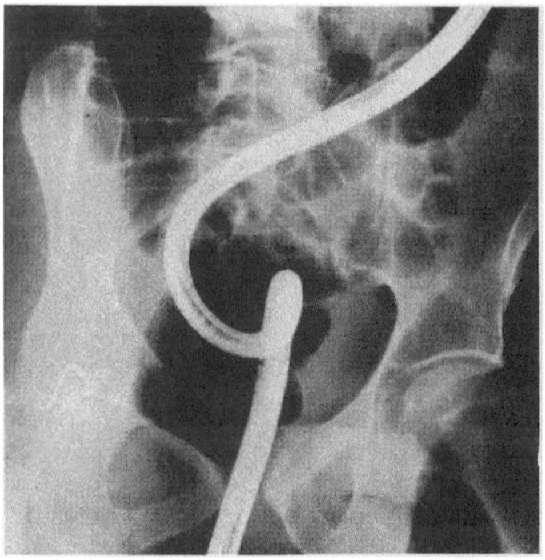
4c

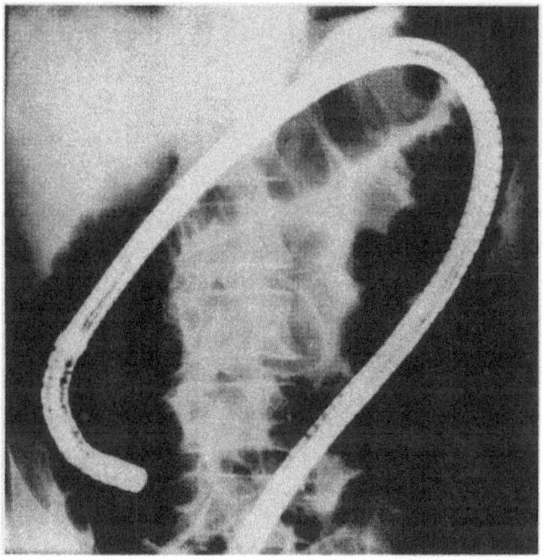
164d

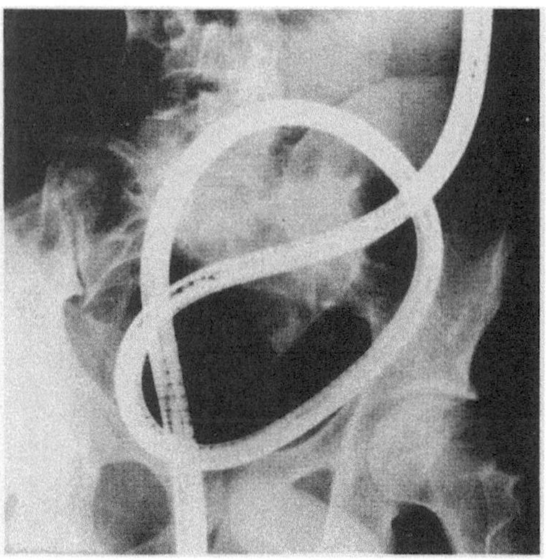
a

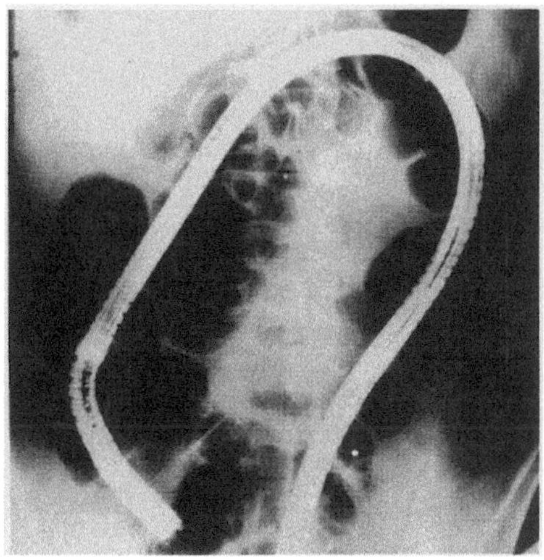
165b

166a Eta-shape

166b Partial straightening of the eta-shape by traction on the coloscope after reaching the distal descending colon

166c Complete straightening

167a Dolichosigmoid with combined phi- and eta-shape

167b Straightening of the dolichosigmoid prior to partial stiffening

167c Straightened sigmoid after partial stiffening

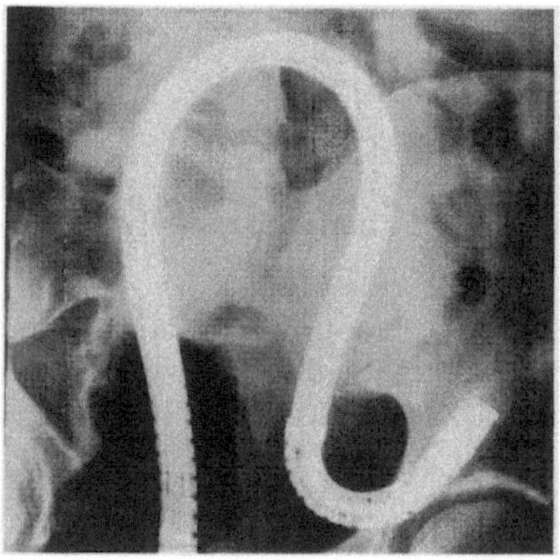
166a

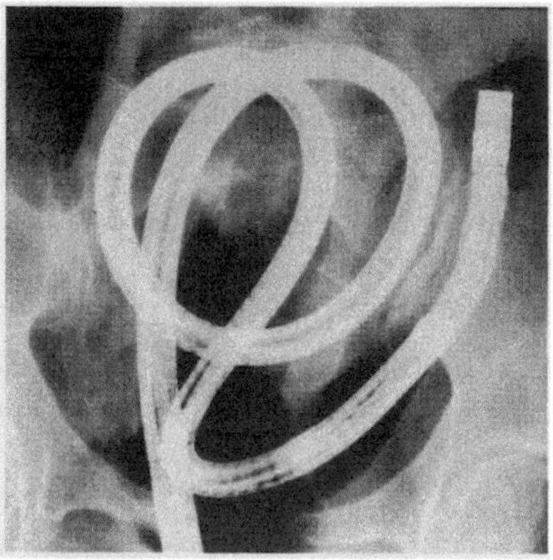
167a

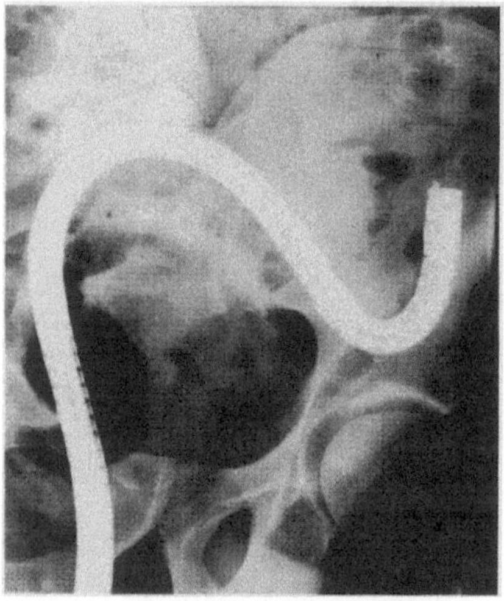
166b

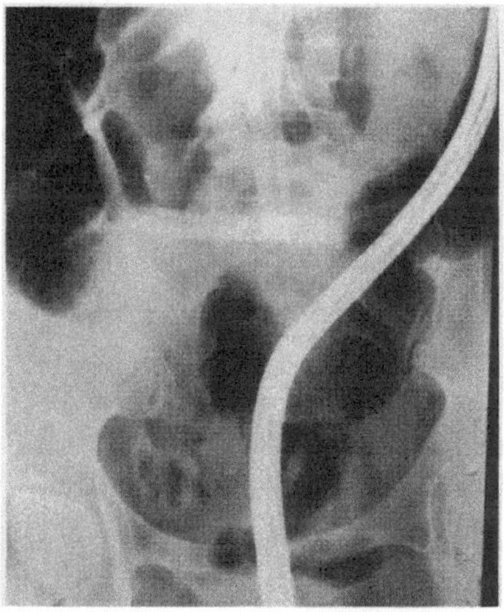
167b

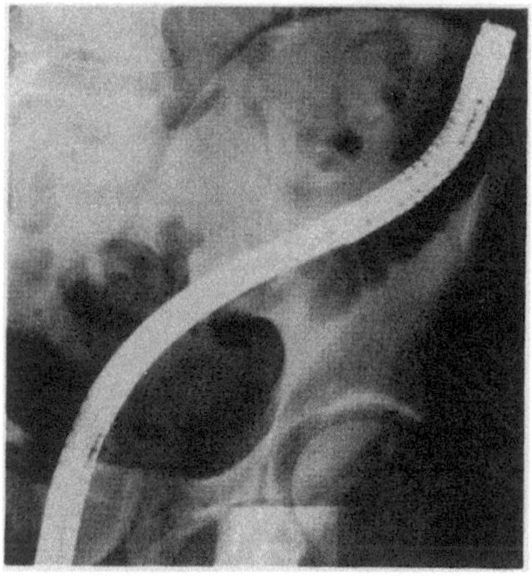
166c

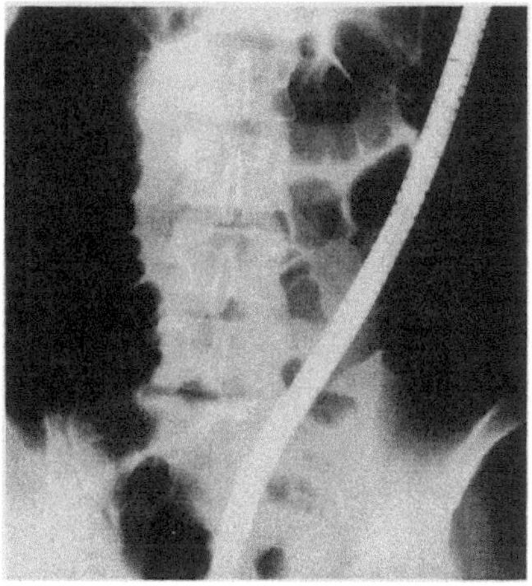
167c

168a Sigmoid with narrow turns: combination phi- and horizontally oriented eta-shape

168b Straightening of the distal loop after reaching the distal one-third of the descending colon by traction and rotation of the coloscope

168c Straightening of the proximal loop by traction on the coloscope

168d Straightened sigmoid prior to partial stiffening

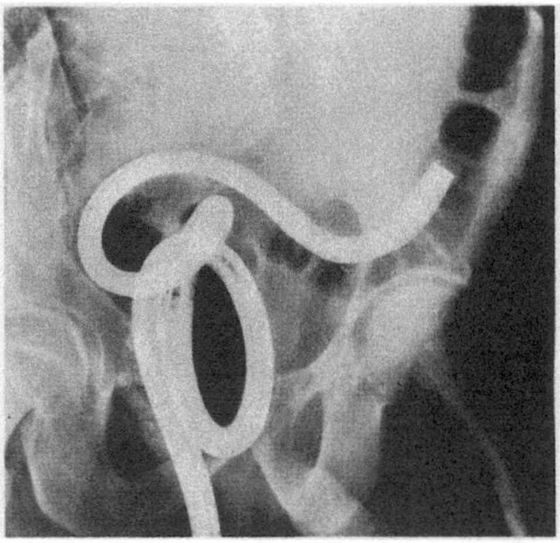

68 a

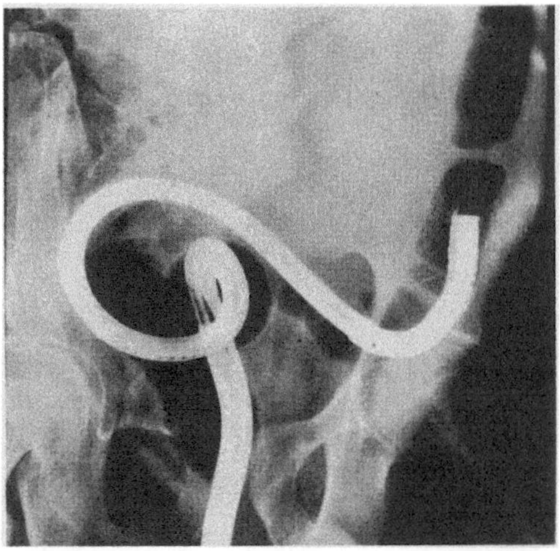

168 b

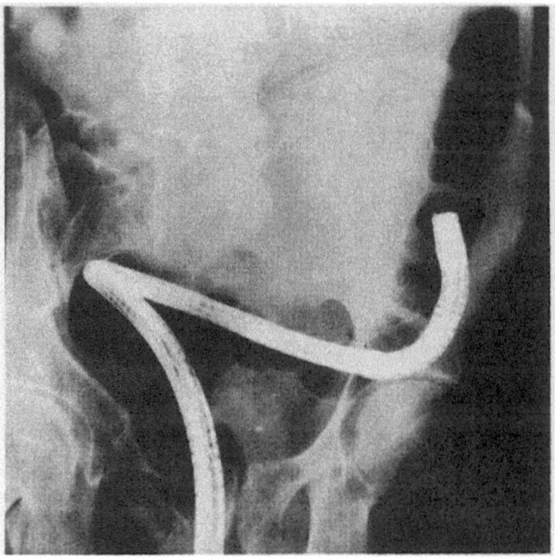

68 c

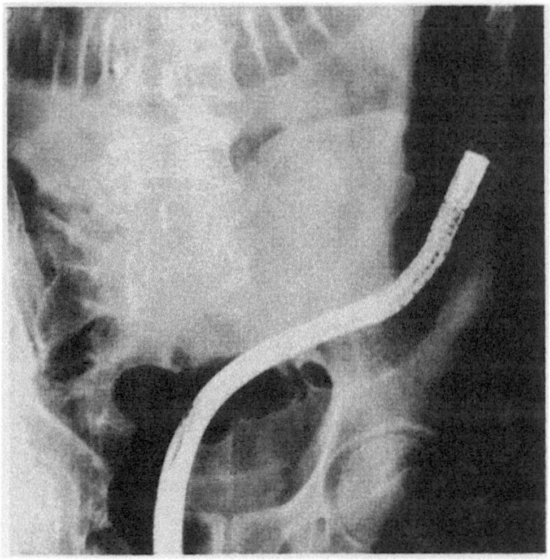

168 d

5.1 Sigmoid Colon (Continuation)

169a Complicated course of the sigmoid: combined phi- and eta-shape

169b Straightening of the distal phi-shape by traction and rotation on the coloscope

169c Straightening of the proximal eta-shape by traction on the coloscope with stiffening of sigmoid and descending colon

170a Eta-shape which could not be straightened by traction on the coloscope in this case

170b Change to the alpha-shape by clockwise rotation of the coloscope

170c Straightening after reaching the splenic flexure

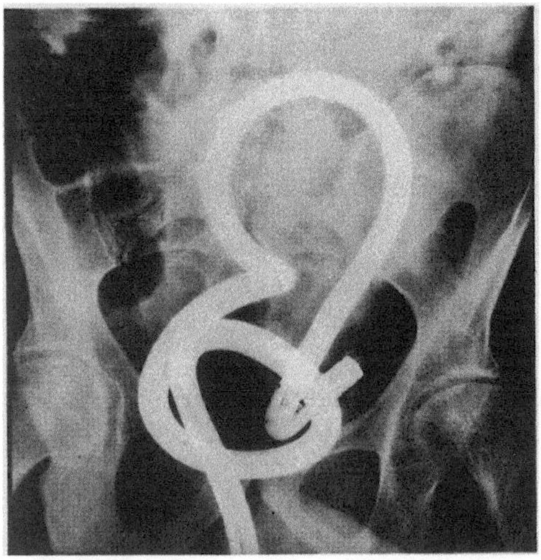
69 a

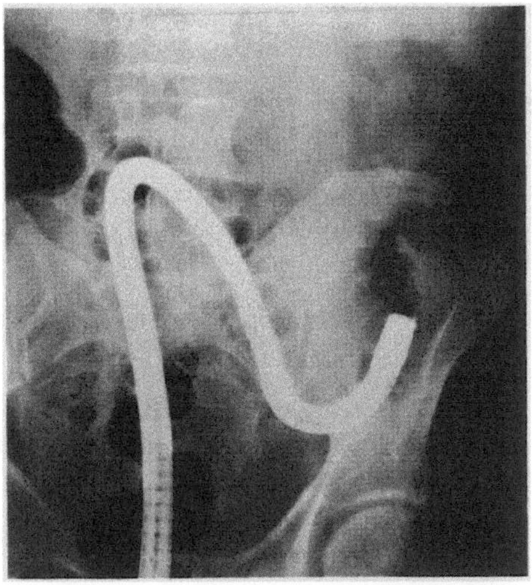
170 a

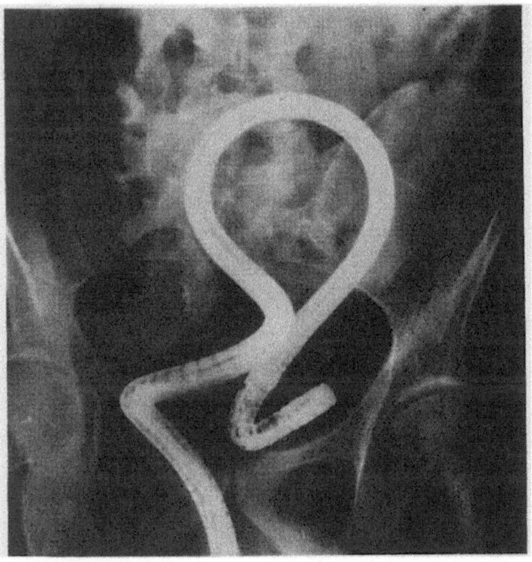
69 b

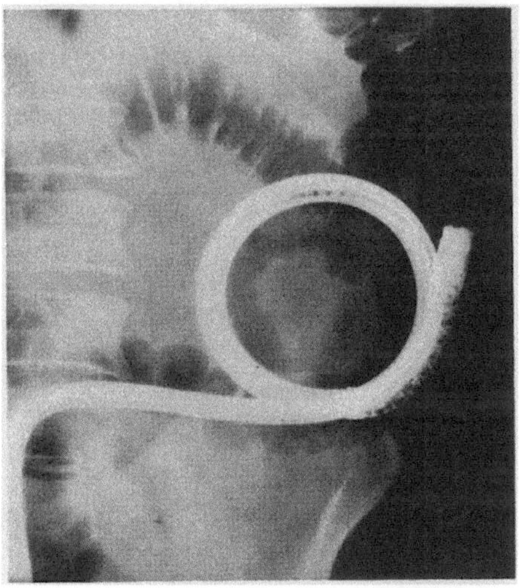
170 b

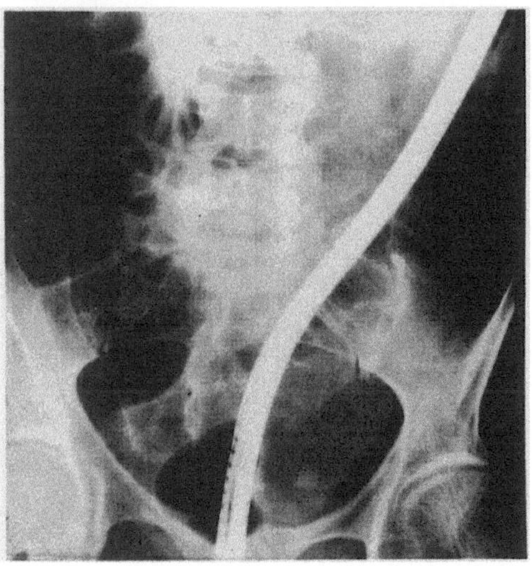
69 c

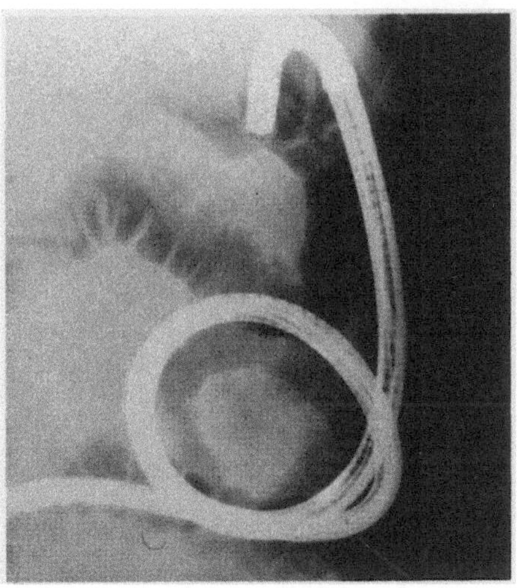
170 c

5.2 Transverse Colon

171 Coloscope advanced to the cecum with U-shaped course of the transverse colon

172a Undulating course of the transverse colon (air insufflation)

172b Straightening of the transverse colon after reaching the hepatic flexure and further advance into the cecum

173a U-shaped course of the transverse colon

173b Fixation of the instrument tip at the hepatic flexure and straightening of the transverse colon by traction on the coloscope

173c Further advance of the coloscope into the cecum

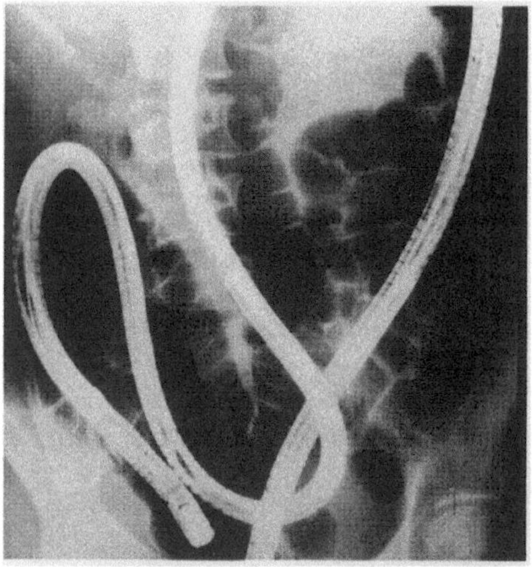
171

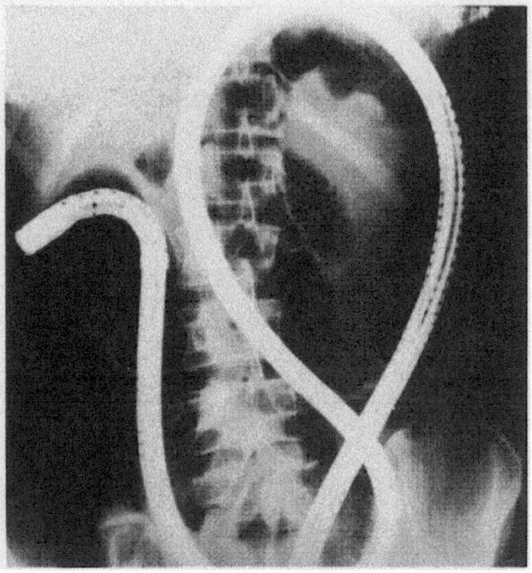
173a

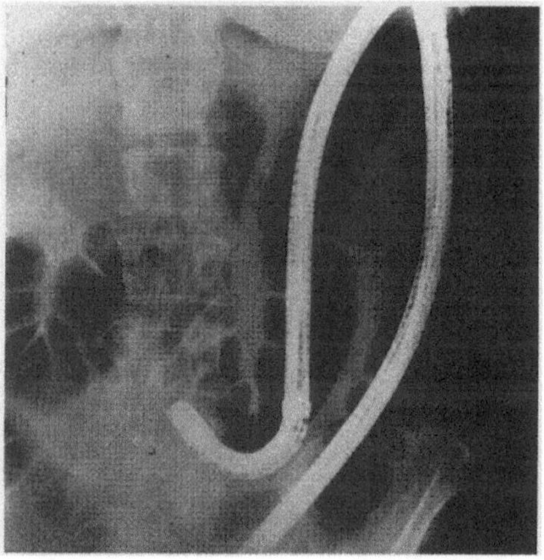
72a

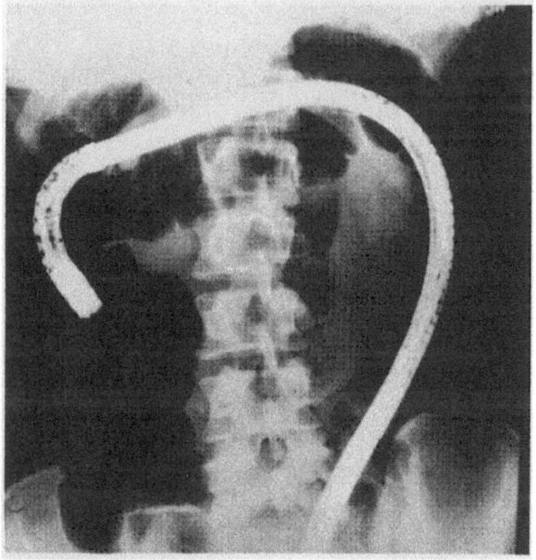
173b

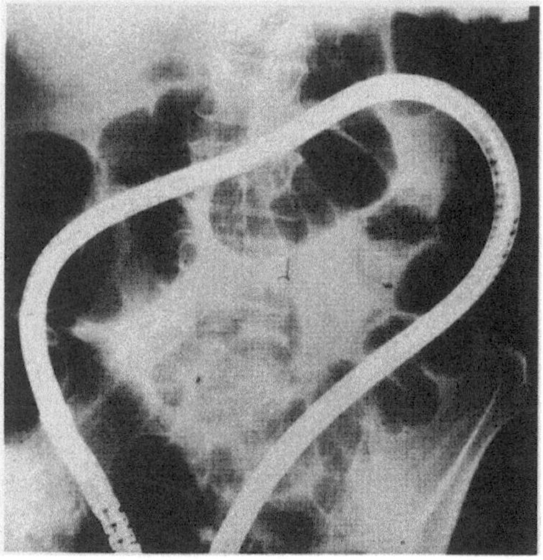
72b

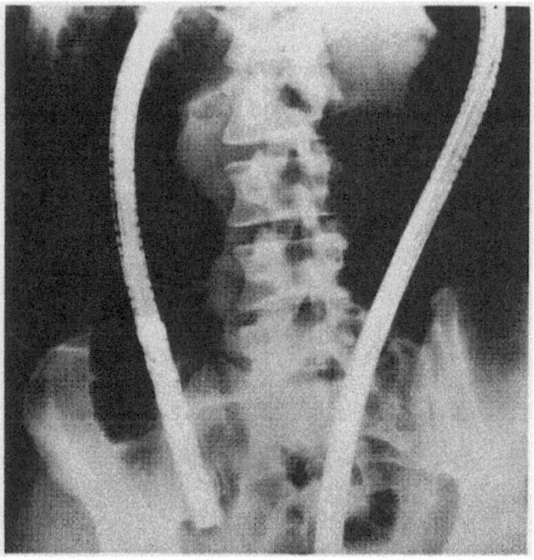
173c

5.2 Transverse Colon (Continuation)

174a Loop formation of the transverse colon

174b Partial straightening by traction on the coloscope after positioning and fixing it in the cecum

174c Complete straightening with ideal position of the endoscope within the colon

175a Combined circular and undulating course of the transverse colon

175b Fixation of the instrument tip after reaching the hepatic flexure

175c Straightening of the transverse colon with the tip located in the cecum by traction and rotation of the coloscope

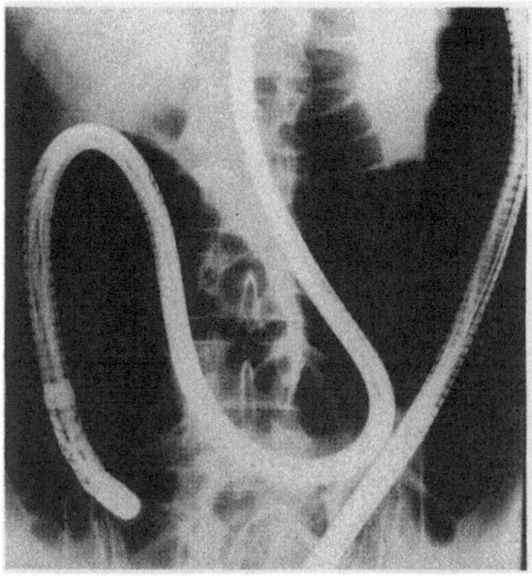
74a

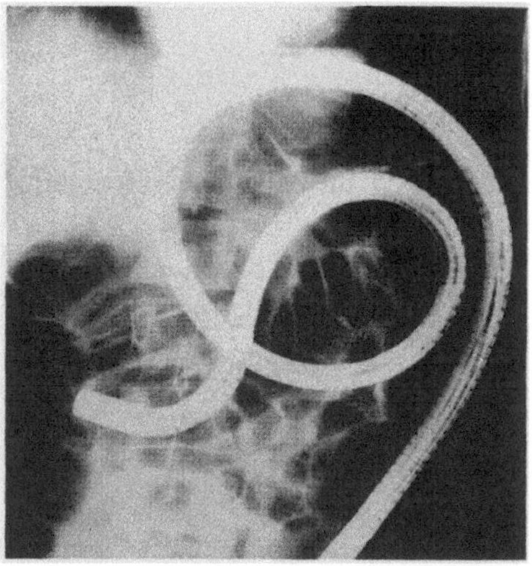
175a

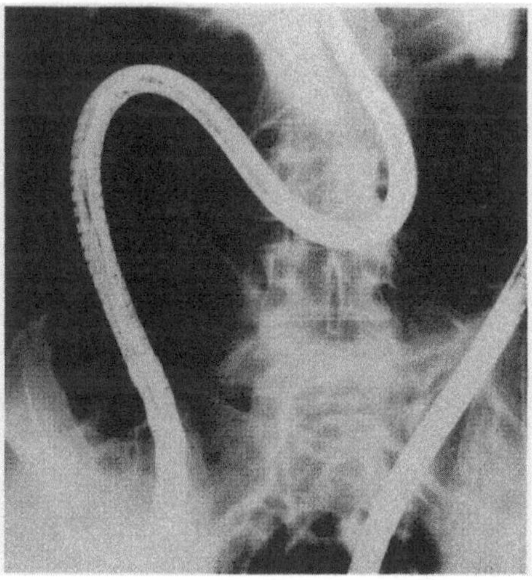
4b

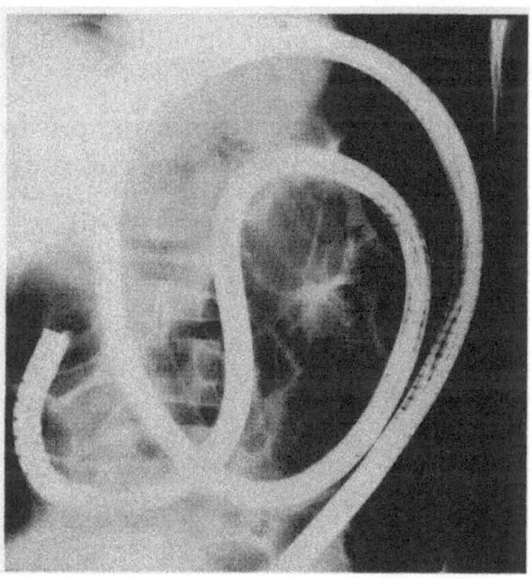
175b

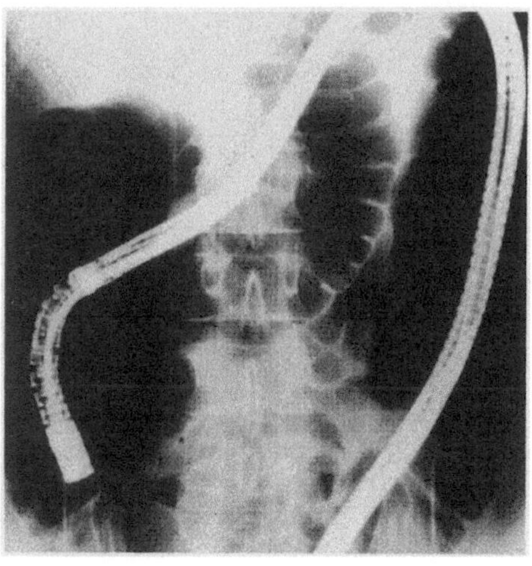
4c

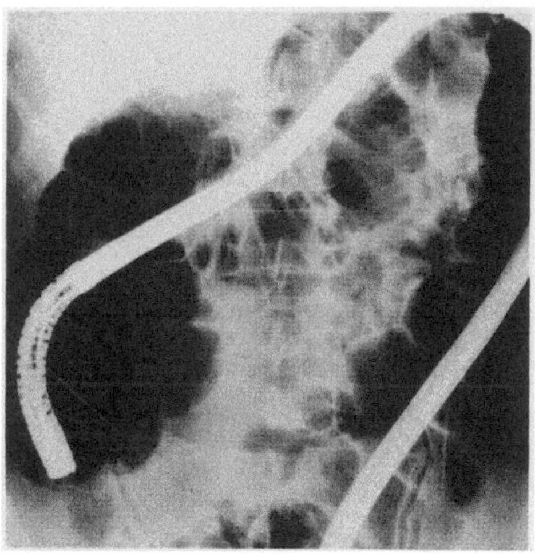
175c

5.3 Inversion

176a In medial direction (cecum)

176b In dorsal direction (cecum)

176c In lateral direction (cecum)

5.4 Ileoscopy

177 Instrument tip in the terminal ileum

178 Instrument tip in the proximal ileum

179 Instrument tip in the proximal ileum in the presence of an ileo-transverse colostomy (Crohn's disease)

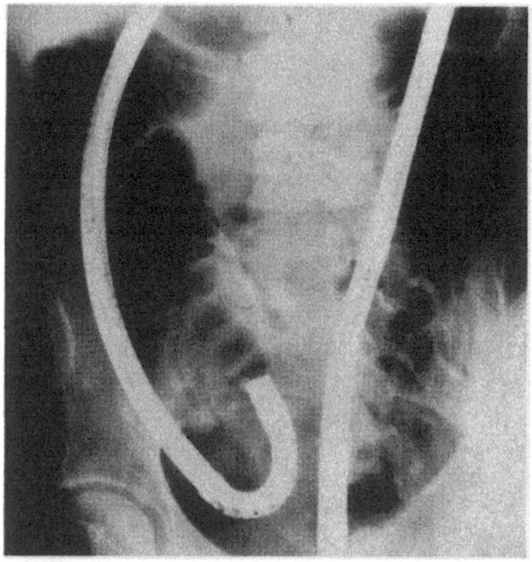
176a

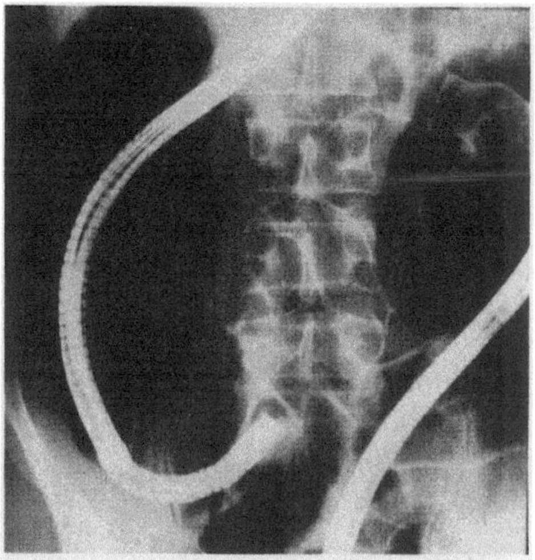
177

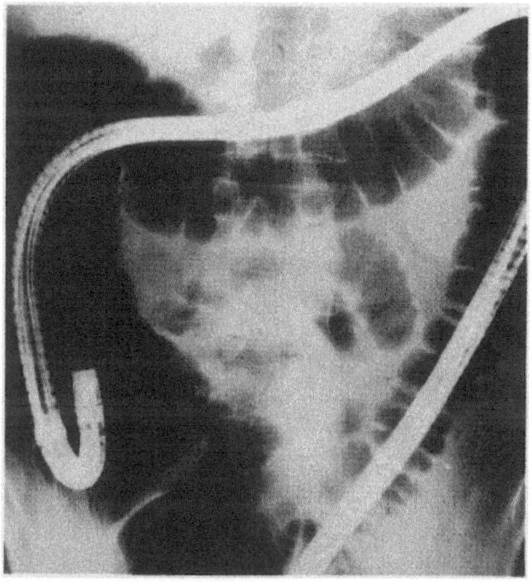
176b

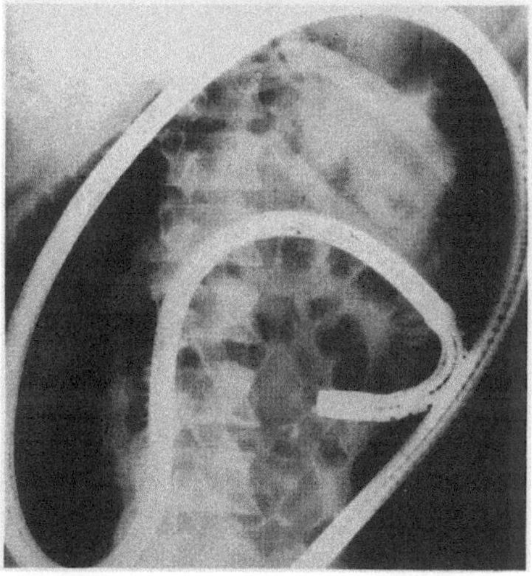
178

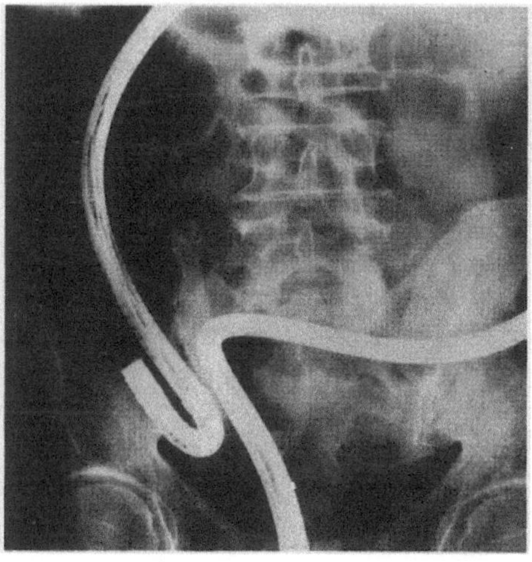
176c

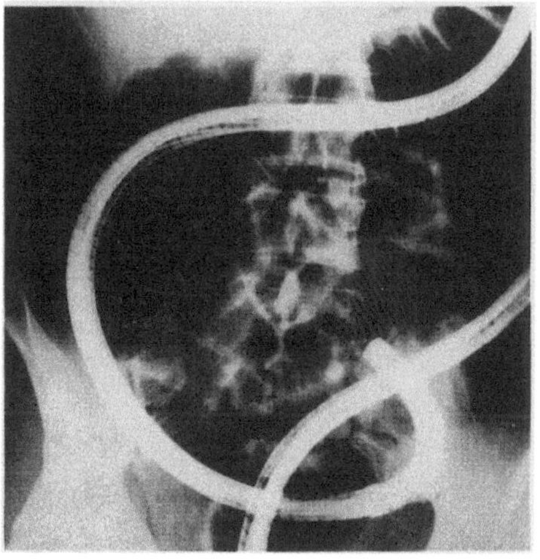
179

6. Findings

6.1 Ileocecal (Bauhin's) Valve

180a Labial shape of the ileocecal valve

180b Papillary shape of the ileocecal valve

180c Intermediate shape of the ileocecal valve

181a–c Physiologic variation in the shape of the ileocecal valve (stages of opening)

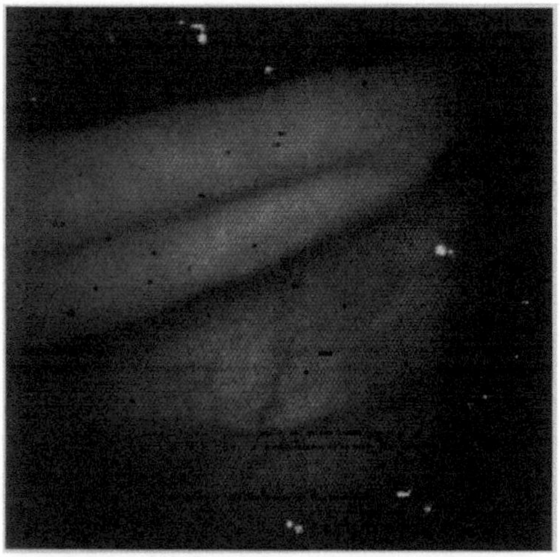

a

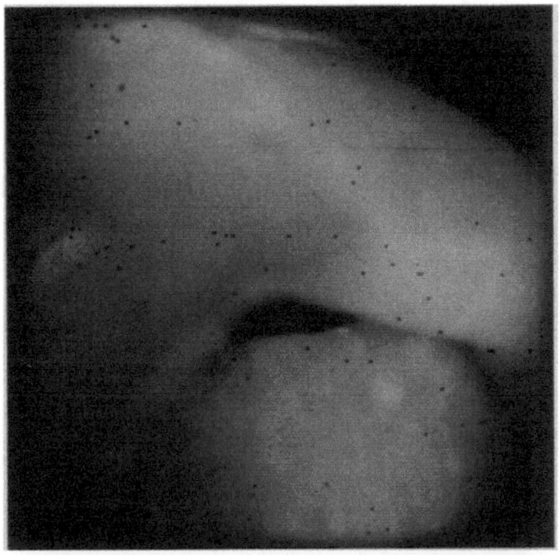

181a

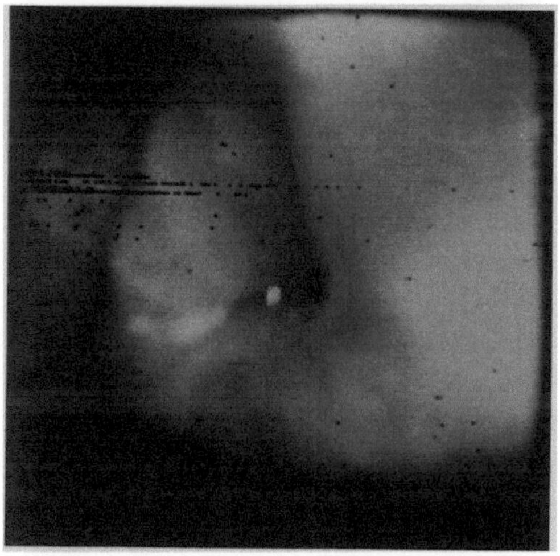

b

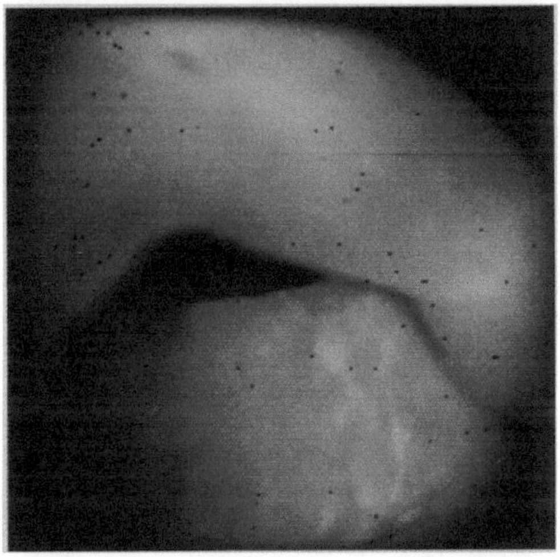

181b

c

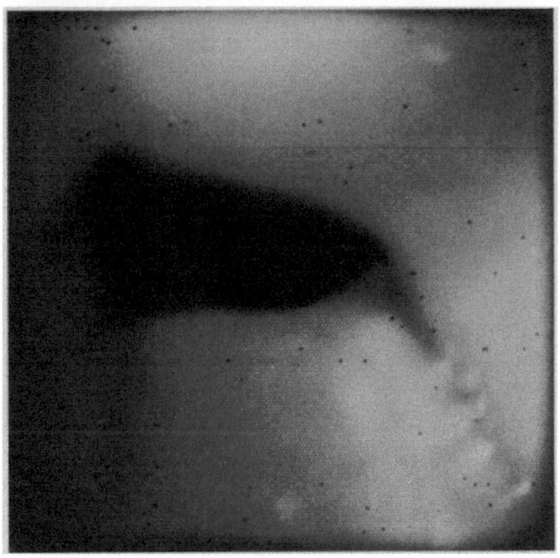

181c

181 d–i Physiologic variation in the shape of the ileocecal valve (complete opening followed by closing)

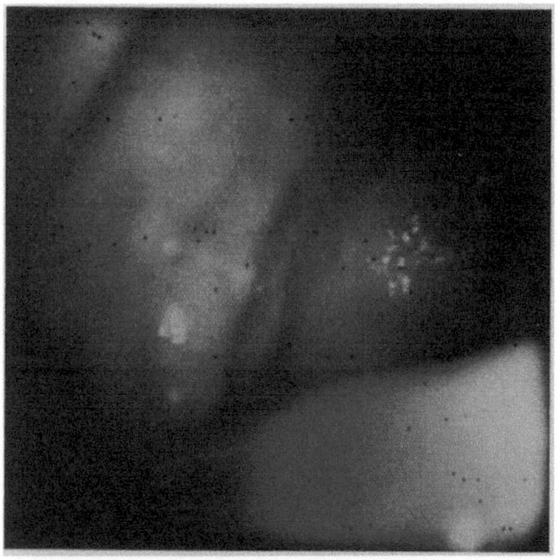

1d

181g

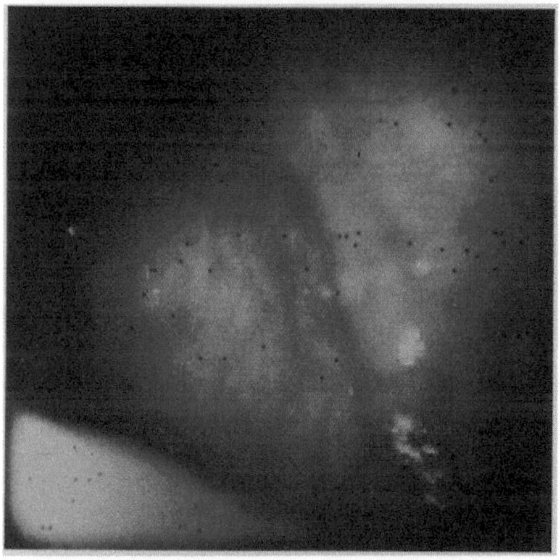

1e

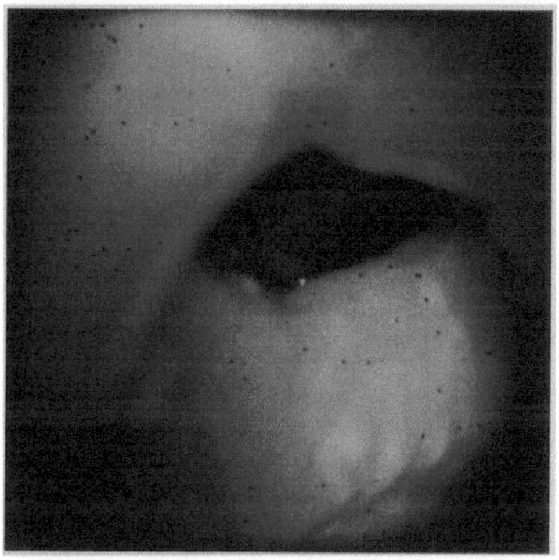

181h

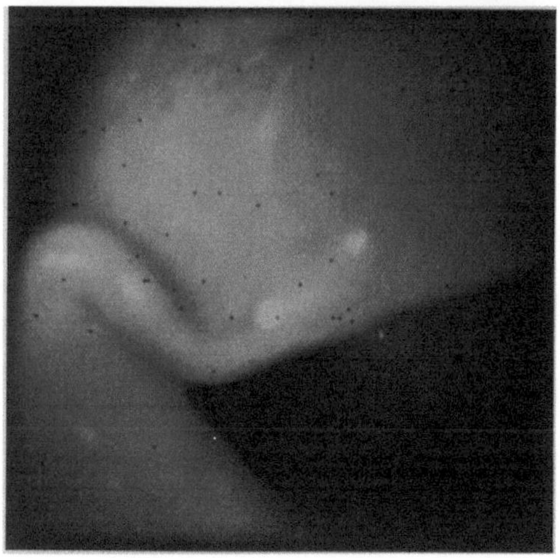

1f

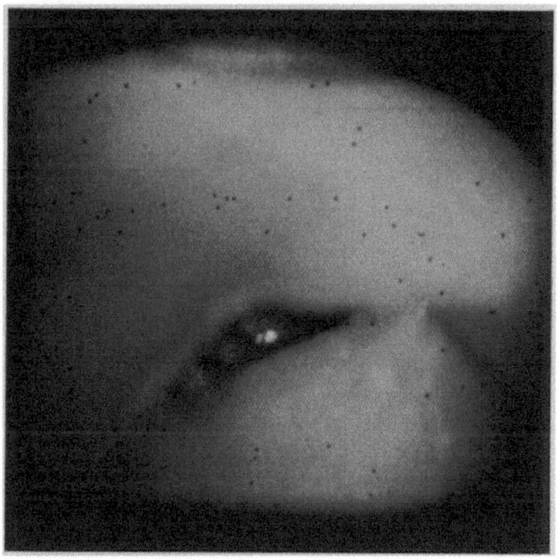

181i

6.2 Ileum

182 Normal mucosal and fold pattern (folds of Kerckring) in the terminal ileum

183 Minor bleeding following forceps biopsy of a lymphoid follicle in the terminal ileum

184a–b Normal mucosal pattern of the proximal ileum

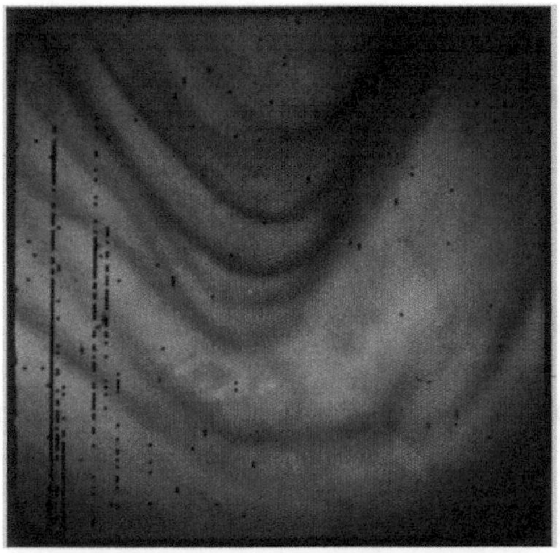

82

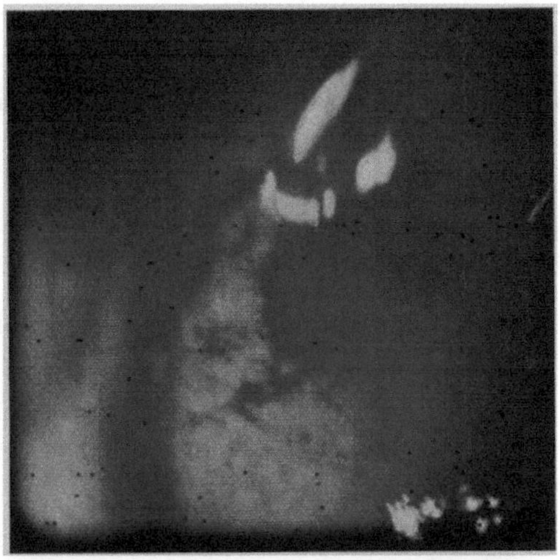

183

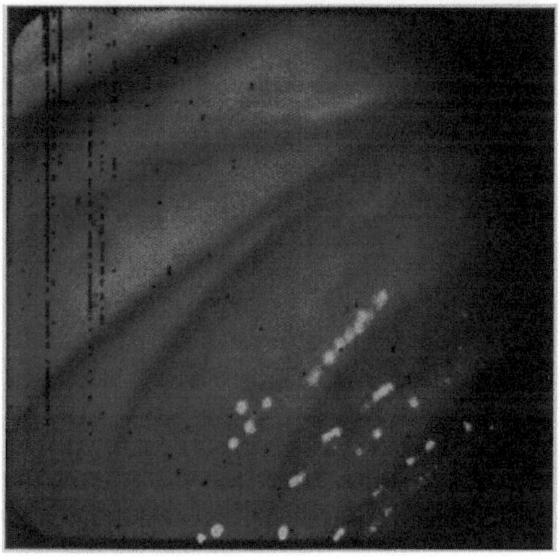

a

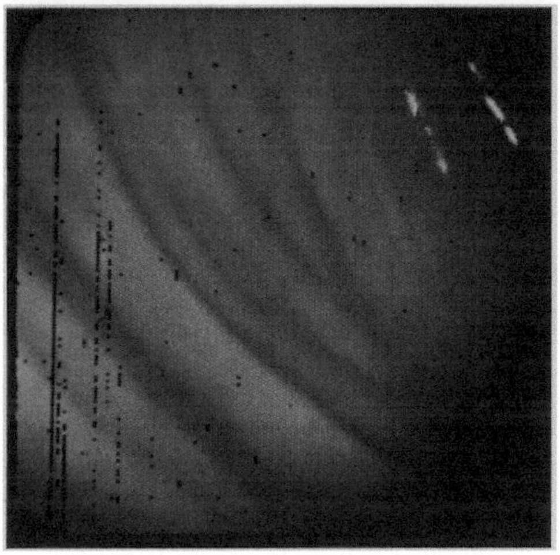

184b

6.3 Selective Coloscopic Visualization of the Appendix

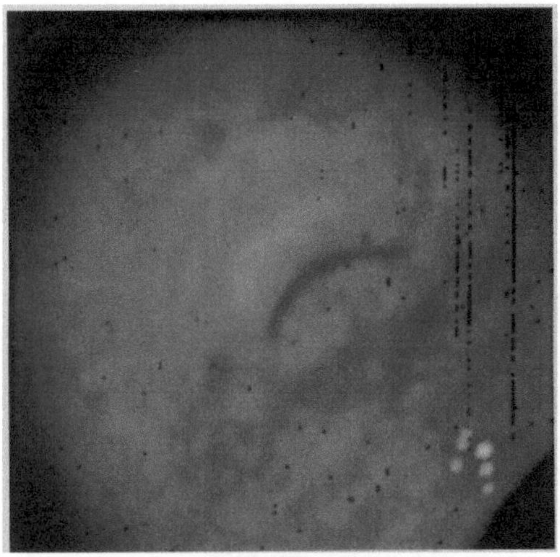
185

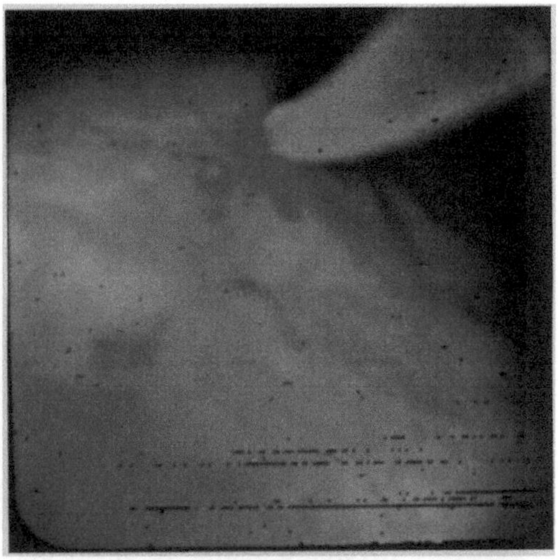
186

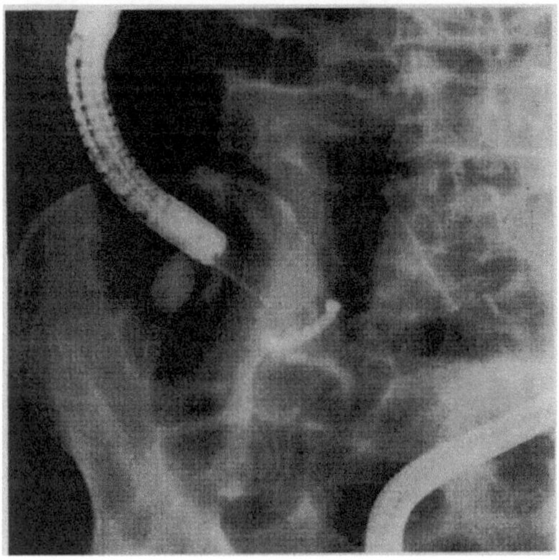
87a

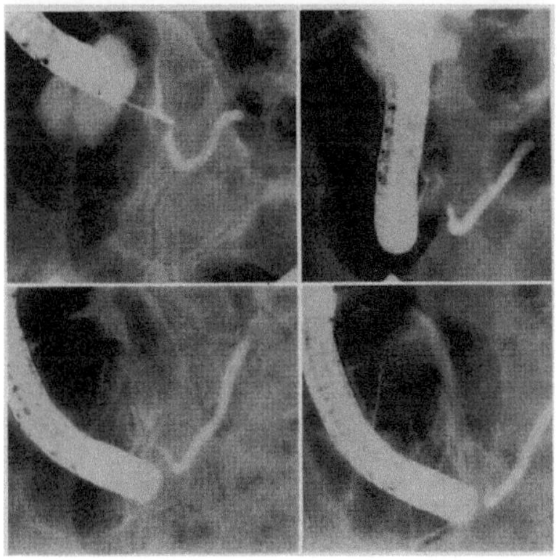
187b

6.4 Findings after Appendectomy

188 Converging folds at the medial aspect of the cecum following appendectomy

189 Inverted mucosal stump, 3×3.5 cm in size, following appendectomy

7. Inversion

190a Inversion of the tip of the coloscope in the cecum

190b Inversion of the tip of the coloscope in the rectal ampulla

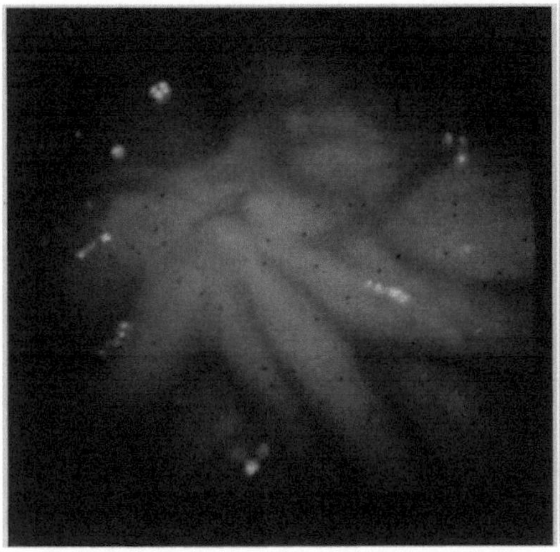

188

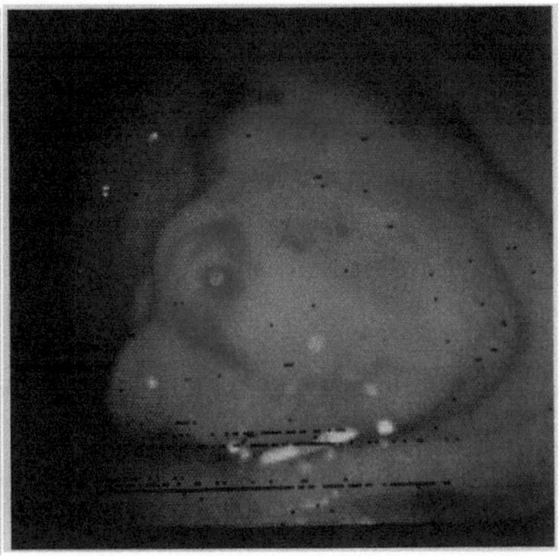

189

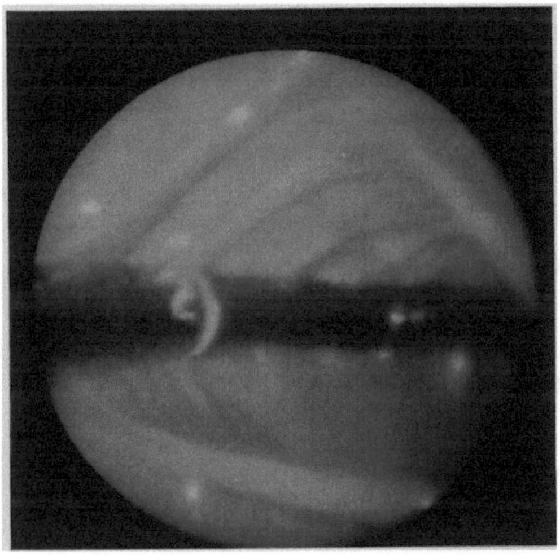

90a

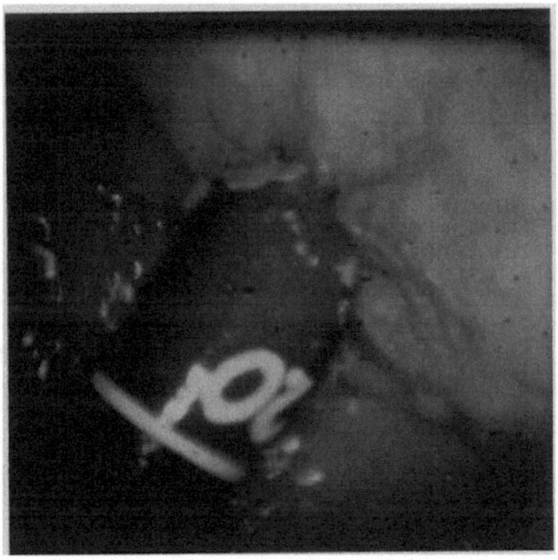

190b

8. Operative Coloscopy

8.1 Mechanical Ablation

191 a Attempted mechanical removal of a 3 cm sigmoid polyp; stalk 6 mm in diameter

191 b Interruption of the procedure because of beginning hemorrhage

191 c Bloodless polypectomy with the high frequency diathermy snare during a second session (adenomatous polyp)

8.2 Electrocoagulation

192 Electrocoagulation (b) of a small polyp (a) and coagulation of its base (c). (TURELL: Diseases of the colon and anorectum)

8.3 High Frequency Currents

193 a Undamped sinusoidal cutting current

193 b Spark gap current: high frequency current with damped oscillations and high voltage peaks: for tissue coagulation

193 c Mixed current: combined cutting and coagulation current

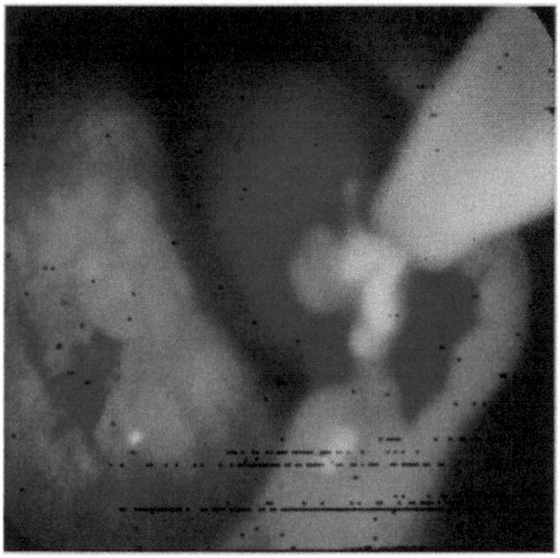

1a

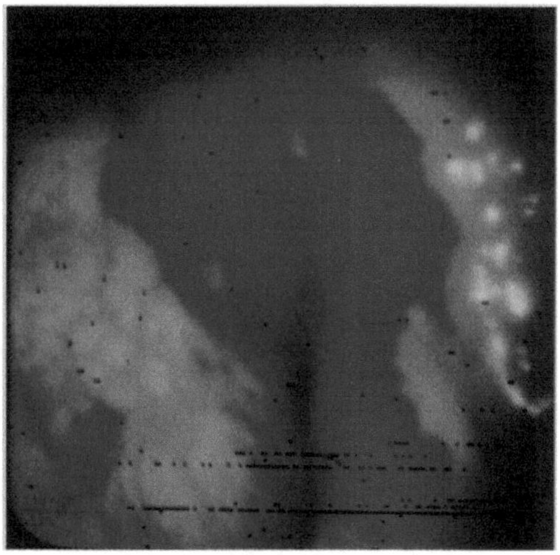

191b

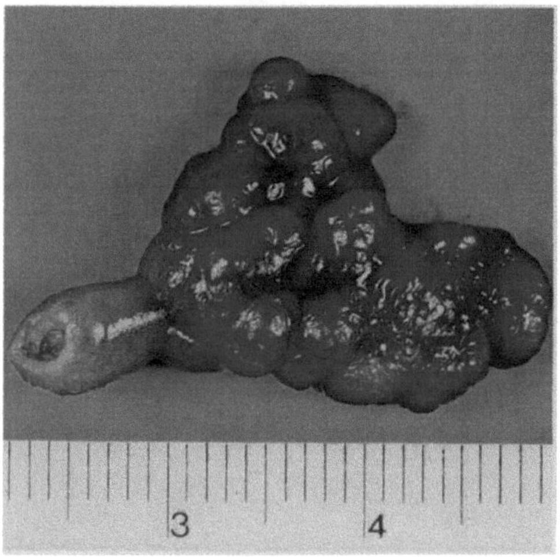

1c

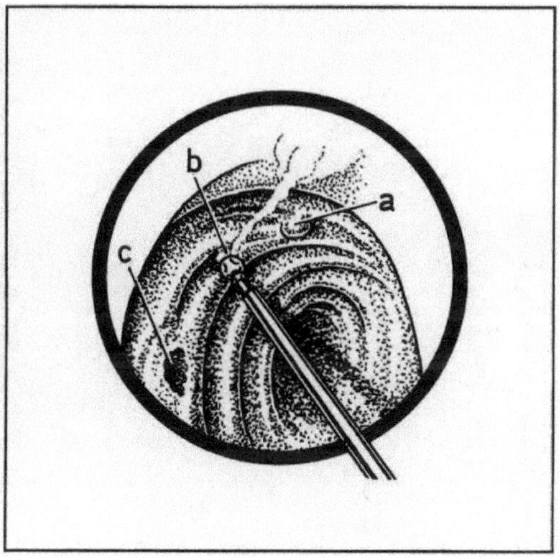

192

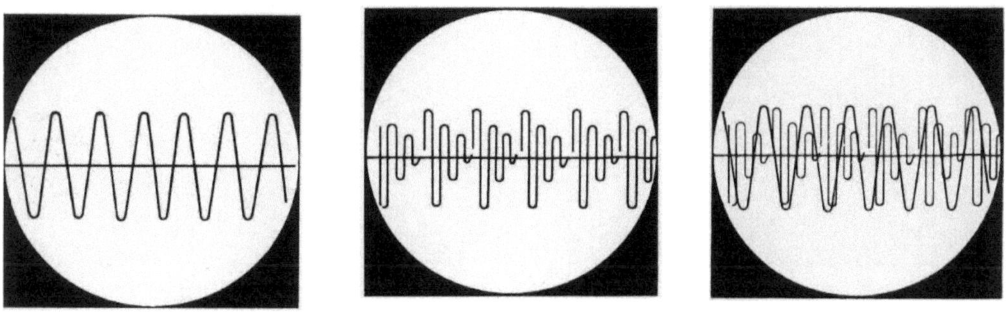

193

a b c

8.4 Resection with the High Frequency Diathermy Snare

194a Pedunculated sigmoid polyp on air contrast barium enema

194b Orientation as to size, position and shape of the polyp with the flexible biopsy forceps

194c–e "Lassoing" of the polyp

194f Base of the polyp being lifted away during excission

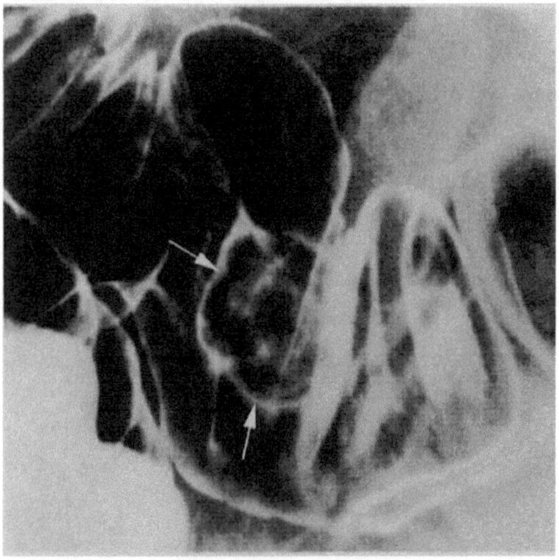
4a

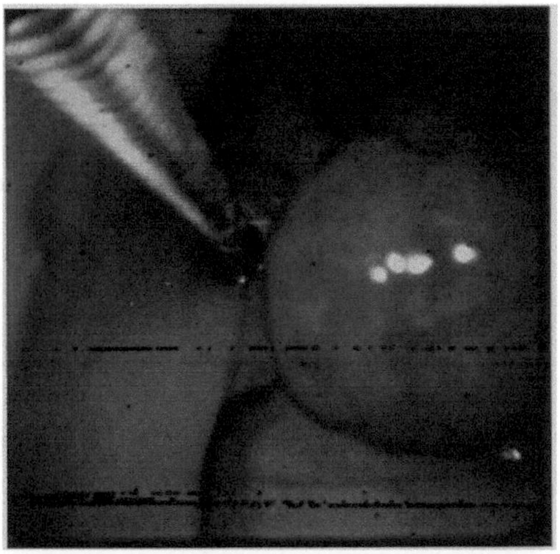
194b

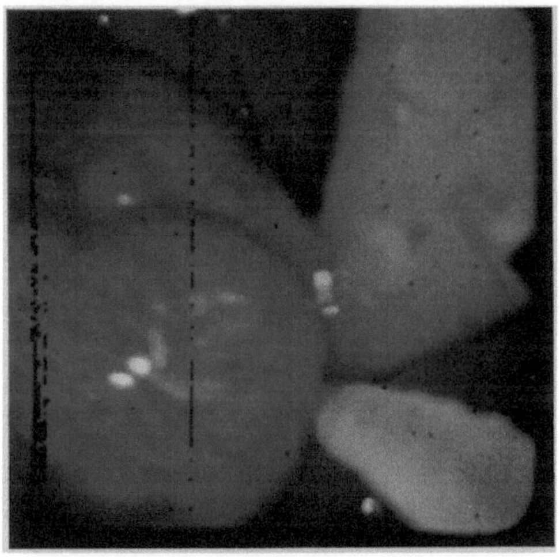
4c

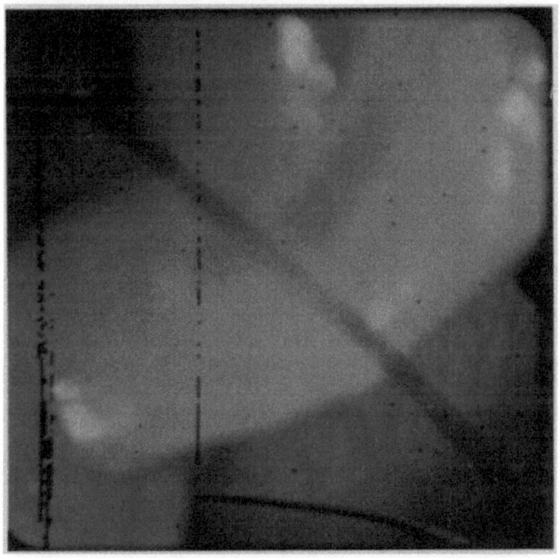
194d

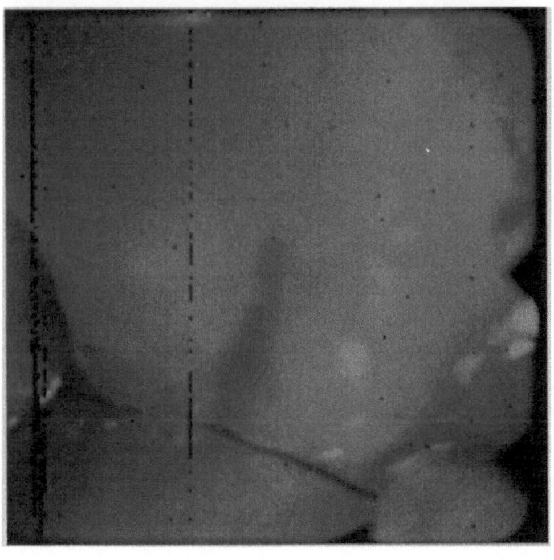
4e

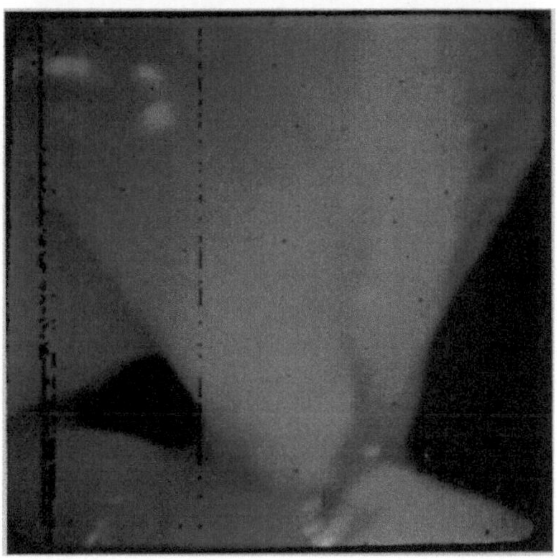
194f

8.4 Resection with the High Frequency Diathermy Snare (Continuation)

194g–h Formation of a small zone of necrosis at the site of excision

194i Polyp removed without bleeding

194k Retrieved polyp with lobulated surface (adenomatous polyp)

194l Small (3 mm) uninflamed scar 10 days following polypectomy

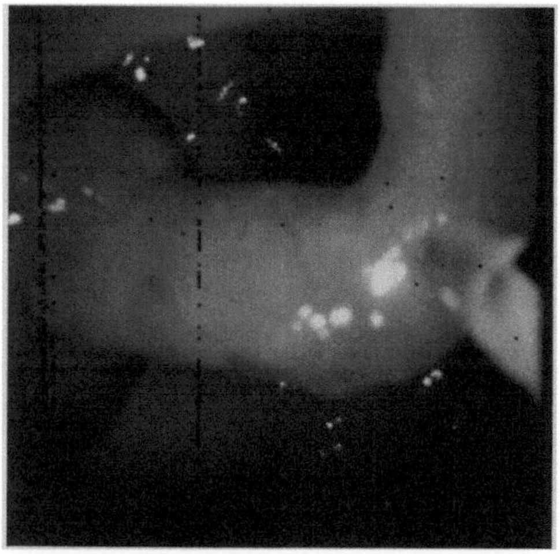

94g

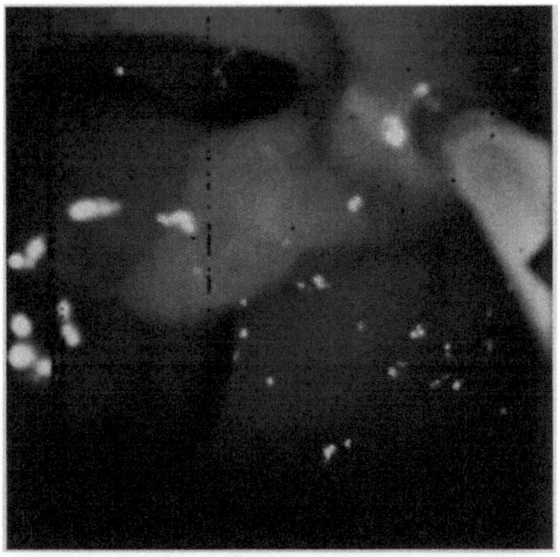

194h

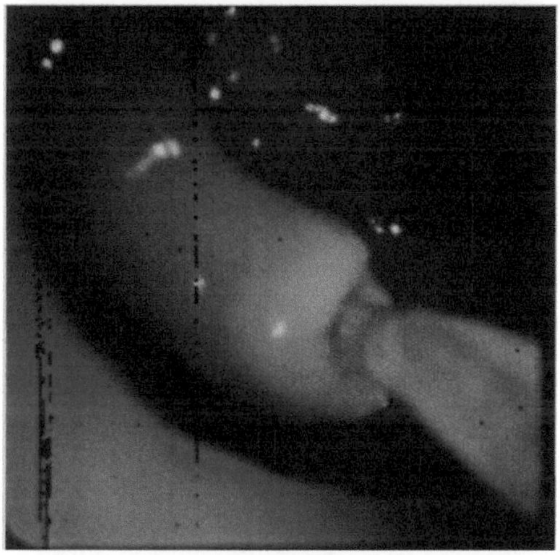

94i

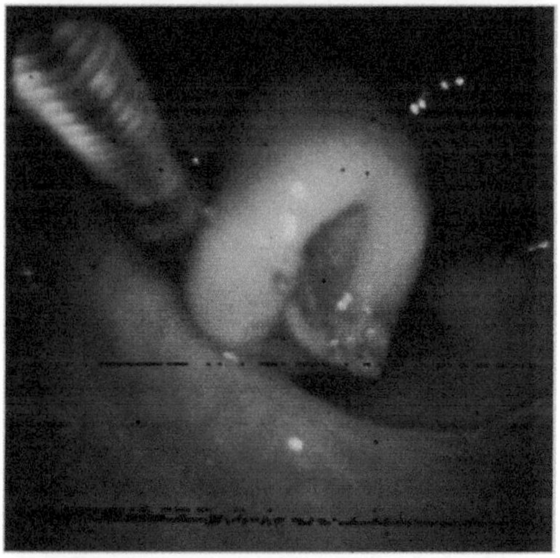

194j

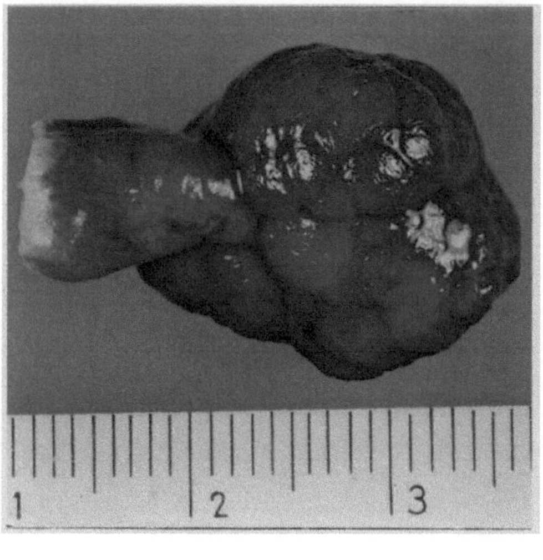

4k

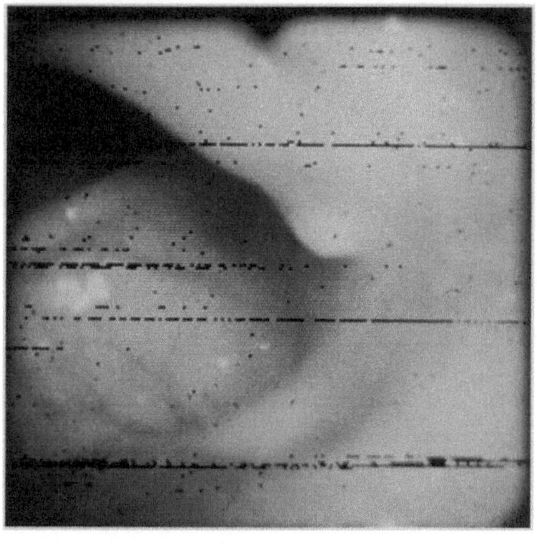

194l

8.4 Resection with the High Frequency Diathermy Snare (Continuation)

195a–d Removal of a lobulated and pedunculated sigmoid polyp (adenomatous polyp)

196a–b Removal of a sessile polyp (base: 6 mm) with the level of excision at the mucosal surface

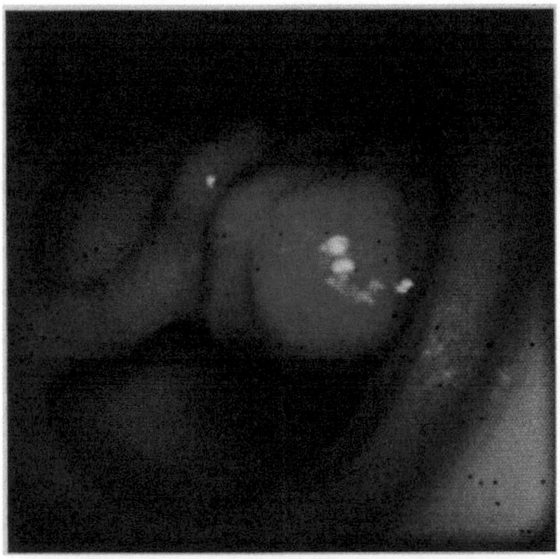

5a

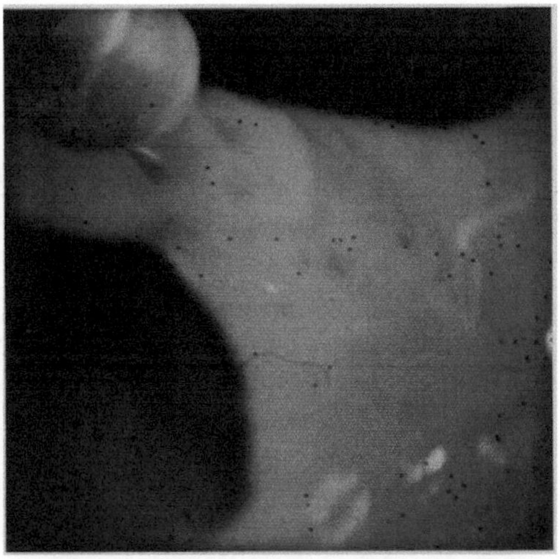

195b

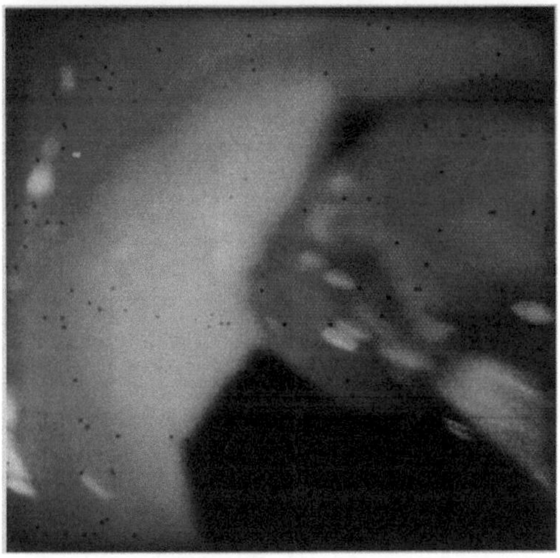

5c

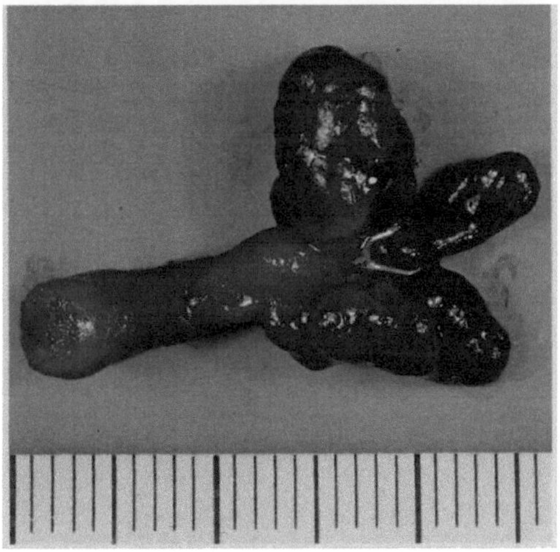

195d

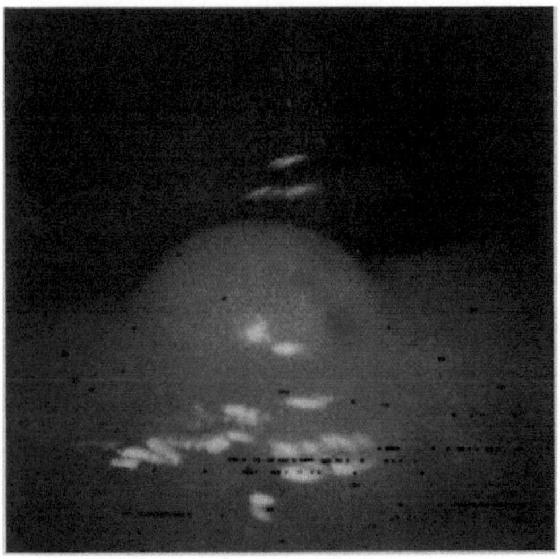

6a

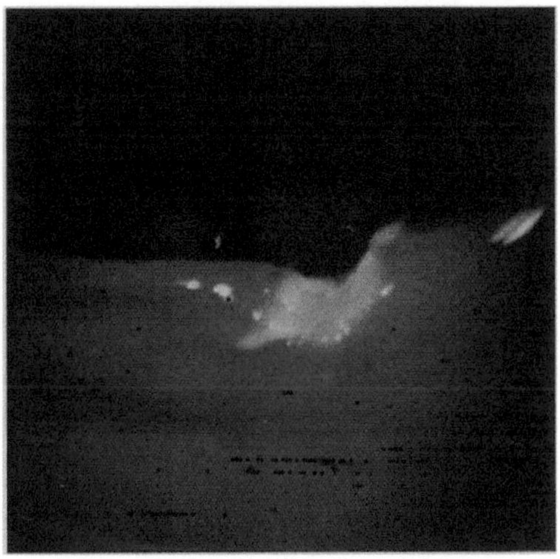

196b

8.4 Resection with the High Frequency Diathermy Snare (Continuation)

197a–c Excision and retrieval of an adenomatous polyp with focal carcinoma on histologic examination

197d–f Follow-up coloscopies
d) Ulcer on the day of polypectomy (6 mm)
e) Ulcer (4 mm) in normal-appearing mucosa 3 days later
f) Stellate scar 6 weeks after polypectomy

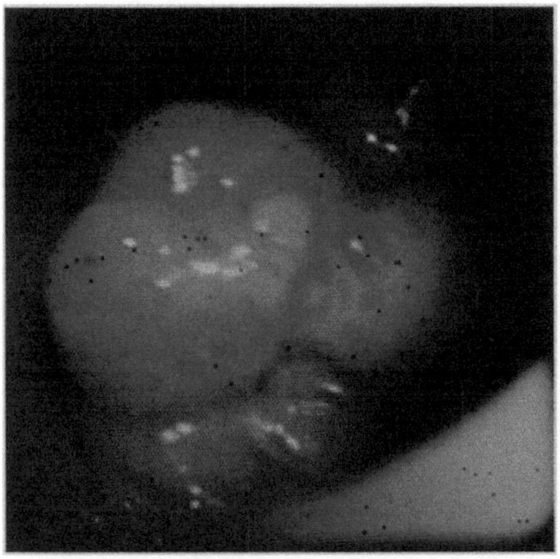

97a

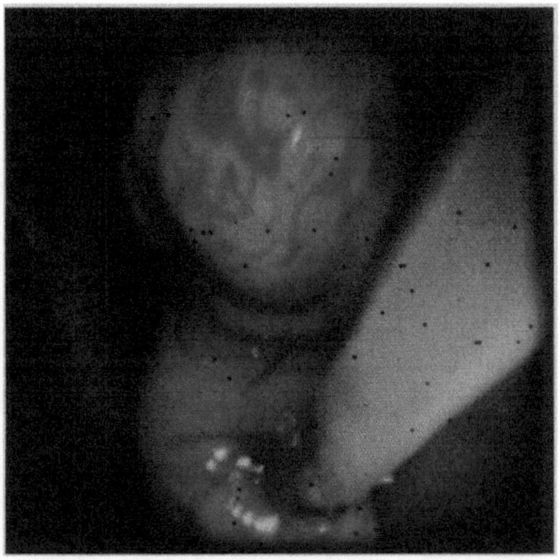

197b

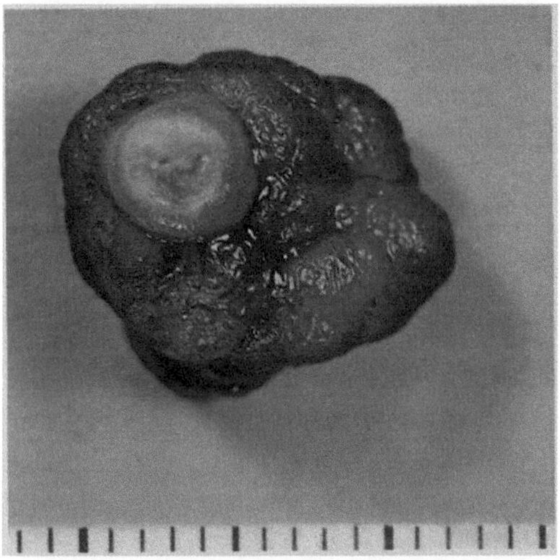

7c

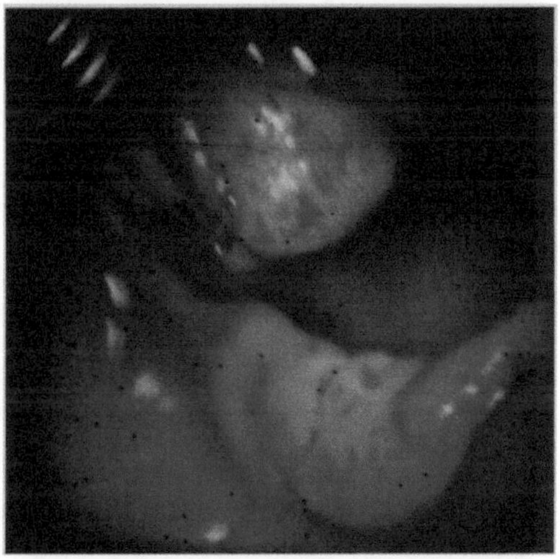

197d

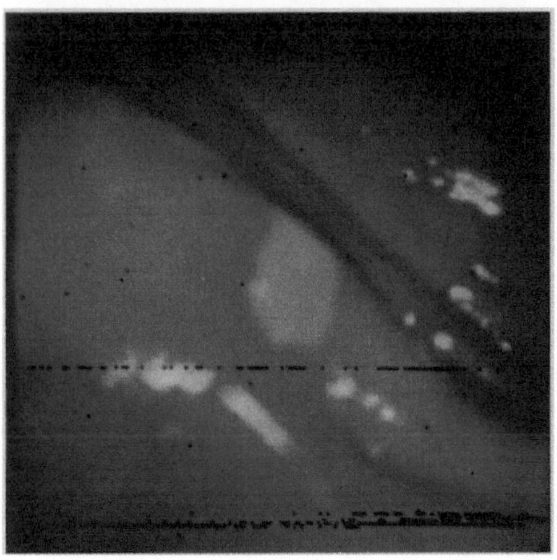

7e

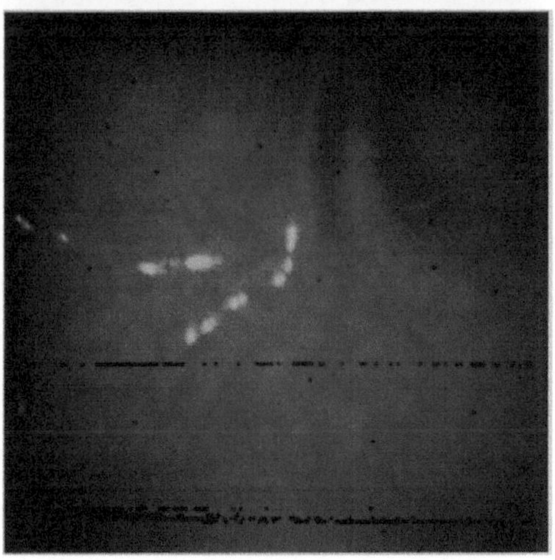

197f

198a–h Electroresection of a large pedunculated and lobulated sigmoid polyp with the open diathermy snare

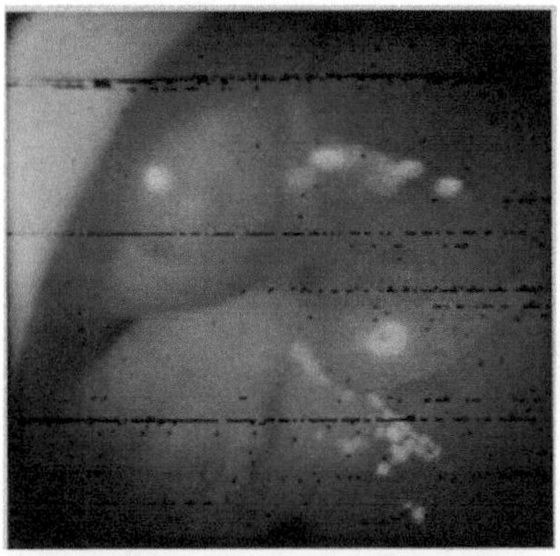
198a

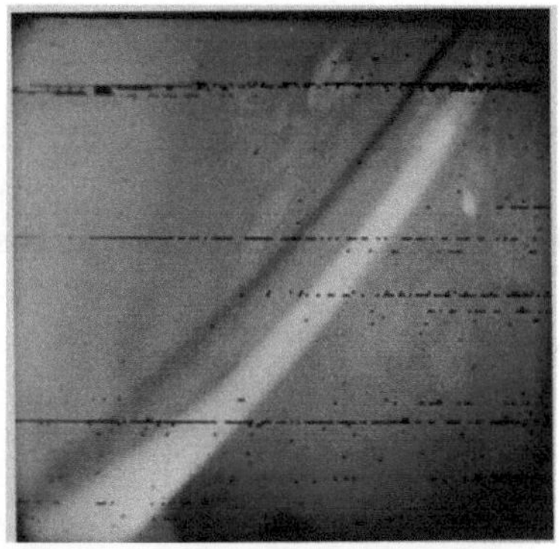
198b

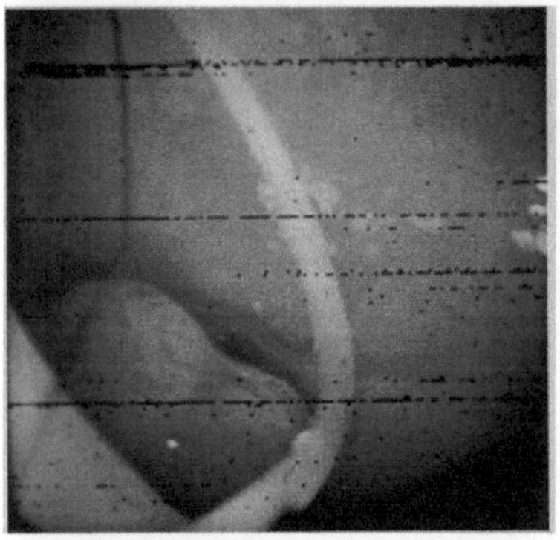
198c

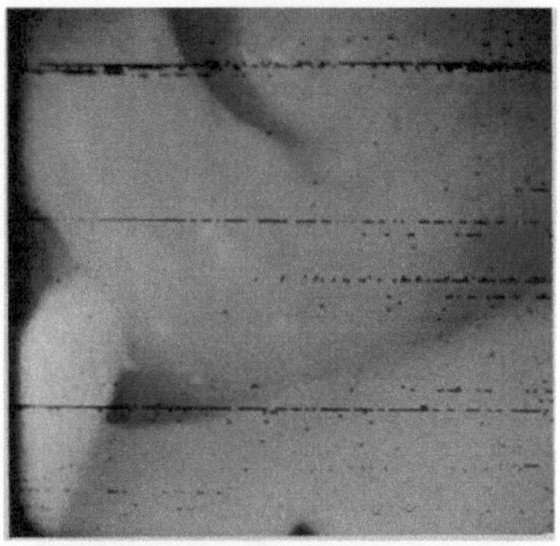
198d

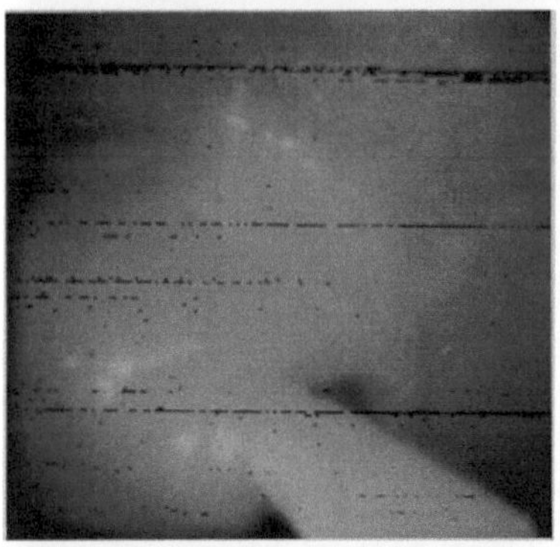
198e

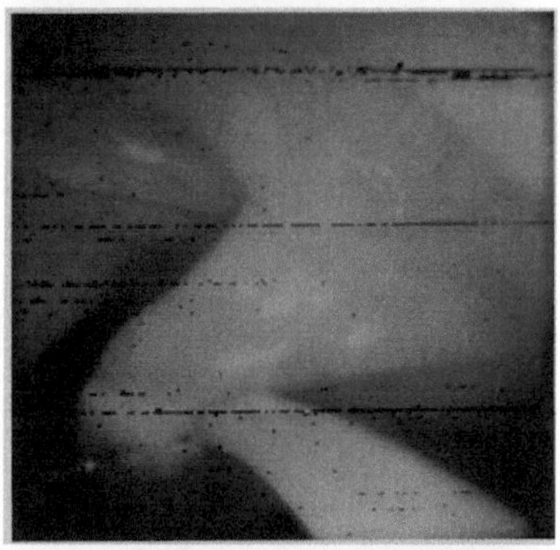
198f

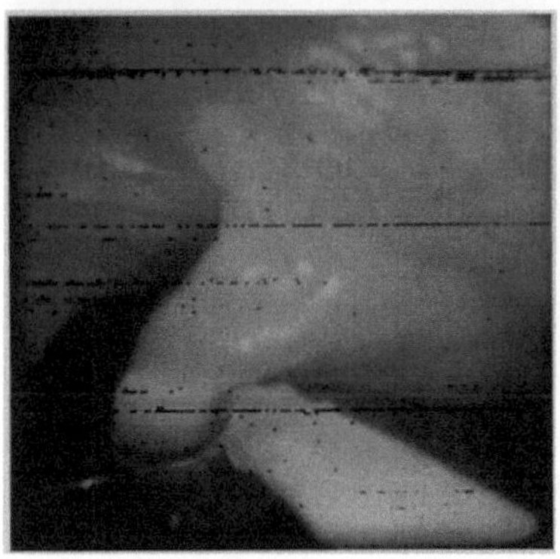
198g

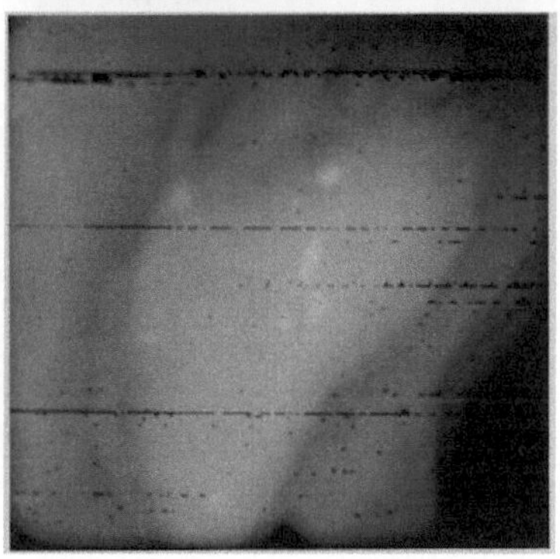
198h

8.5 Sessile Colonic Polyps

199 a–b Adenomatous polyps (base: 1.5×2.0 cm)

200 a–b Papillary adenoma (base: 3.0 cm)

9a

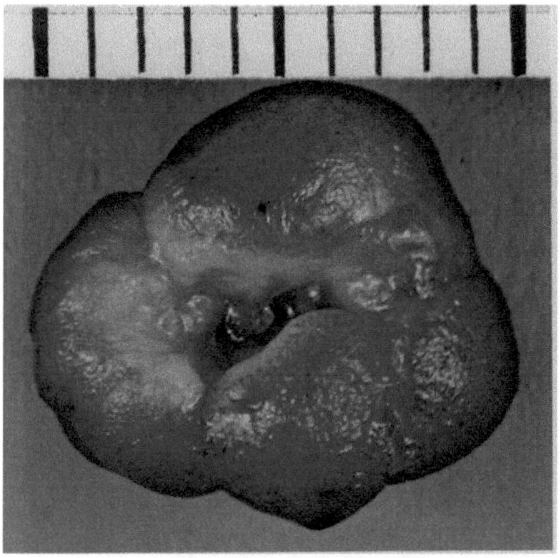

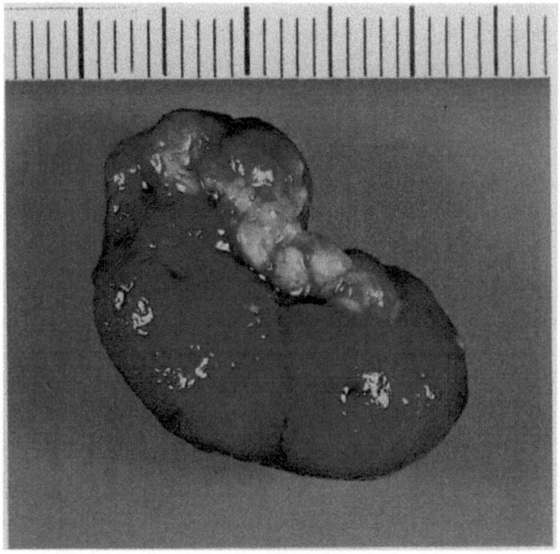

199b

)a

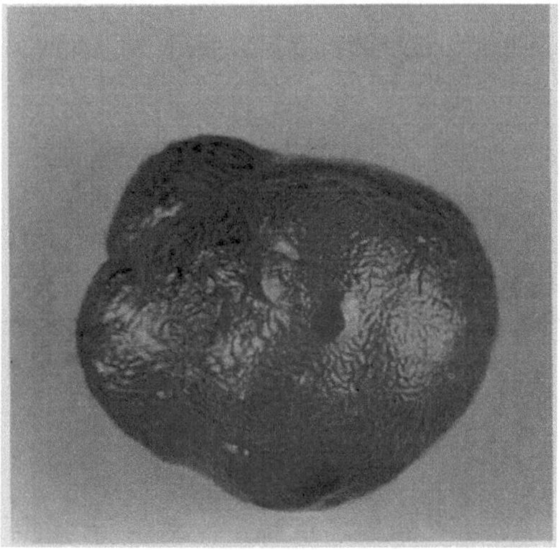

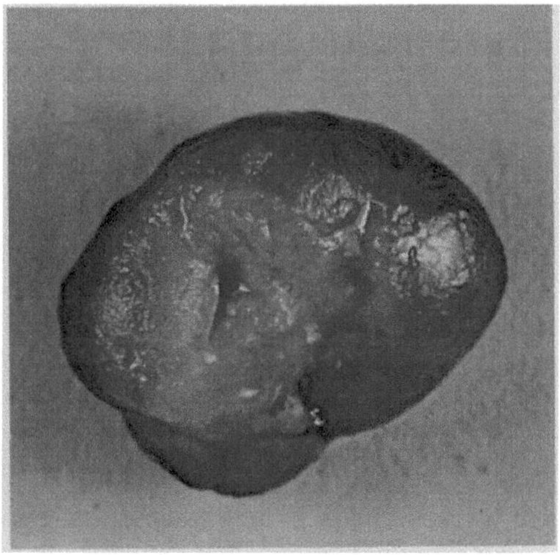

200b

8.5 Sessile Colonic Polyps (Continuation)

201 a–b Villous papilloma (surface)
Villous papilloma (base: 2.0 cm)

202 a–b Adenomatous polyp with focal carcinoma

8.6 Peutz-Jeghers Polyps

203 a Large pedunculated polyp in the ascending colon. (Tip: 3.0 cm; base: 1.0 cm)

203 b Retrieved polyp

203 c Histology: papillomatous polyp with feathery arrangement of the muscularis mucosae (Peutz-Jeghers polyp)

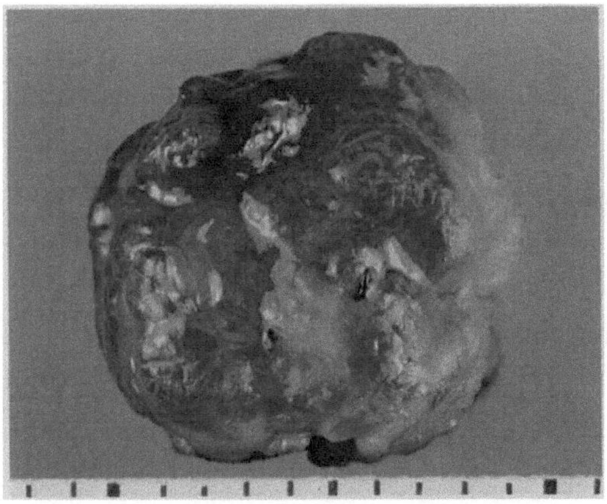

1a

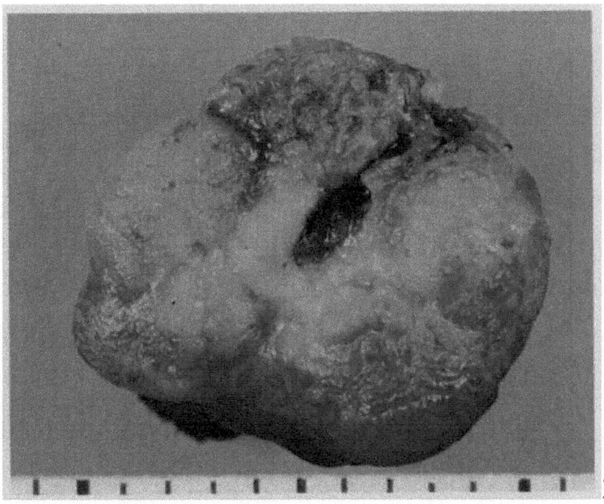

201 b

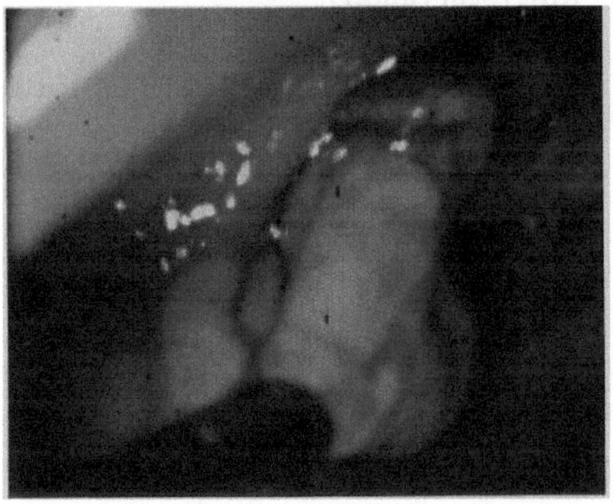

2a

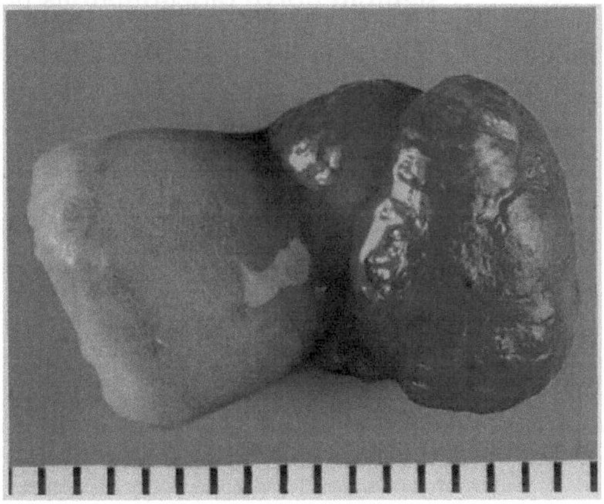

202 b

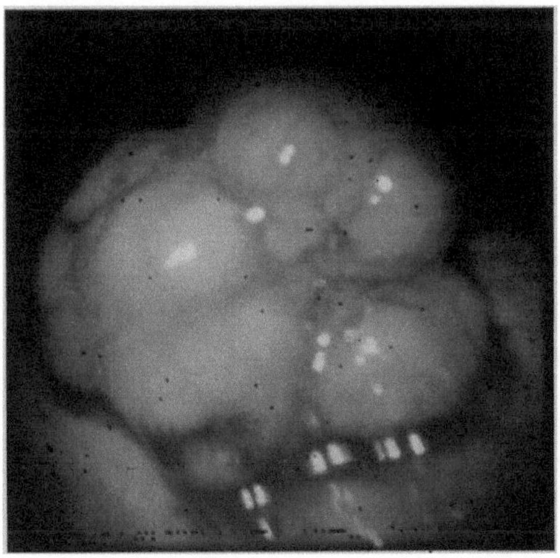

03

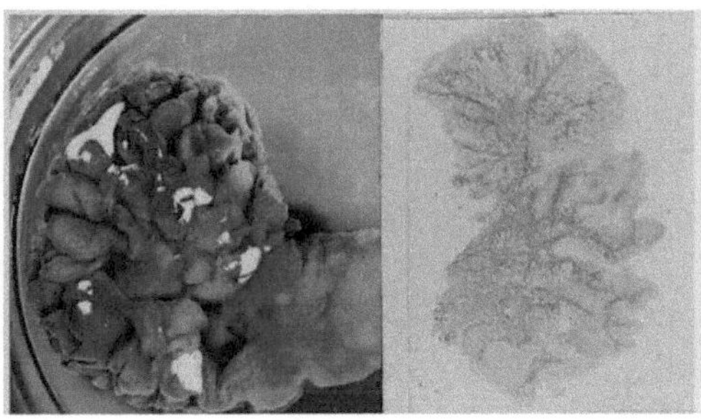

203

a b c

8.7 Follow-up Observations after Polypectomy

204a Pedunculated polyp in the proximal sigmoid (tip: 2 × 2.5 cm; base: 1 cm)

204b Flat residual ulcer with smooth margins (4 mm) after 5 weeks

204c Small scar with converging folds after 12 weeks

205a Polypectomy ulcer immediately following excision of a broadbased (1.5 cm) sigmoid polyp (adenomatous polyp with focal cancer)

205b Follow-up after 3 days. Sharply demarcated area of necrosis (1 cm) with slightly elevated margin

205c Follow-up after 5 days. Oval ulcer (10 × 6 mm). Complete healing in 18 days

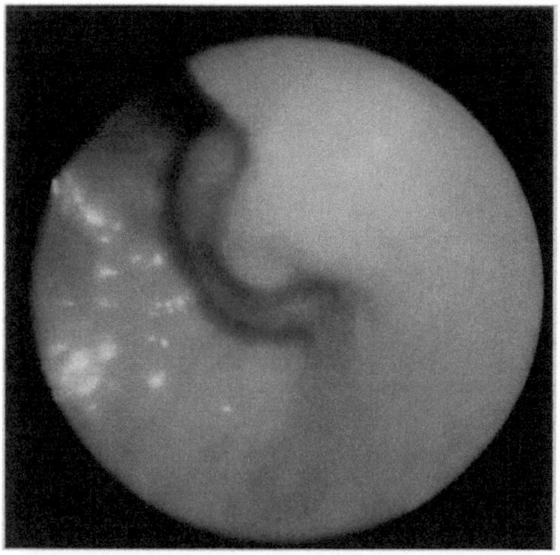

204a

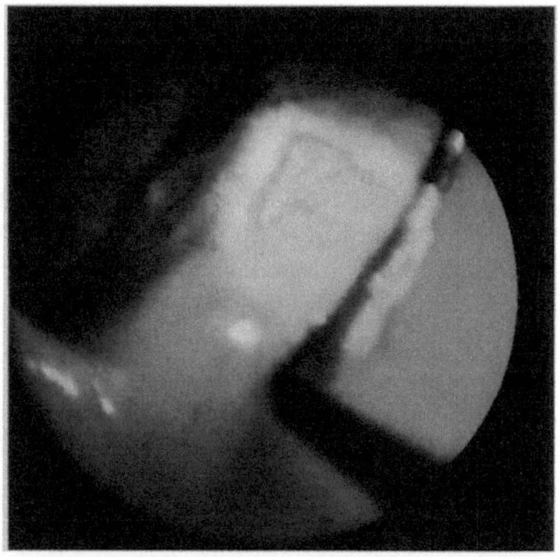

205a

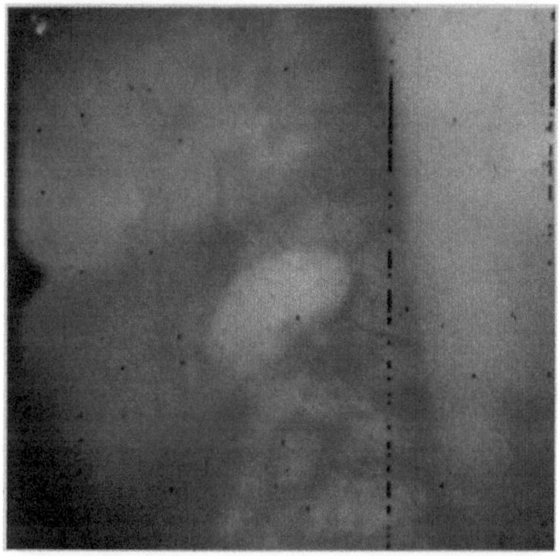

204b

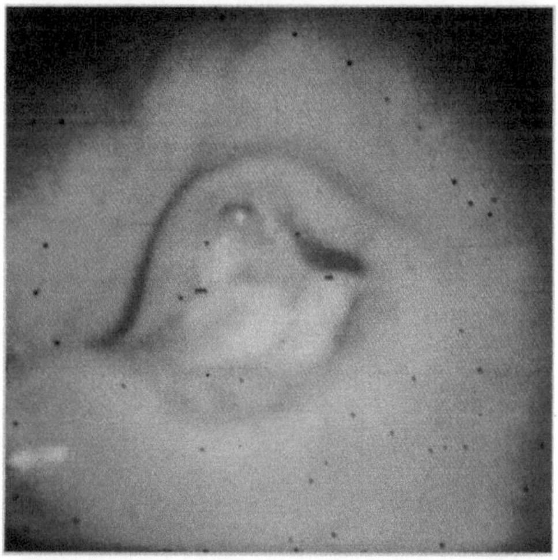

205b

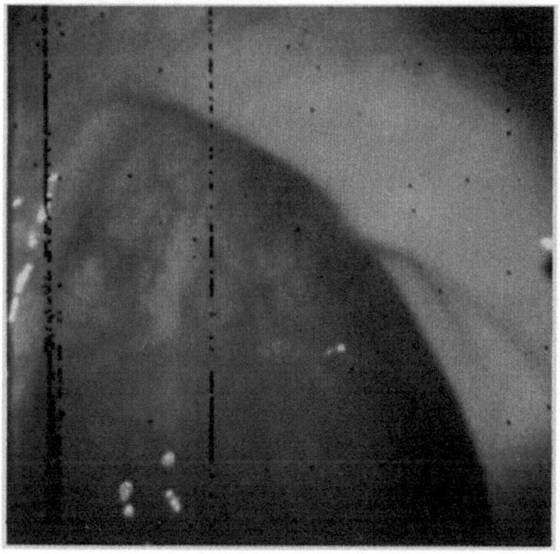

204c

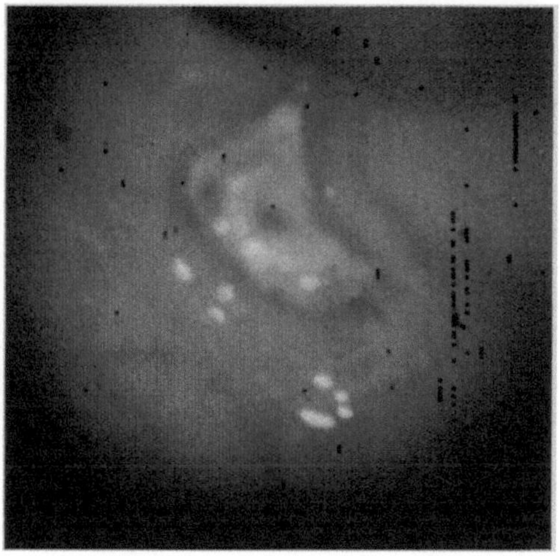

205c

8.8 Foreign Body Removal

206 a–c Extraction of a transintestinal tube with attached rubber balloon filled with lead shot from the proximal sigmoid

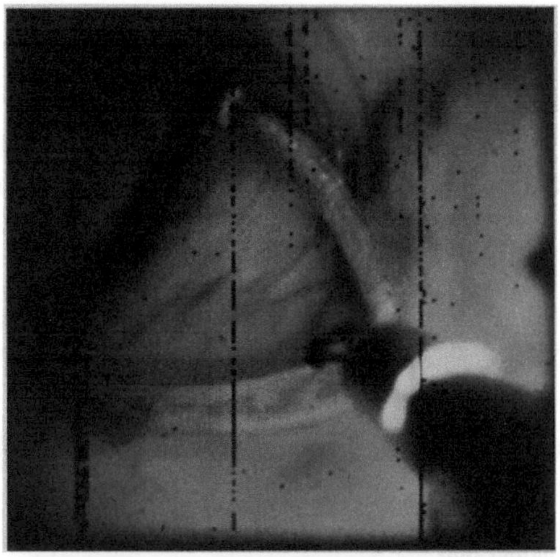

206a

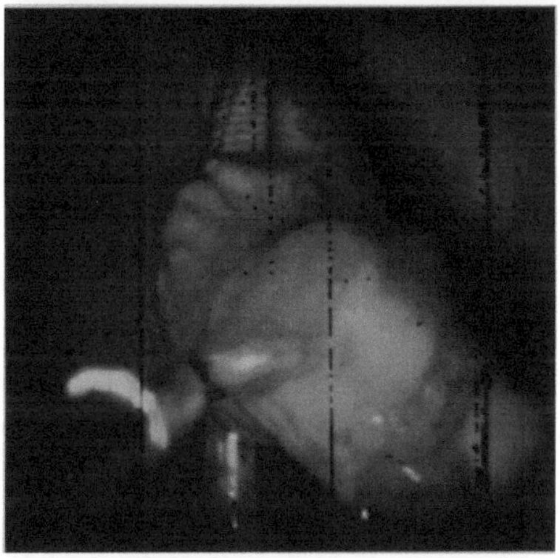

206b

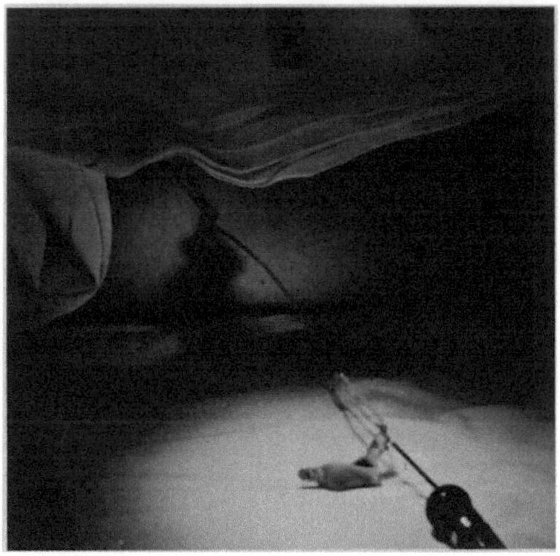

206c

8.9 Injections

207a–b Sclerosing injection of a small hemangioma in the transverse colon
a) Before injection
b) Fibrotic change after 14 days

8.10 Electrocoagulation

208a–b Bleeding hemangioma (ascending colon) before and after electrocoagulation

8.11 Angiography

209a–b Endoscopic-angiographic demonstration of varices in the descending colon

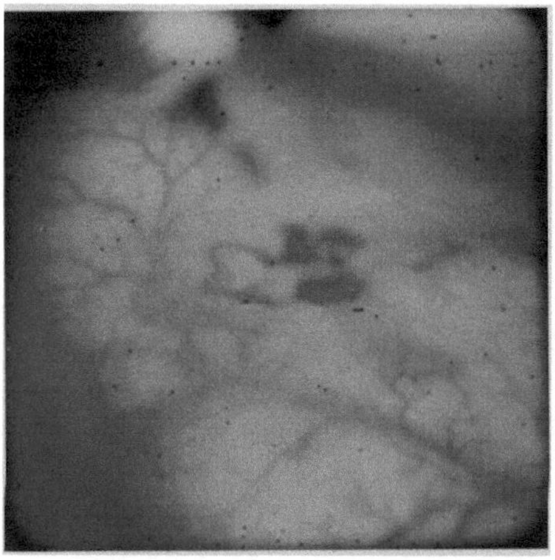
207a

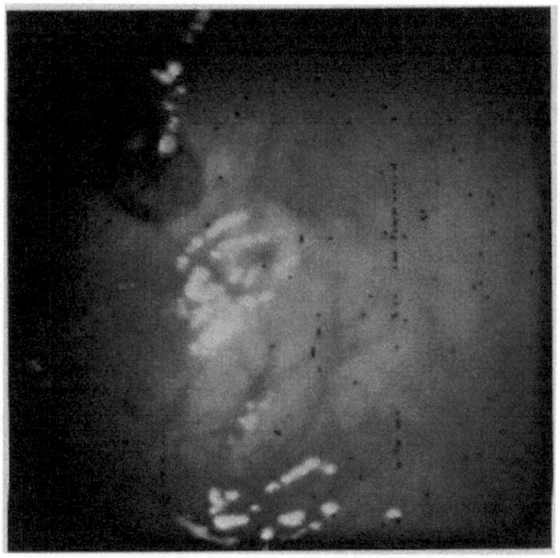
207 b

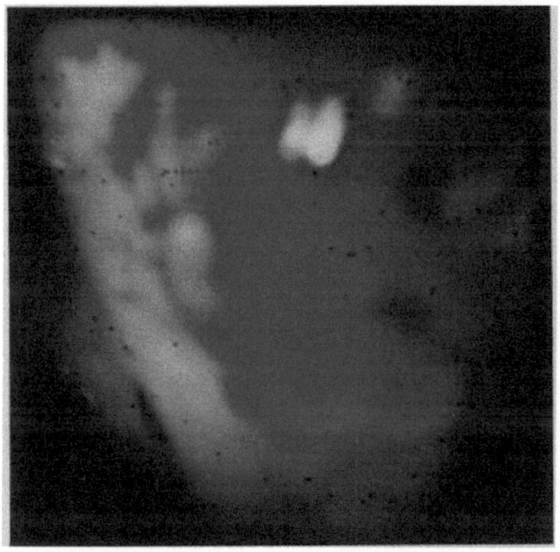
208a

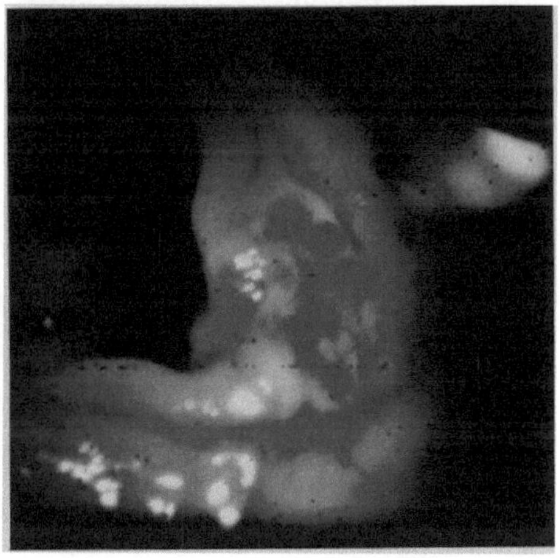
208 b

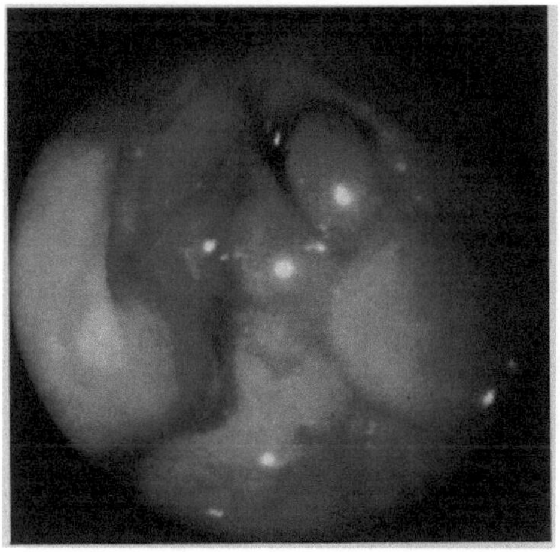
209a

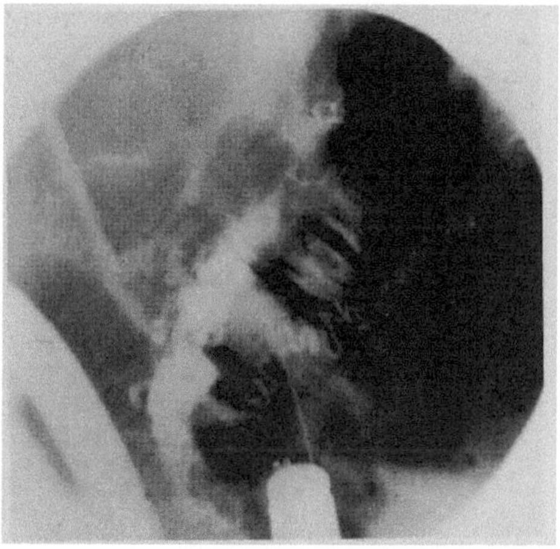
209 b

9. Tumors of the Colon

9.1 Benign Tumors

210a–c Adenomatous polyp (10 mm) in the presence of extensive diverticulosis of the sigmoid

211 Longitudinal-oval sessile adenomatous polyp of the cecum (20 × 5 mm)

212 Pedunculated adenomatous polyp in the sigmoid (stalk 1.5 cm; tip 2 × 3 cm)

213 Two papillary adenomas of the sigmoid on a common stalk

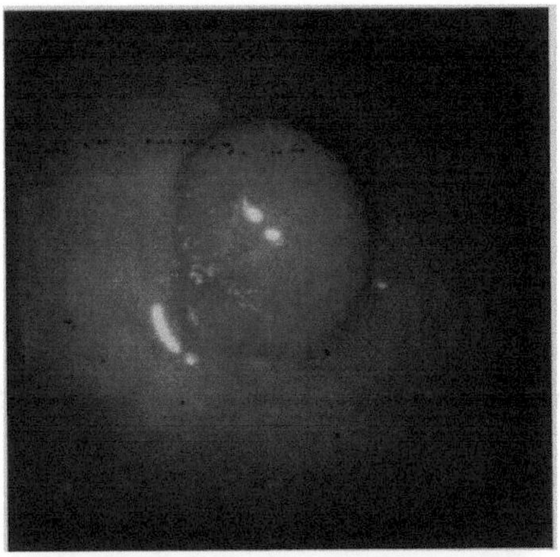

210a

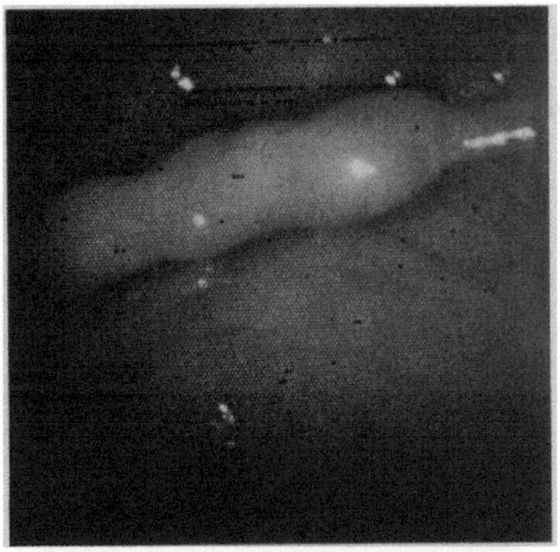

211

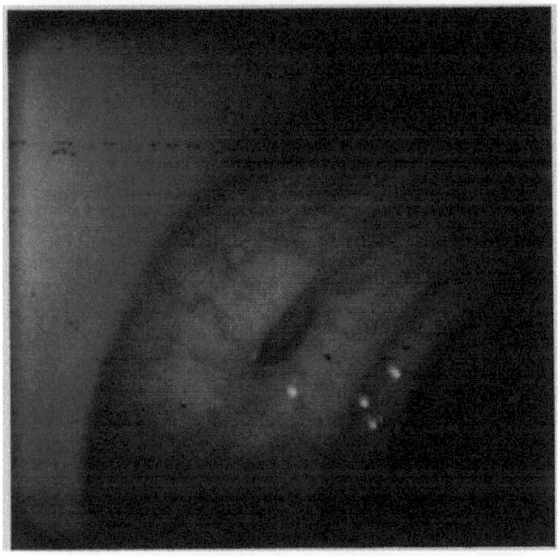

210b

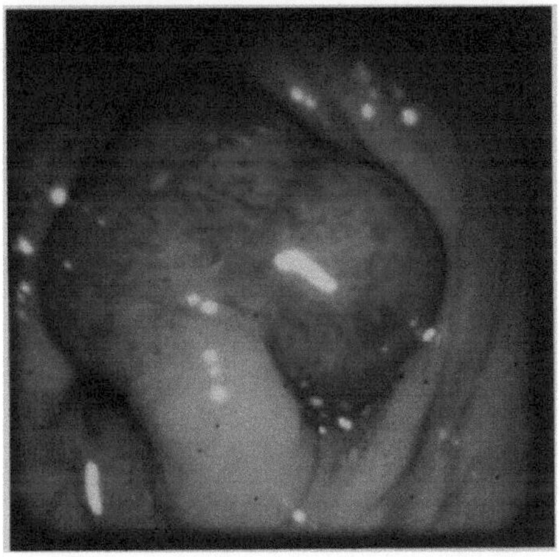

212

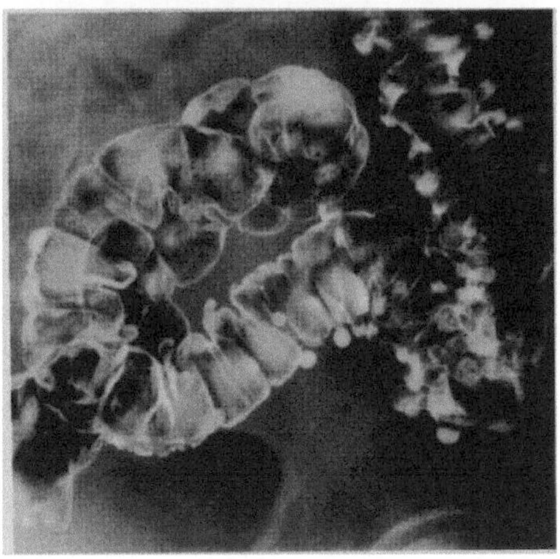

210c

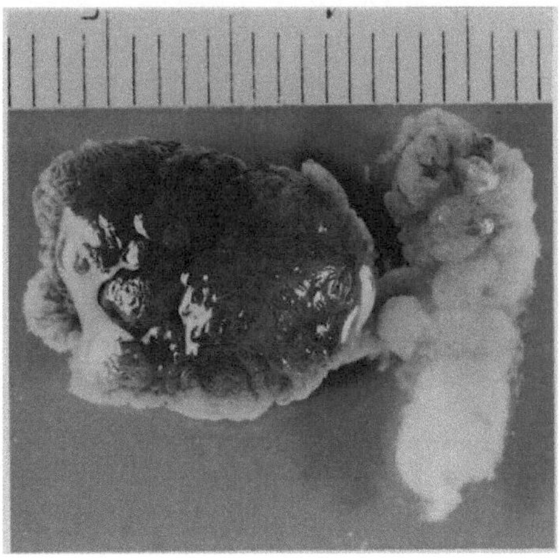

213

9.1 Benign Tumors (Continuation)

214 Villous papilloma of the rectum (40 × 40 mm)

215 Two vascular hamartomas of the cecum

216 Carcinoid (7 mm) near the margin of excision (5 o'clock) of an adenomatous polyp

217 Polyposis coli

218a–b Gardner syndrome: polyposis of the colon with soft tissue tumors

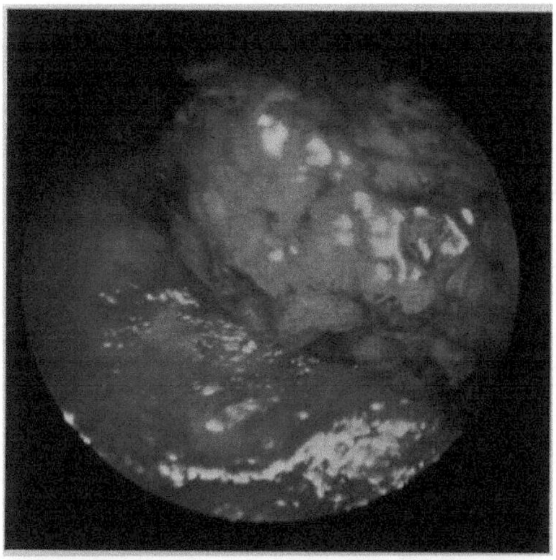

214

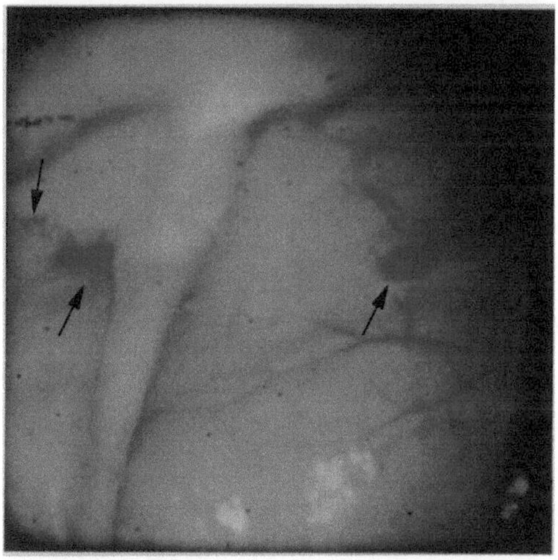

215

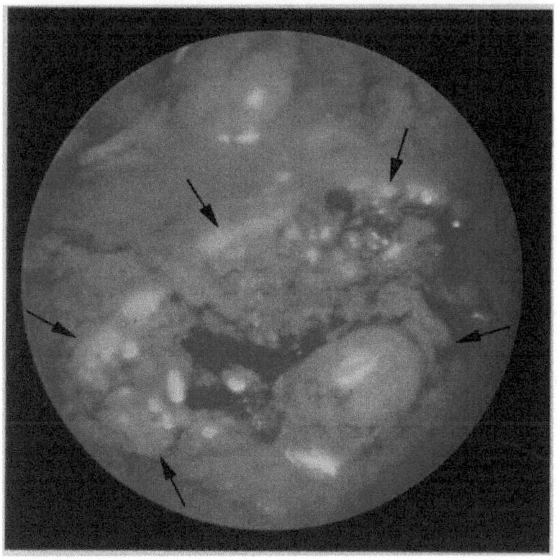

216

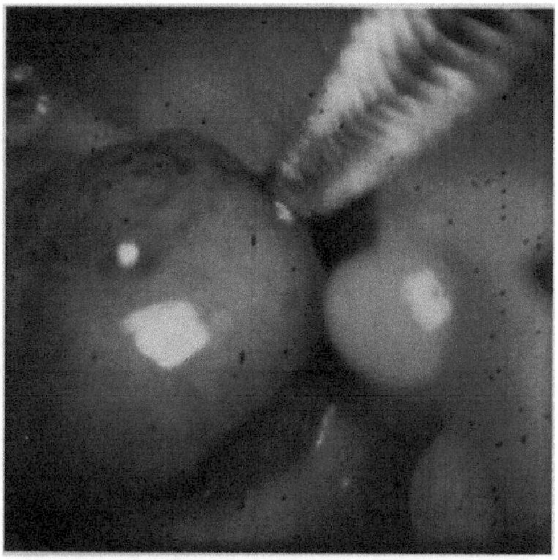

217

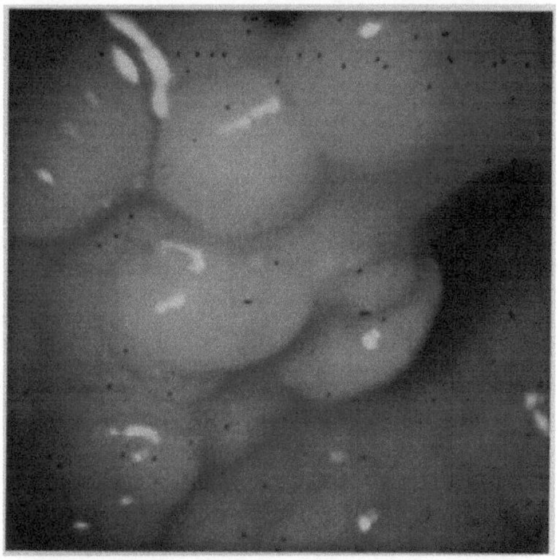

218a

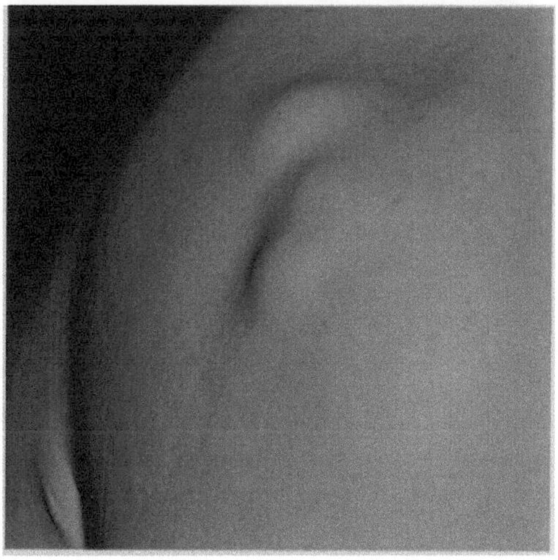

218b

9.2 Malignant Tumors

219 Large pedunculated lesion in the proximal sigmoid (adenocarcinoma)

220 Polypoid adenocarcinoma of the transverse colon

221 Tumor in the transverse colon with central ulceration (lymphosarcoma)

222 Circular, stenosing adenocarcinoma of the sigmoid with partial ulceration

223 Stenosing adenocarcinoma of the cecum

224 Polypoid recurrence of carcinoma of the sigmoid at the line of anastomosis

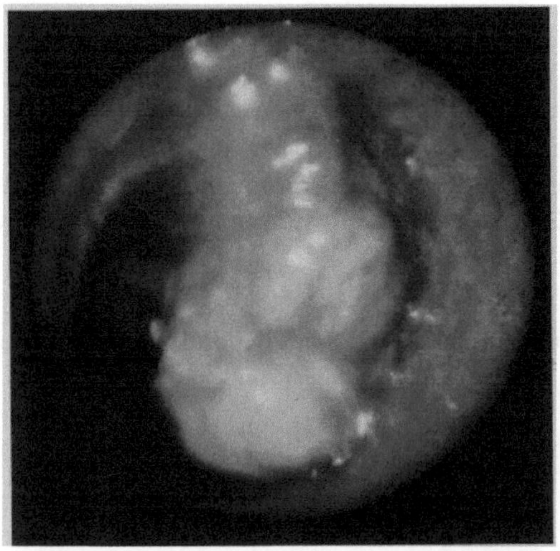
219

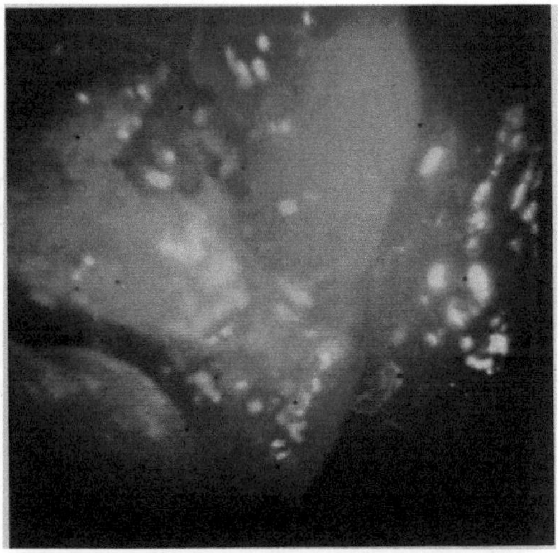
222

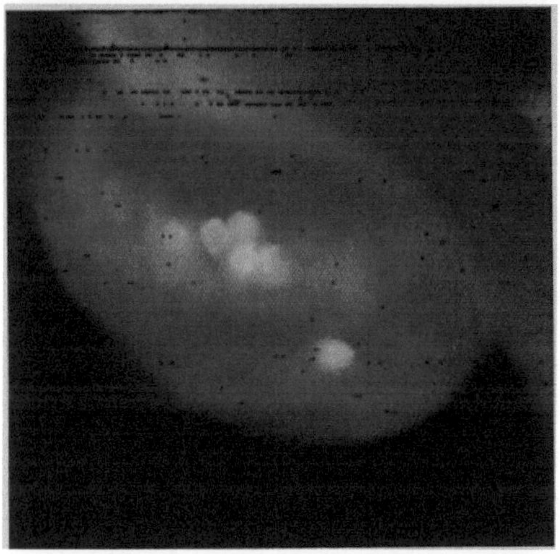
220

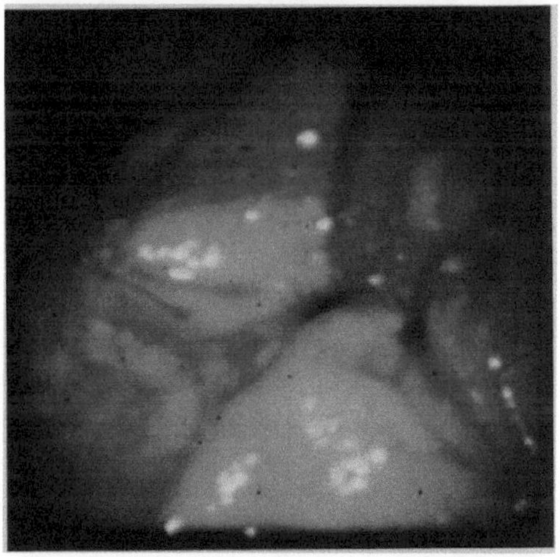
223

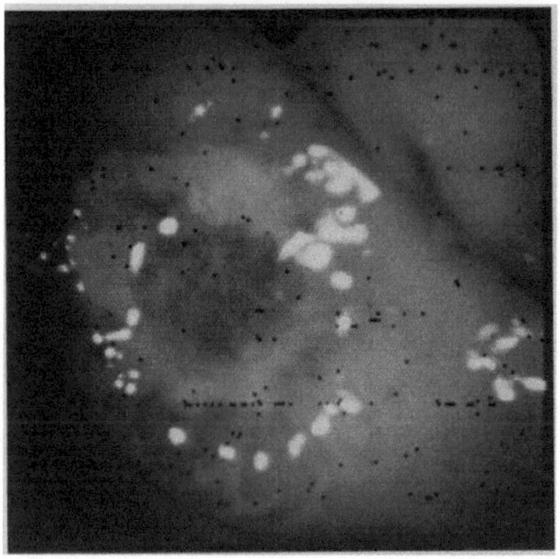
221

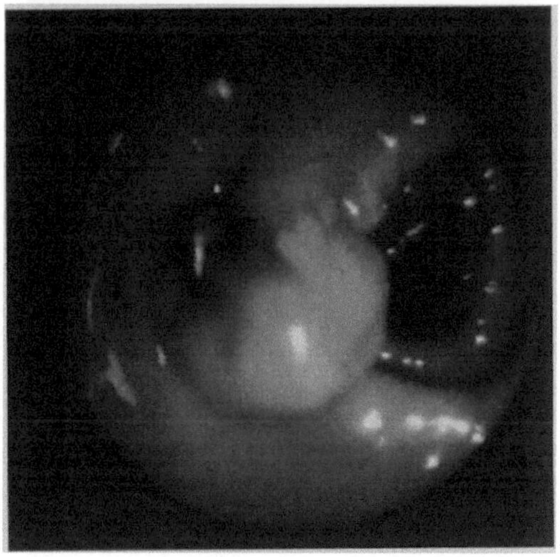
224

9.2 Malignant Tumors (Continuation)

225a–b Polypoid adenocarcinoma of the sigmoid with central ulceration (225a) with 2 sessile adenomatous polyps (225b) 10 cm distal to the malignancy (sentinel polyps)

226a–b Recurrence of a carcinoma of the sigmoid (226a) 8 cm beyond the anstomotic line (226b)

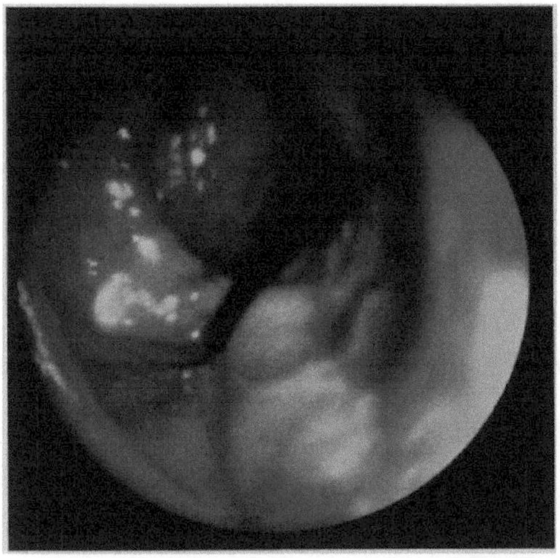
25a

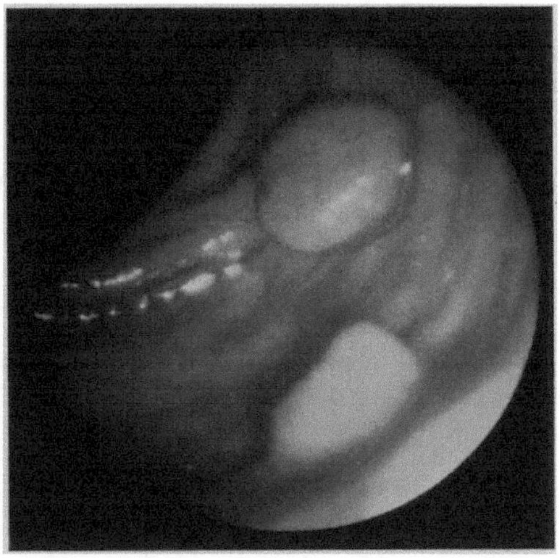
225b

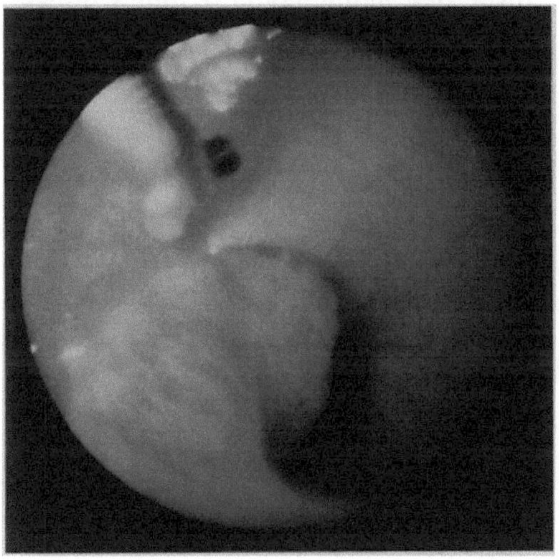
6a

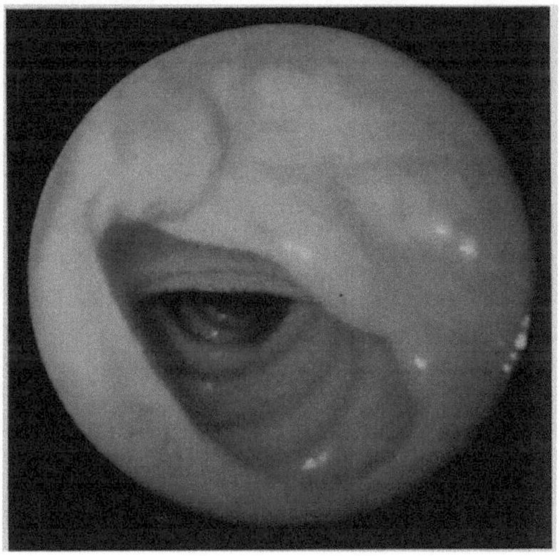
226b

9.3 Stenosis of the Sigmoid Colon

227 Circular, stenosing carcinoma of the sigmoid with partial ulceration

228 Exophytic stenosing carcinoma of the sigmoid

229 Nonspecific inflammatory stenosis of the sigmoid with polypoid formations (Crohn's disease)

230 Extrinsic hemispheric indentation of the sigmoid with intact mucosa (fist-sized myoma of the uterus)

231 a–b High-grade scarred stenosis of the distal descending colon (Crohn's disease)

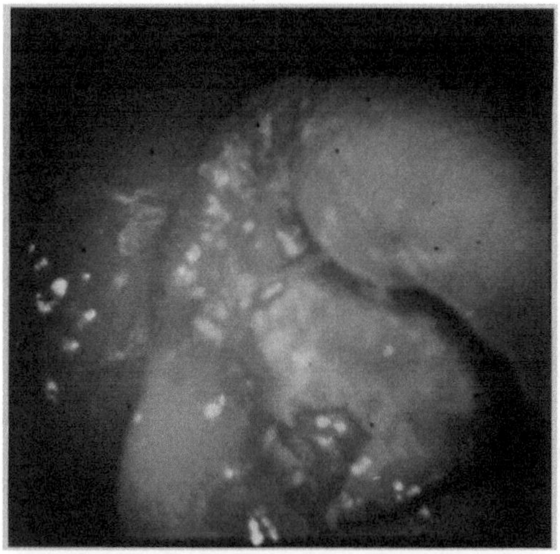

:27

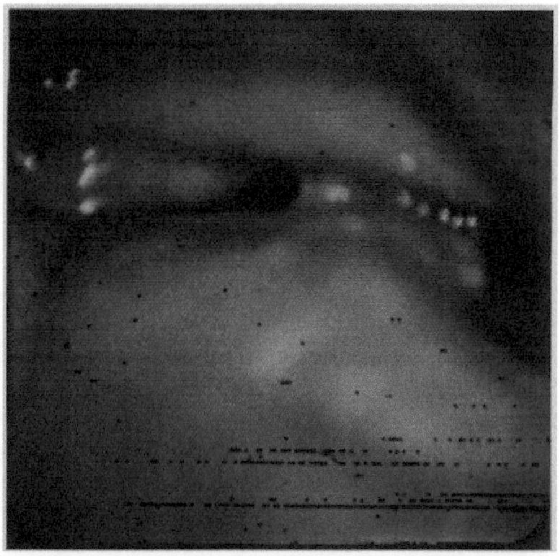

228

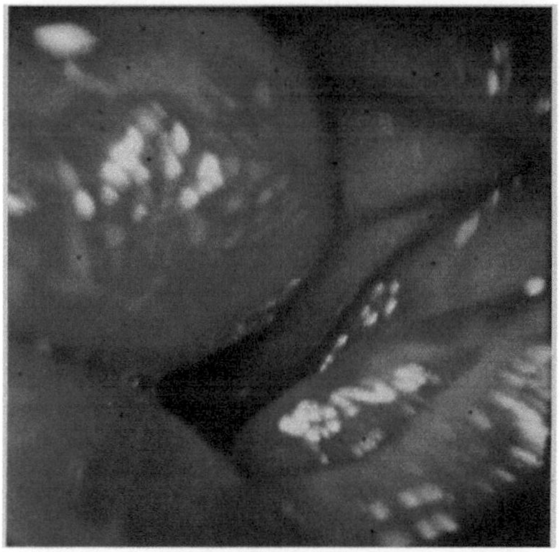

29

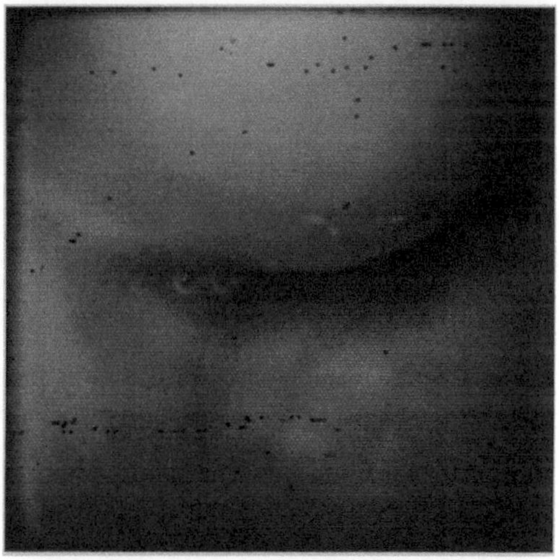

230

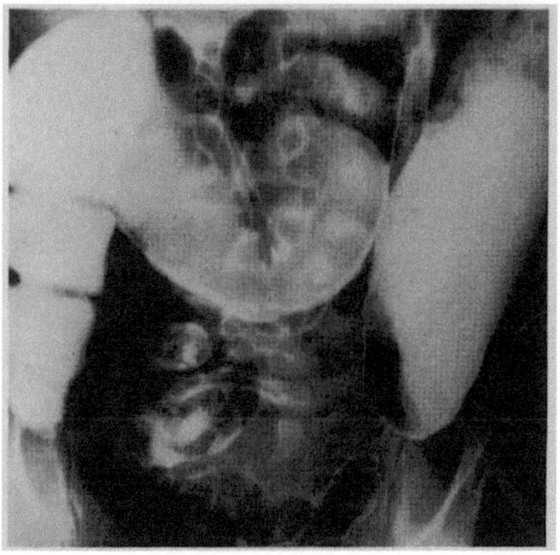

1a

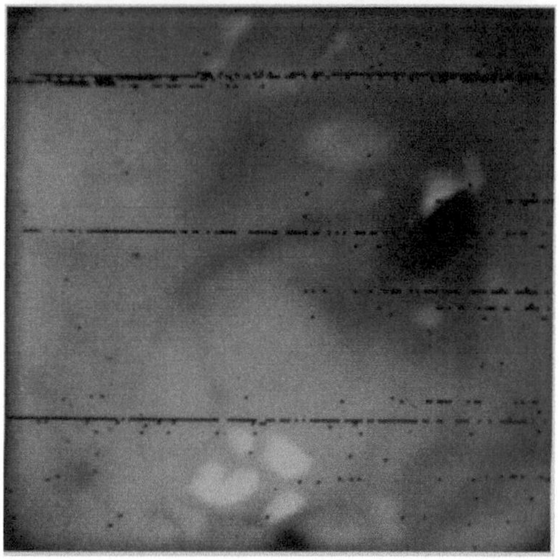

231b

9.4 Pseudotumors

232 Benign lymphoid polyposis of the terminal ileum

233 Sessile hyperplastic (metaplastic) polyp in the descending colon

234 Sessile hyperplastic (metaplastic) polyp in the cecum

235 Pseudopolyp with active ulcerative colitis

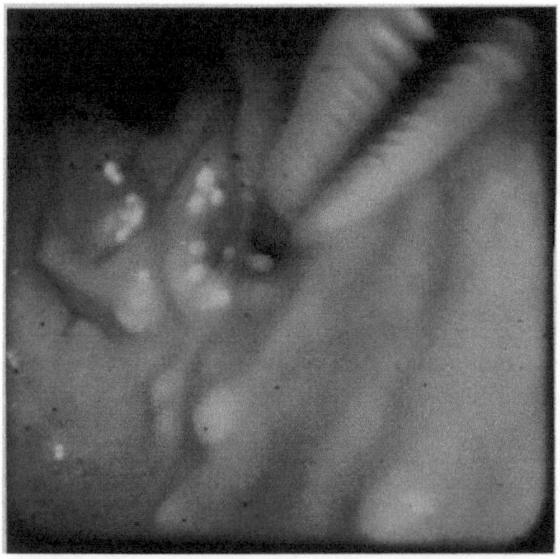

232

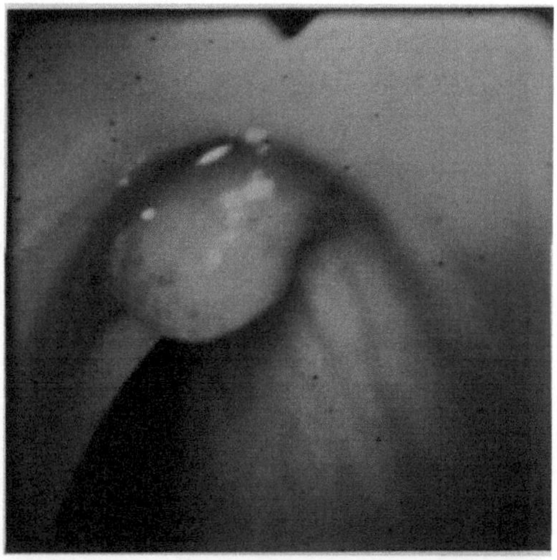

233

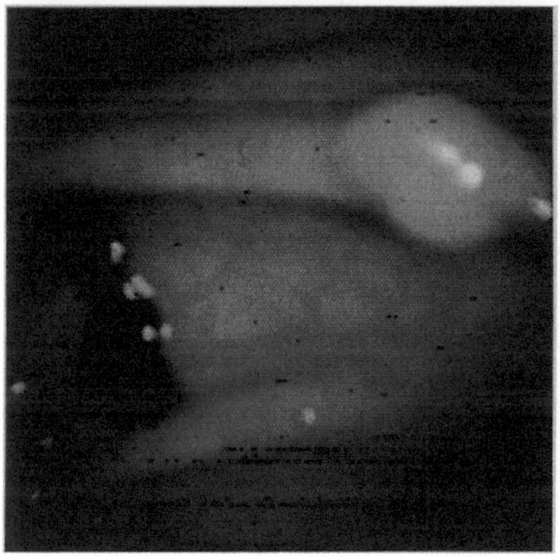

234

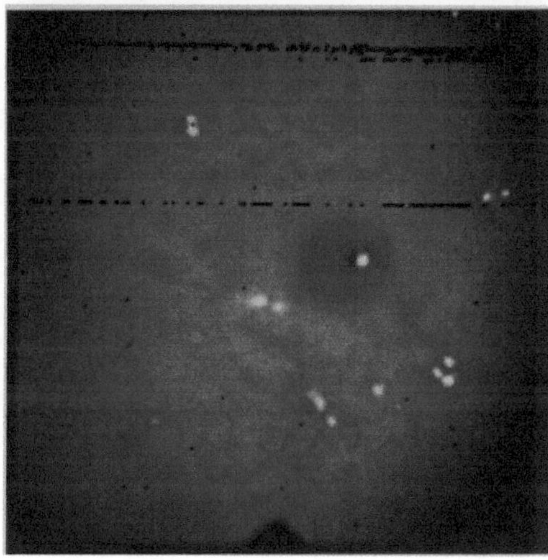

235

10. Idiopathic Ulcerative Colitis

236 Normal mucosa (transverse colon)

237 Prominent vascular pattern following thorough cleansing of the colon

238 a–b Ulcerative colitis (early stage): diffuse reddening, absent vascular pattern, edema, mucosal friability, no ulcerations

240 a Ulcerative colitis (acute stage): partly confluent ulcers, mucosal edema

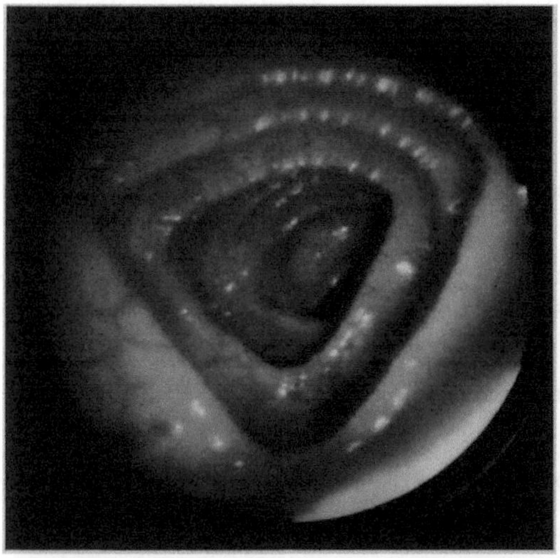

236

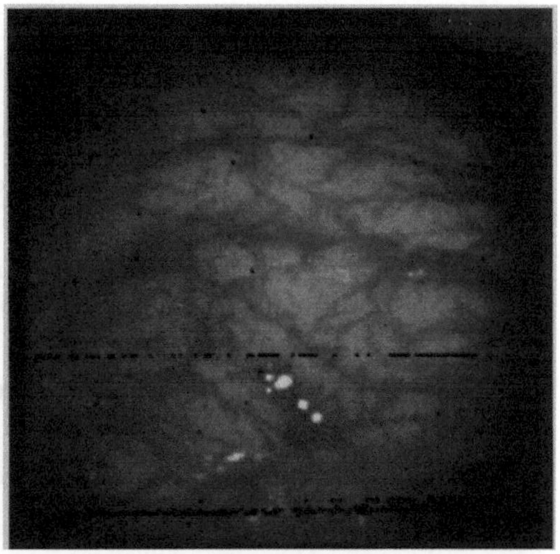

237

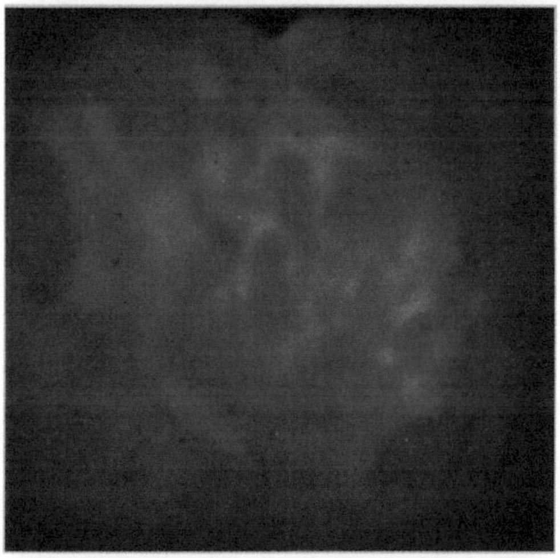

38a

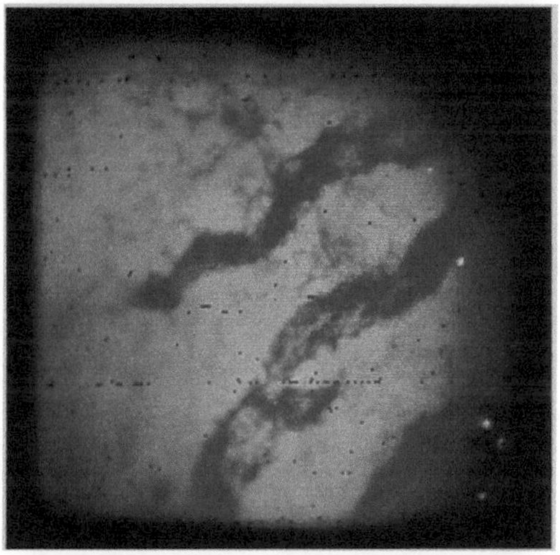

238b

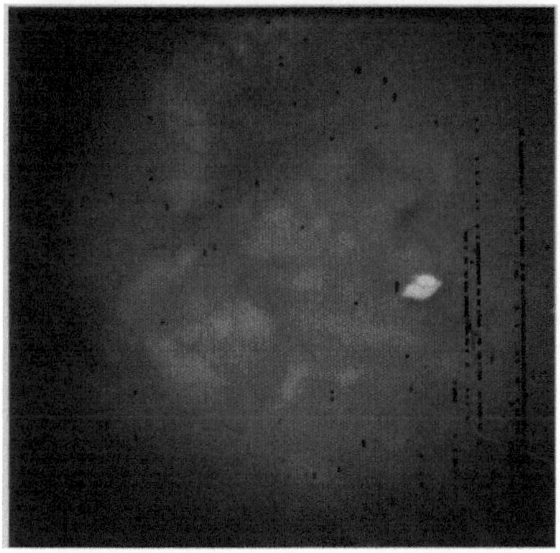

39

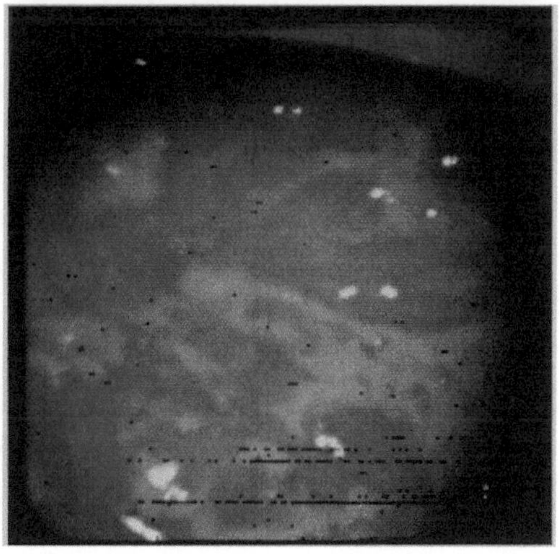

240a

10. Idiopathic Ulcerative Colitis (Continuation)

240 b Ulcerative colitis (acute stage): confluent ulcers, mucosal edema

241 a–b Ulcerative colitis (acute stage): numerous confluent ulcers with a few edematous islands of remaining mucosa

242 Ulcerative colitis (acute stage): massive coating by pus

243 Ulcerative colitis (acute stage): confluent ulcerations with beginning pseudopolyposis

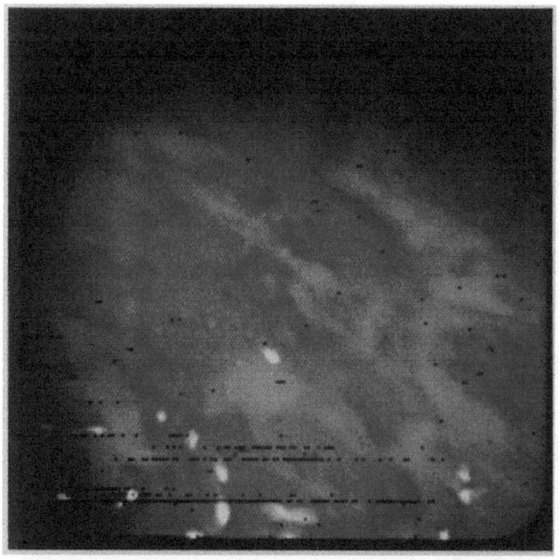

0b

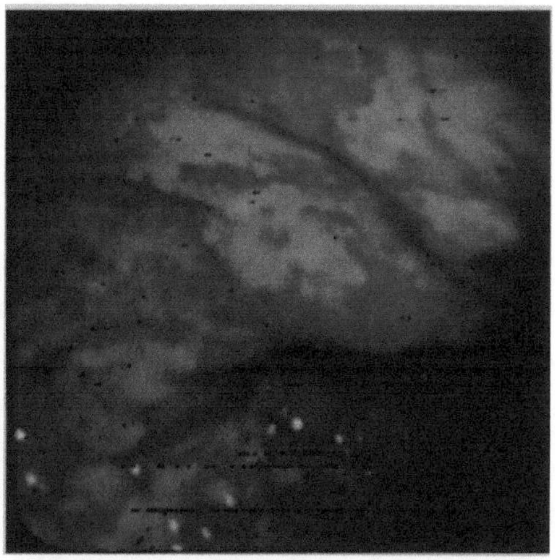

241a

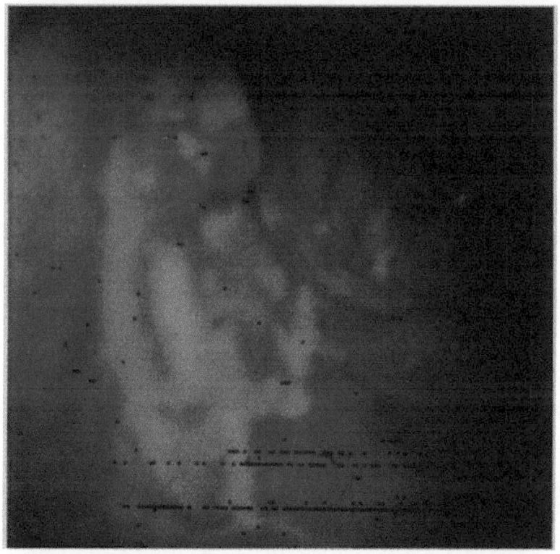

1b

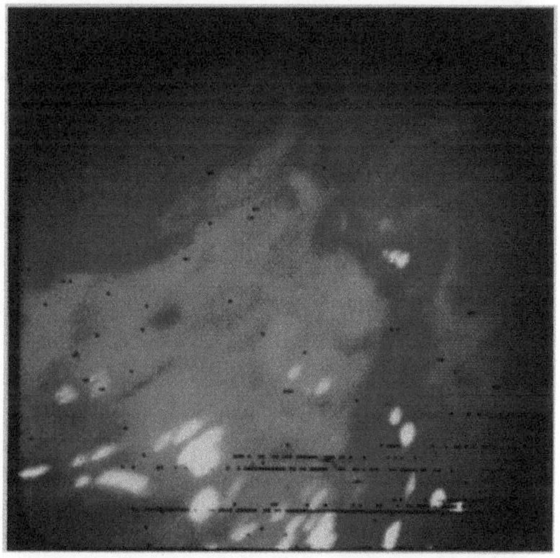

241c

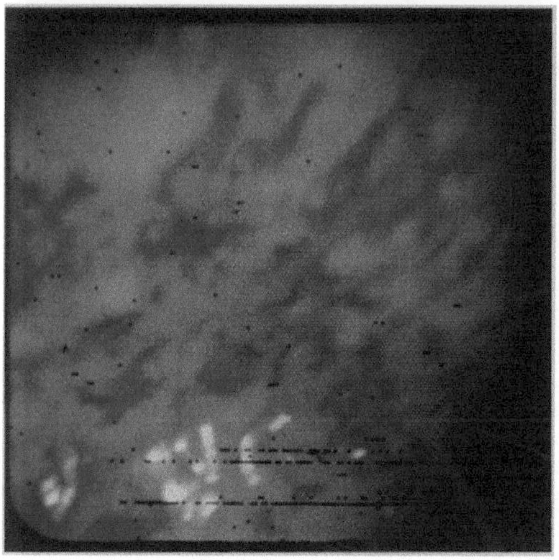

2

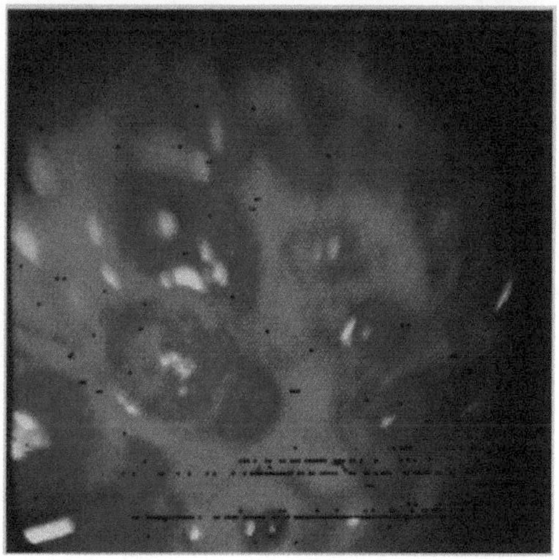

243

10. Idiopathic Ulcerative Colitis (Continuation)

244 Ulcerative colitis (chronic stage): sail-like mucosal bridges

245 Ulcerative colitis (chronic stage): absent haustrations, fine mucosal granularity

246 Ulcerative colitis (chronic stage): pseudopolyposis

247 Ulcerative colitis (chronic stage): pale-red atrophic mucosa

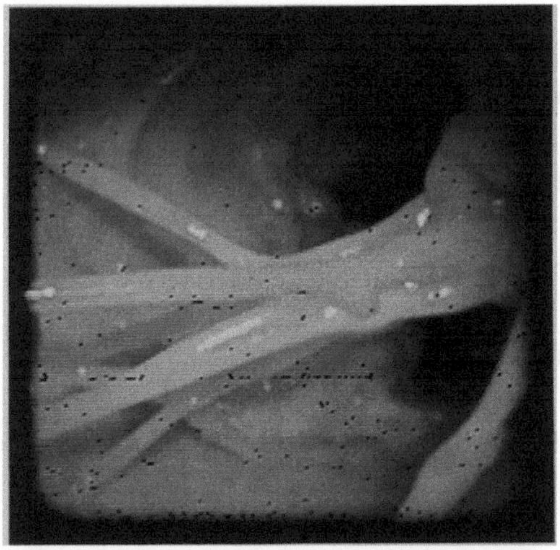
244

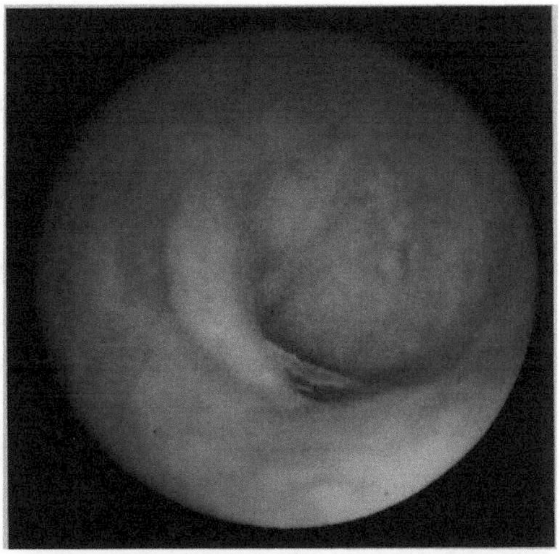
245

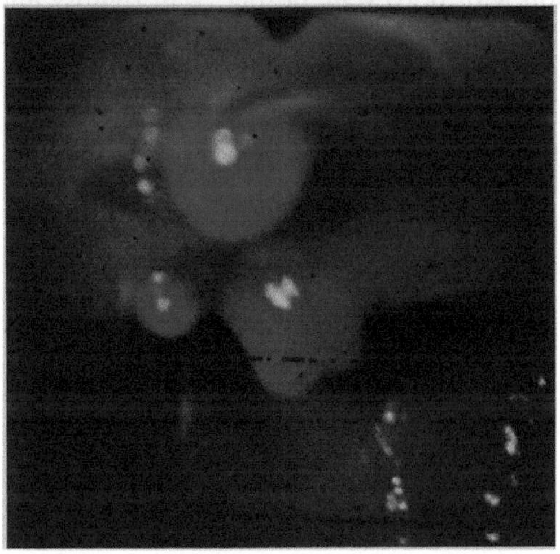
246

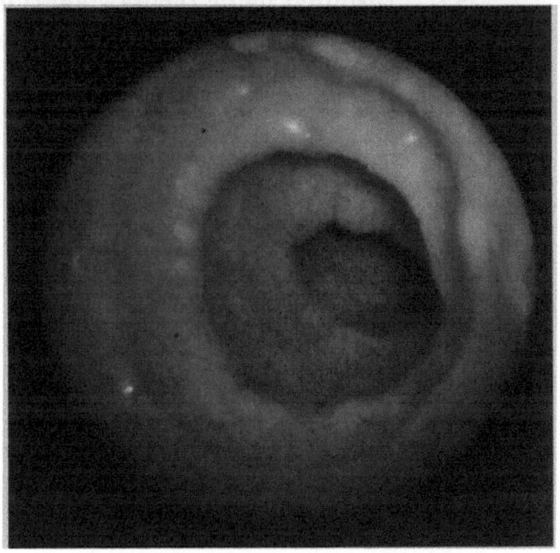
247

11. Crohn's Disease of the Colon and Terminal Ileum

248 Multiple perianal fissures and fistulas (Crohn's disease)

249 Erosions surrounded by normal mucosa (skip lesions) in the rectum

250 Crohn's disease of the colon (fissures, edema)

251 Terminal ileitis (acute stage): thickened ileocecal valve protruding into the lumen

252 Terminal ileitis (acute stage): lesion with polycyclic border, wall rigidity and narrowing of the lumen in the terminal ileum, surrounded by normal mucosa (skip lesion)

253 Irregular erosion with mucosal edema in the cecum (skip lesion)

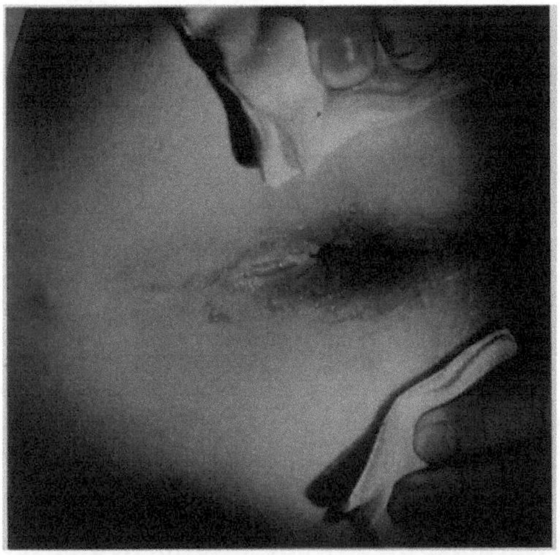

248

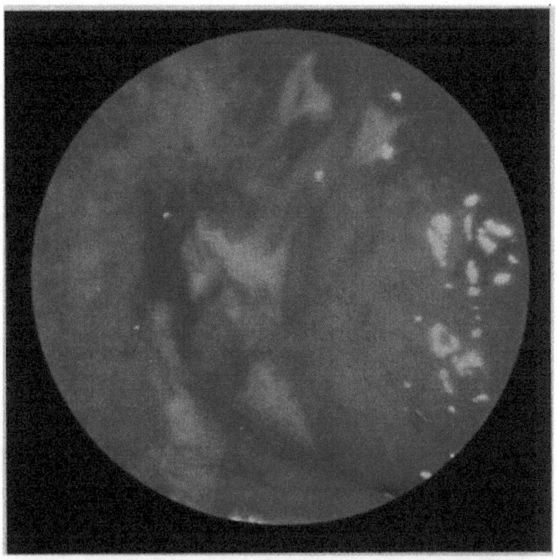

249

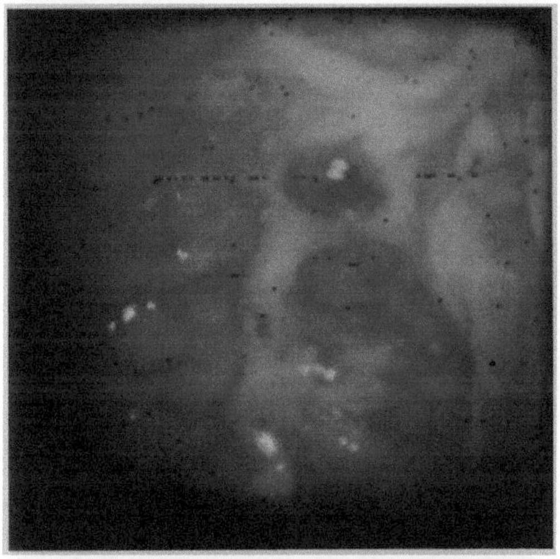

50

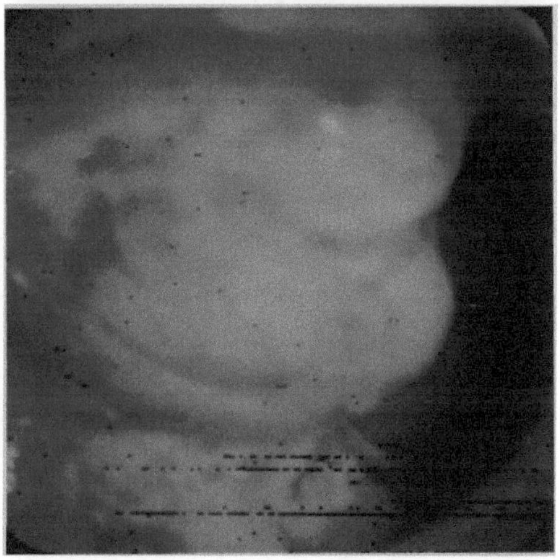

251

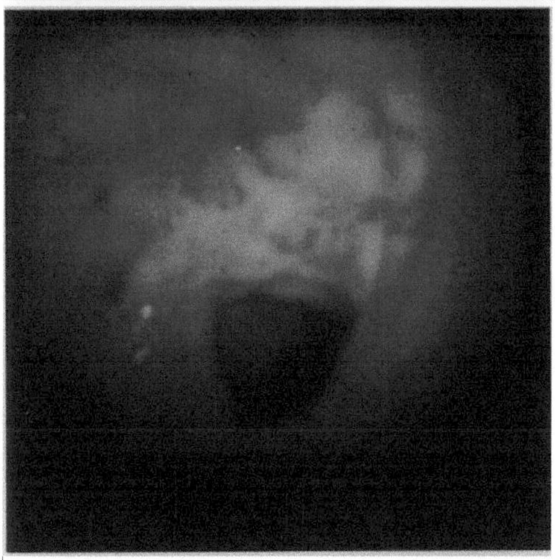

52

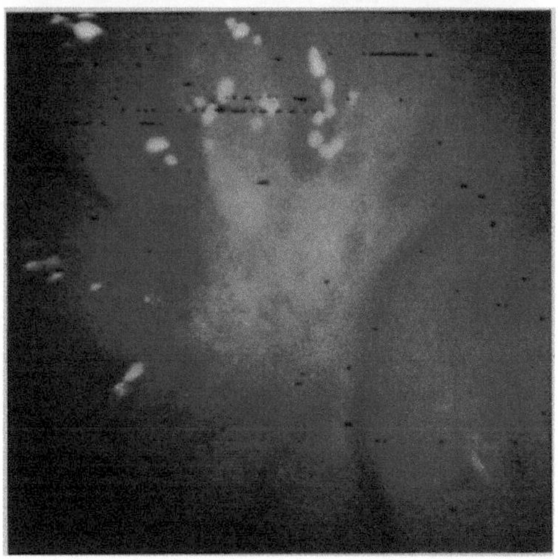

253

11. Crohn's Disease of the Colon and Terminal Ileum (Continuation)

254 Crohn's disease (acute stage): firm, diffusely thickened and nodular wall of the cecum with isolated ulcers and fissures

255 Crohn's disease: solitary ulcer in markedly thickened, rigid and deformed wall of the cecum

256 Crohn's disease (acute stage): isolated small ulcers in the transverse colon surrounded by normal mucosa (skip lesions)

257 Crohn's disease (chronic stage): thickening, rigidity and deformation of the transverse colon

258 a–b Crohn's disease: cobblestone pattern of cecum and transverse colon

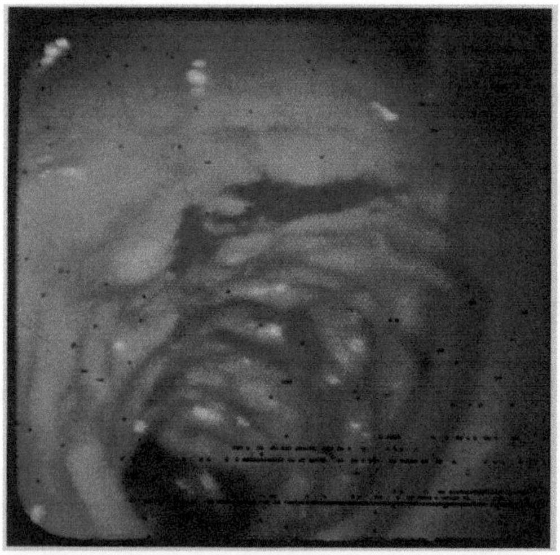

254

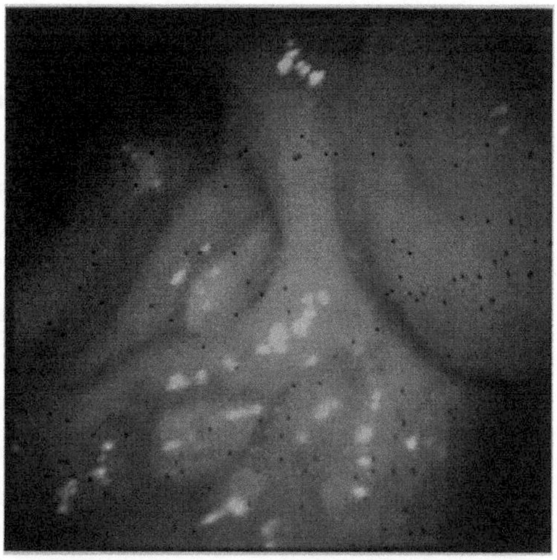

255

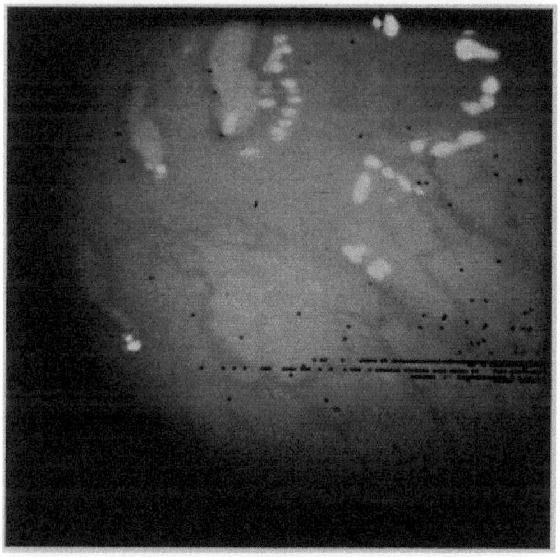

56

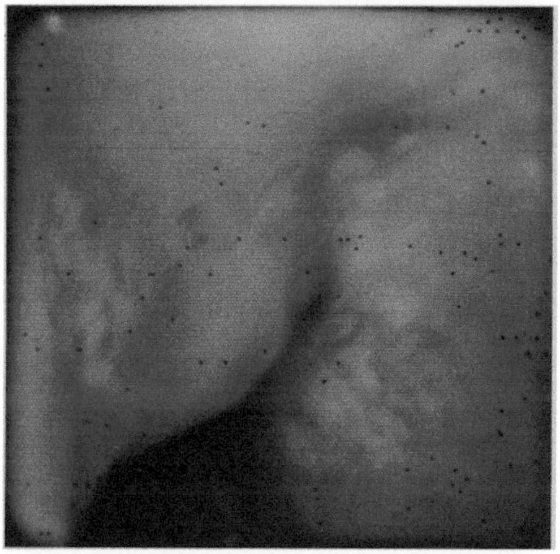

257

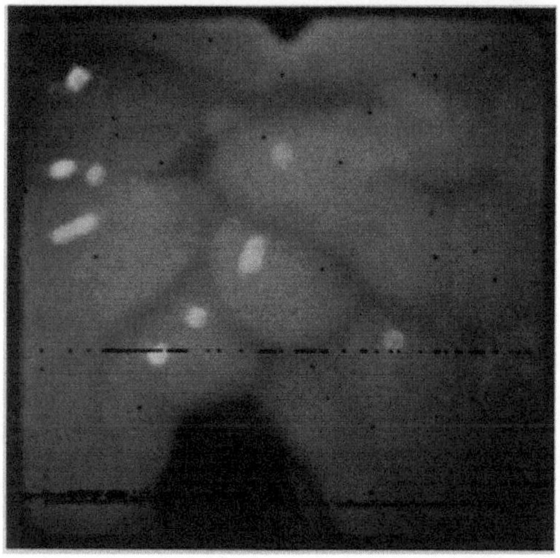

8a

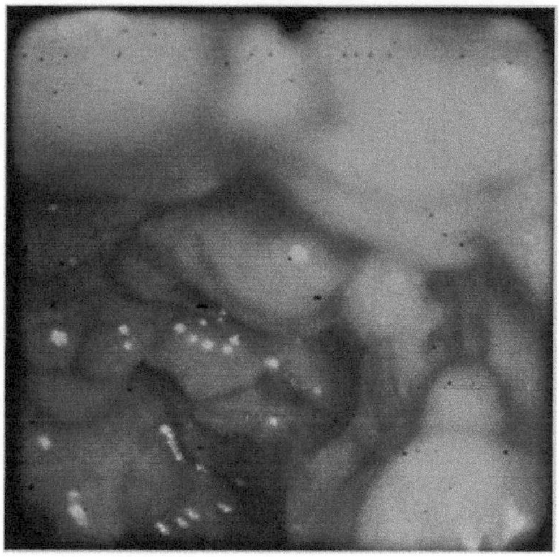

258b

11. Crohn's Disease of the Colon and Terminal Ileum (Continuation)

259a–b Status post ileo-transverse colostomy: no recurrence

260a–b Disseminated ulcerations (skip lesions) in the area of anastomosis: postoperative recurrence of Crohn's disease

261 Status post ileo-transverse colostomy. Early stage of recurrent Crohn's disease in the ileum: aphthoid mucosal lesion

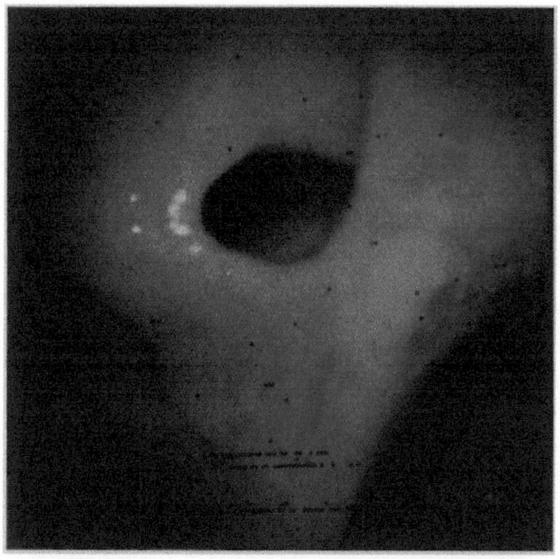
9a

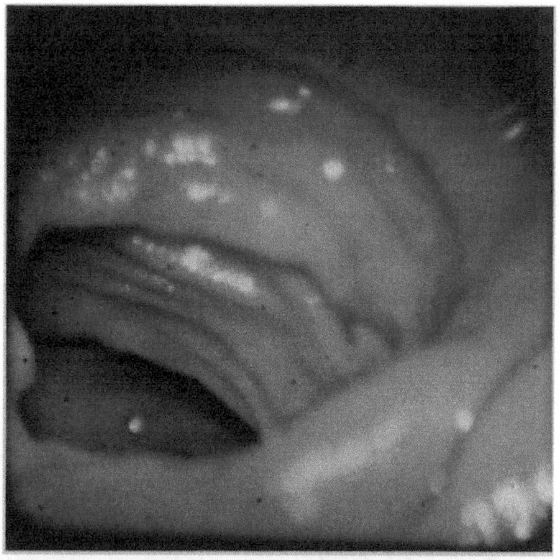
259b

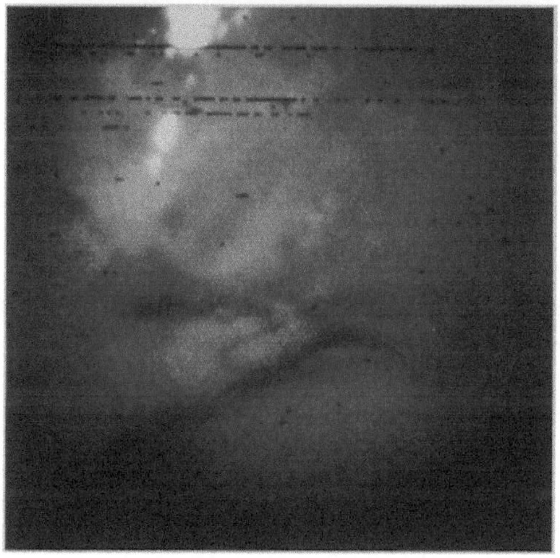
0a

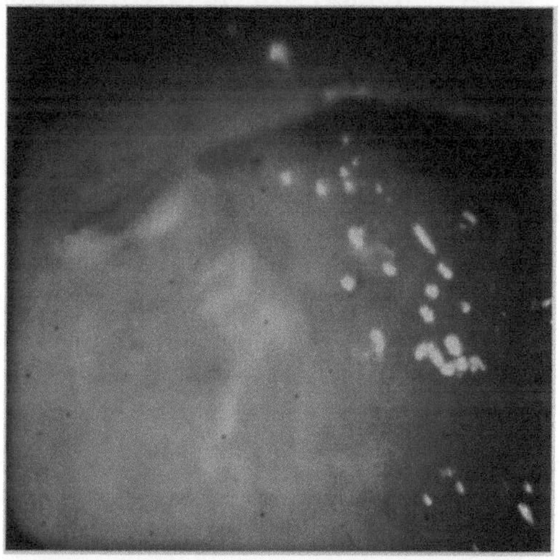
260b

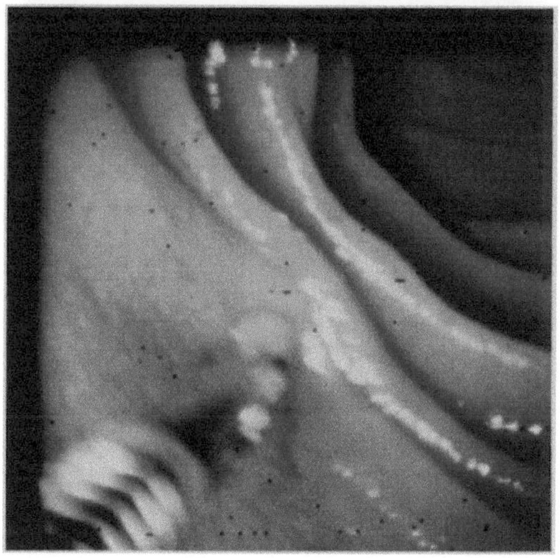
261

12. Radiation Colitis

262 Radiation proctitis: local edema, mucosal bleeding and fibrosis

13. Melanosis Coli

263 Melanosis coli: reticular pigmentation of the mucosa

14. Diverticula

264 Multiple sigmoid diverticula without evidence of inflammation

265 Sigmoid diverticulum with fecal contamination and rigidity of the adjoining wall (chronic diverticulitis)

15. Enteric Parasites

266a–b Trichiuris trichiura: worm attached to the cecal mucosa by its filiform whip (266a). Low magnification photograph of a worm removed intact (266b)

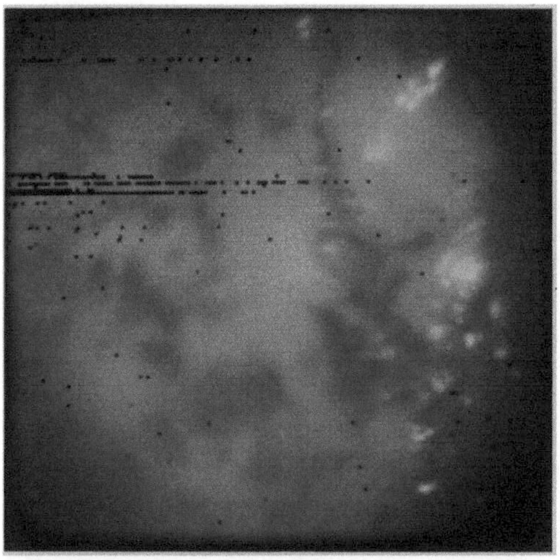

262

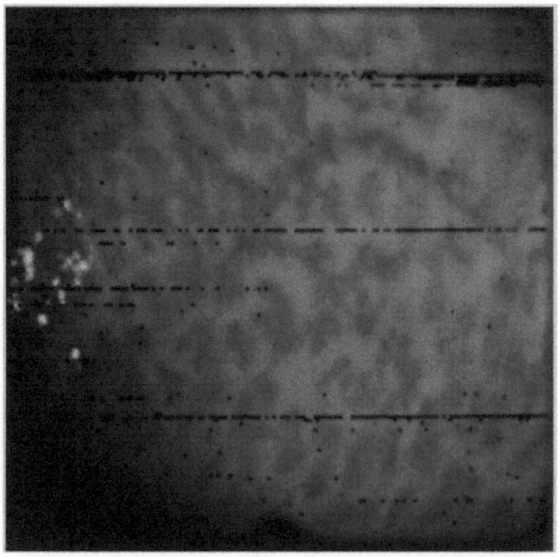

263

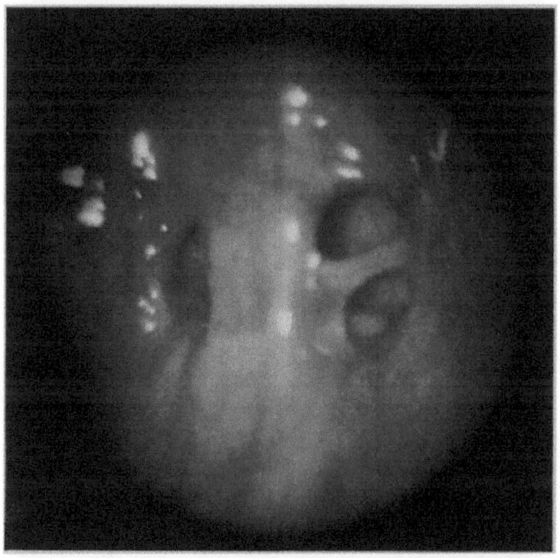

264

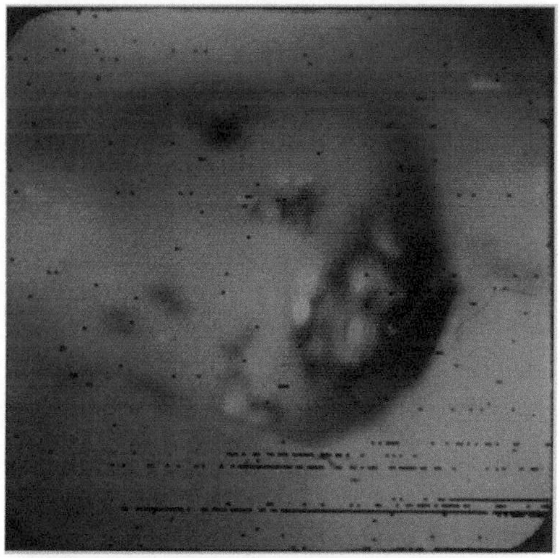

265

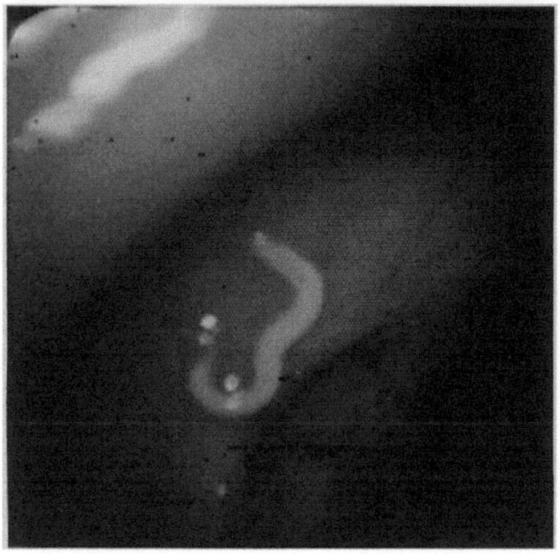

266a

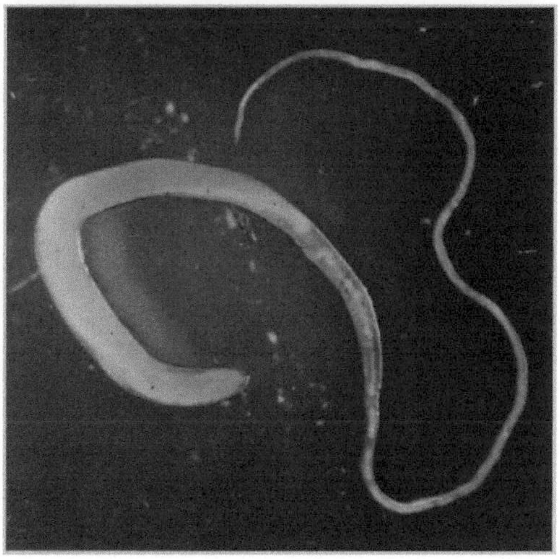

266b

Subject Index

Page numbers in **boldface** refer to illustration pages

Early Gastric Cancer

Current Status of Diagnosis
Editors: E. Grundmann, H. Grunze, S. Witte
82 figures. VIII, 206 pages. 1974
ISBN 3-540-06802-3 DM 48,—
ISBN 0-387-06802-3 (North America) $19.70

K. Kawai, H. Tanaka

Differential Diagnosis of Gastric Diseases

102 color photos, 422 black and white photos, 31 figures. VI, 262 pages. 1974
ISBN 3-540-06579-2 Cloth DM 168,—
ISBN 0-387-06579-2 (North America) Cloth $68.90
Published by Igaku Shoin Ltd., Tokyo
Distribution rights for Europe (including United Kingdom): Springer-Verlag

W. Wenz

Abdominal Angiography

In collaboration with G. van Kaick, D. Beduhn, F.-J. Roth
183 figures, some in color, comprising 351 radiographs and 34 drawings
VIII, 217 pages. 1974
ISBN 3-540-06508-3 Cloth DM 72,—
ISBN 0-387-06508-3 (North America) Cloth $27.80
Distribution rights for Japan: Igaku Shoin Ltd., Tokyo

Angiography/ Scintigraphy

Symposium of the European Association of Radiology, Mainz 1-3 October, 1970. Editor: L. Diethelm
262 figures. XVIII, 445 pages. 1972
ISBN 3-540-05804-4 Cloth DM 96,—
ISBN 0-387-05804-4 (North America) Cloth $30.10

Clinical Oncology

A Manual for Students and Doctors
Editor: Committee on Professional Education of UICC International Union Against Cancer
89 figures. XVII, 321 pages. 1973
ISBN 3-540-05851-6 DM 26,—
ISBN 0-387-05851-6 (North America) $9.90

Prices are subject to change without notice

Springer-Verlag Berlin Heidelberg New York

MIX
Papier aus verantwortungsvollen Quellen
Paper from responsible sources
FSC® C105338

If you have any concerns about our products,
you can contact us on
ProductSafety@springernature.com

In case Publisher is established outside the EU,
the EU authorized representative is:
Springer Nature Customer Service Center GmbH
Europaplatz 3, 69115 Heidelberg, Germany

Printed by Libri Plureos GmbH
in Hamburg, Germany